DERMOSCOPY
The Essentials

DERMOSCOPY
The Essentials
THIRD EDITION

H. Peter Soyer, MD, FACD
Professor and Chair,
Dermatology Research Centre,
The University of Queensland Diamantina
Institute,
The University of Queensland
and
Princess Alexandra Hospital,
Brisbane, Australia

Giuseppe Argenziano, MD
Professor of Dermatology,
Dermatology Unit,
University of Campania, Naples, Italy

Rainer Hofmann-Wellenhof, MD
Professor of Dermatology,
Research Unit for Teledermatology, Prevention
and
Innovative Diagnostic Technologies in Dermato-
Oncology,
Department of Dermatology,
Medical University Graz,
Graz, Austria

Iris Zalaudek, MD
Professor of Dermatology,
Department of Dermatology and Venereology,
University of Trieste,
Trieste, Italy

ELSEVIER

1600 John F. Kennedy Blvd.
Ste 1600
Philadelphia, PA 19103-2899

Notice

Practitioners and researchers must always rely on their own experience and knowledge in evaluating and using any information, methods, compounds or experiments described herein. Because of rapid advances in the medical sciences, in particular, independent verification of diagnoses and drug dosages should be made. To the fullest extent of the law, no responsibility is assumed by Elsevier, authors, editors or contributors for any injury and/or damage to persons or property as a matter of products liability, negligence or otherwise, or from any use or operation of any methods, products, instructions, or ideas contained in the material herein.

Previous editions copyrighted 2012 and 2004.

Library of Congress Control Number: 2019950369

Content Strategist: Charlotta Kryhl, Nancy Duffy
Content Development Manager: Kathryn DeFrancesco
Content Development Specialist: Kevin Travers
Publishing Services Manager: Deepthi Unni
Project Manager: Haritha Dharmarajan
Design: Ryan Cook

Printed in India

Last digit is the print number: 9   8   7   6

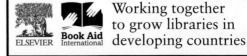

Preface to the Third Edition

As we prepare the third edition of *Dermoscopy: The Essentials*, it has been 14 years since the first edition and 6 years since we last updated our guidebook to dermoscopy. With dermoscopy continuing to grow in popularity as a physician's tool, we are pleased to revamp our book and bring it to a new generation of dermoscopists. As always, it is a pleasure to collaborate with old colleagues and peers, though we are scattered around the world. We are able to work hand-in-glove despite the vast distances with the miracle of modern technology and with the advantage of having known each other and worked together for many years (over 20 years in some cases), and having been through many highs and lows together.

This third edition continues to use the traffic light system to help practitioners quickly review lesion categories during regular use and consolidate their knowledge, and to help new users absorb the skill of evaluating a whole lesion as well as its component parts. We have substituted nearly 30% of the dermoscopic and clinical images to bring a fresh set of clinically relevant examples to both novice and experienced dermoscopists.

We are especially indebted to the Elsevier Editorial Team, Caroline Dorey-Stein and Charlotta Kryhl, for their flexible support and patience during the slow process of revising the book. We also thank our colleagues Dr Teresa Russo, Glen Wimberley and Katie Lee for their assistance in selecting and preparing the updated images and text.

As with the earlier editions, we consign our book to all those interested in the science and art of dermoscopy and hope that we contribute to the lofty goal of eradicating melanoma.

H. Peter Soyer
Brisbane, Australia
Giuseppe Argenziano
Naples, Italy
Rainer Hofmann-Wellenhof
Graz, Austria
Iris Zalaudek
Trieste, Italy
2018

KEY TO TRAFFIC LIGHT SYMBOLS

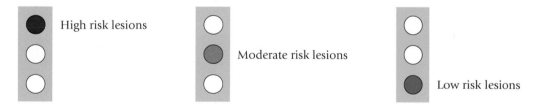

High risk lesions

Moderate risk lesions

Low risk lesions

Acknowledgements

To my Oz-based team, Zoja and Niko, for both their support and welcome distraction from my work.

H. Peter Soyer

To my patients…to whom I have dedicated my life.

Giuseppe Argenziano

To my teacher in dermoscopy and to my friends in the field of dermoscopy. Special thanks go to my wife Andrea and my children Elisabeth, Paul, Martin and Georg, who have given me the strength to joyfully work on the book.

Rainer Hofmann-Wellenhof

To my "dermoscopy" friends and colleagues, to my patients, and to my parents Ilse and Gunter, my sister Karin, my niece Lilith, and my nephew Arthur for their love.

Iris Zalaudek

Contents

Introduction: The 3-point checklist

The short, easy way to avoid missing a melanoma using dermoscopy

Other names for dermoscopy
Dermatoscopy
Epiluminescence microscopy (ELM)
Skin surface microscopy

Dermoscopy is an in vivo noninvasive diagnostic technique that magnifies the skin in such a way that color and structure in the epidermis, dermoepidermal junction, and papillary dermis become visible. This color and structure cannot be seen with the naked eye. With training and experience, dermoscopy has been shown to significantly increase the clinical diagnosis of melanocytic, non-melanocytic, benign and malignant skin lesions, with a 10–27% improvement in the diagnosis of melanoma compared to that achieved by clinical examination alone. There is, however, a learning curve to mastering dermoscopy, and it is essential to spend time perfecting it—practice makes perfect!

Technique

In classic dermoscopy, oil or fluid (mineral oil, immersion oil, KY jelly, alcohol, water) is placed over the lesion to be examined. Fluid eliminates surface light reflection and renders the stratum corneum transparent, allowing visualization of subsurface colors and structures. Using handheld dermoscopes that exploit the properties of cross-polarized light (polarized dermoscopy), visualization of deep skin structures can be achieved without the necessity of a liquid interface or direct skin contact with the instrument.

The list of dermoscopy instrumentation is long and continues to grow and evolve with the development of better and more sophisticated handheld instruments and computer systems. Depending on the budget and goals for the evaluation and management of patients with pigmented skin lesions, there is a wide variety of products to choose from.

The 3-point checklist

To encourage clinicians to start using dermoscopy, simplified algorithms for analyzing what is seen with the technique have been developed.

For the novice dermoscopist, the primary goal of dermoscopy is to determine whether a suspicious lesion should be biopsied or excised. The bottom line is that no patient should leave the clinic with an undiagnosed melanoma.

For the general physician, dermoscopy can be used to determine whether a suspicious lesion should be evaluated by a more experienced clinician.

Dermoscopy is not just for dermatologists; any clinician who is interested can master this potentially life-saving technique.

Triage of suspicious pigmented skin lesions

The 3-point checklist was developed specifically for novice dermoscopists with little training to help them not to misdiagnose melanomas while improving their skills.

Results of the 2001 Consensus Net Meeting on Dermoscopy (Argenziano G, *J Am Acad Dermatol* 2003) showed that the following three criteria were especially important in distinguishing melanomas from other benign pigmented skin lesions:

- dermoscopic asymmetry of color and structure;
- atypical pigment network; and
- blue-white structures (a combination of the previous categories of blue-white veil and regression structures).

Statistical analysis showed that the presence of any two of these criteria indicates a high likelihood of melanoma. Using the 3-point checklist, one can have a sensitivity and specificity result comparable with other algorithms requiring much more training. In a preliminary study of 231 clinically equivocal pigmented skin lesions, it was shown that, after a short introduction of 1-h duration, six inexperienced dermoscopists were able to classify 96.3% of melanomas correctly using this method.

This first chapter provides 60 examples of benign and malignant pigmented skin lesions to demonstrate how the 3-point checklist works and the practical value of this simplified diagnostic algorithm.

The 3-point checklist was designed to be used as a screening method. The sensitivity is much higher than the specificity to ensure that melanomas are not misdiagnosed. We recommend that all lesions with a positive test (3-point checklist score of 2 or 3) are excised (Table 1).

Table 1.1 Definition of dermoscopic criteria for the 3-point checklist. The presence of two or three criteria is suggestive of a suspicious lesion

3-Point checklist	Definition
1. Asymmetry	Asymmetry of color and structure in one or two perpendicular axes
2. Atypical network	Pigment network with irregular holes and thick lines
3. Blue-white structures	Any type of blue and/or white color

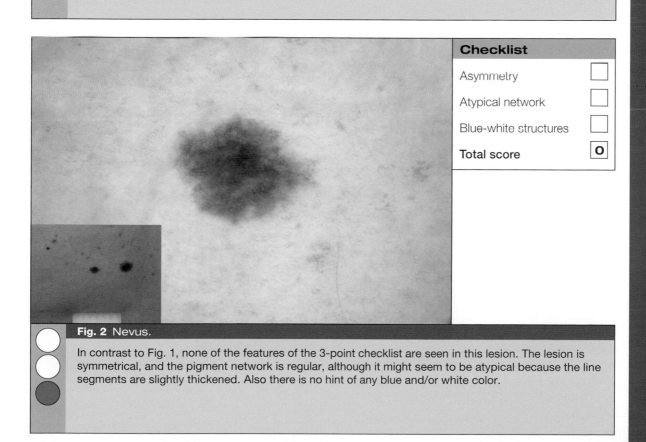

Checklist	
Asymmetry	☑
Atypical network	☑
Blue-white structures	☑
Total score	**3**

Fig. 1 Melanoma.

Criteria to diagnose melanoma can be very subtle or obviously present as in this case. This lesion clearly demonstrates all of the 3-point checklist criteria, namely asymmetry in all axes, an atypical pigment network (*circle*), and blue-white structures (*asterisks*).

Checklist	
Asymmetry	☐
Atypical network	☐
Blue-white structures	☐
Total score	**0**

Fig. 2 Nevus.

In contrast to Fig. 1, none of the features of the 3-point checklist are seen in this lesion. The lesion is symmetrical, and the pigment network is regular, although it might seem to be atypical because the line segments are slightly thickened. Also there is no hint of any blue and/or white color.

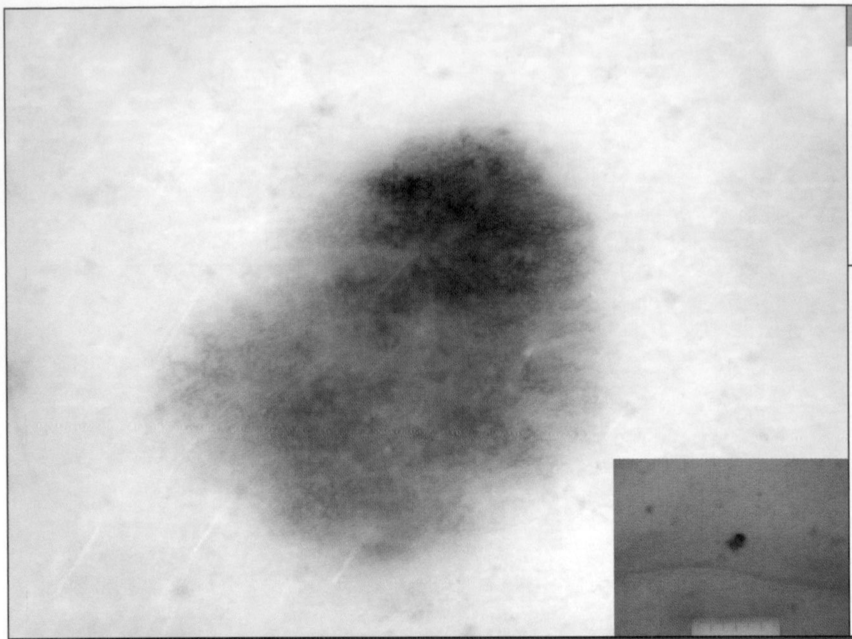

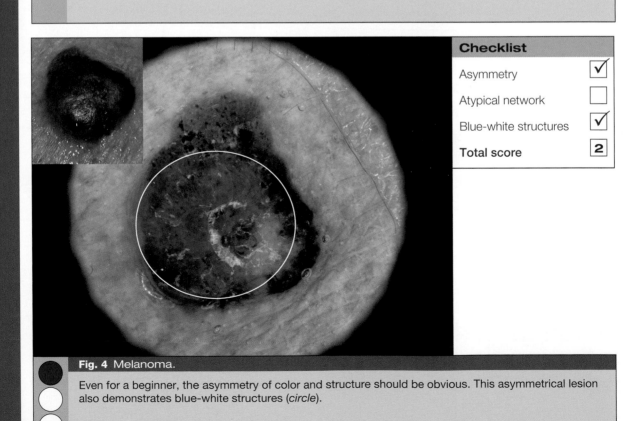

Checklist	
Asymmetry	☑
Atypical network	☐
Blue-white structures	☐
Total score	1

Fig. 3 Nevus.

The novice might find this lesion difficult to diagnose. If in doubt, cut it out! With experience, the clinician will excise fewer of these banal nevi. There is asymmetry; however, neither an atypical pigment network nor subtle blue-white structures are present.

Checklist	
Asymmetry	☑
Atypical network	☐
Blue-white structures	☑
Total score	2

Fig. 4 Melanoma.

Even for a beginner, the asymmetry of color and structure should be obvious. This asymmetrical lesion also demonstrates blue-white structures (*circle*).

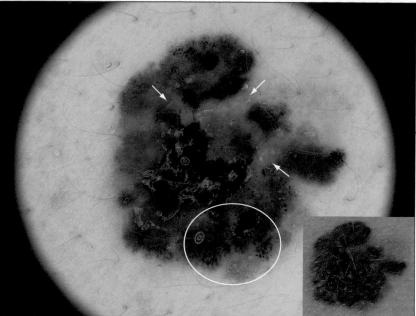

Checklist	
Asymmetry	☑
Atypical network	☑
Blue-white structures	☑
Total score	3

Fig. 5 Melanoma.

The color and structure in the lower half is not a mirror image of the upper half; therefore, there is asymmetry. An atypical pigment network with thickened and broken-up line segments (*circle*) and a large area of blue-white structures (*arrows*) are also seen.

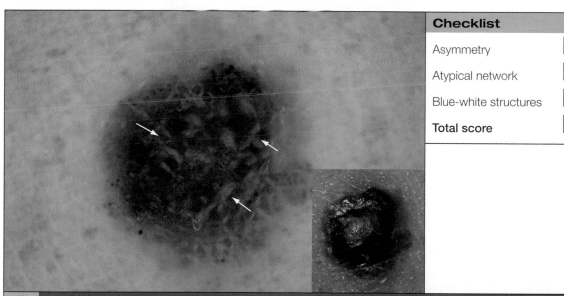

Checklist	
Asymmetry	☑
Atypical network	☐
Blue-white structures	☑
Total score	2

Fig. 6 Melanoma.

This lesion is slightly asymmetric in shape and more in structure, and therefore, a red flag should be raised. No pigment network is present, but there are numerous shiny white streaks (also called chrysalis-like structures) (*arrows*) representing a variation on the theme of blue-white structures.

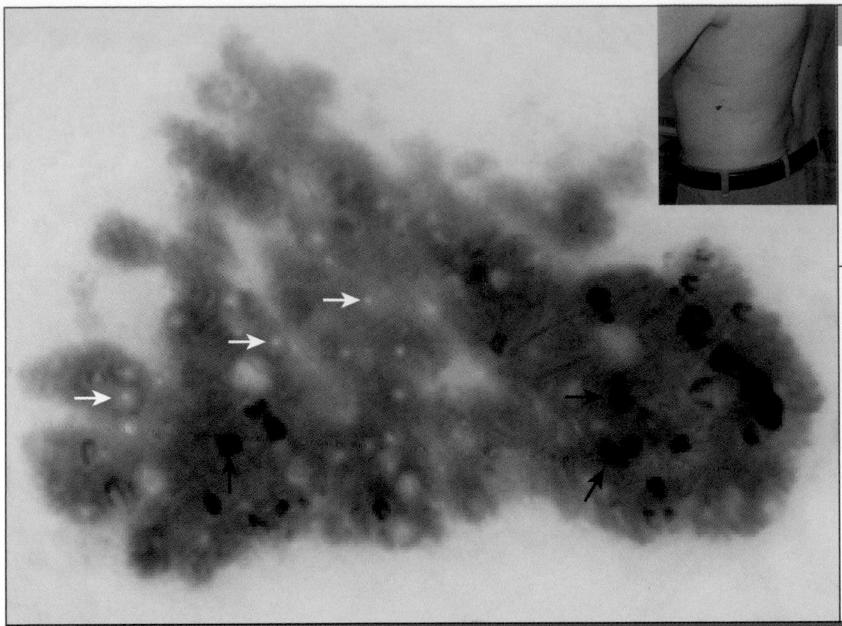

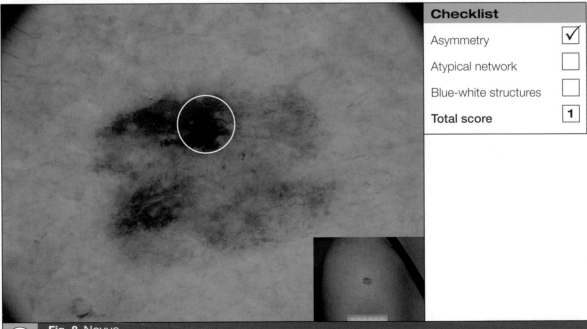

Checklist	
Asymmetry	☑
Atypical network	☐
Blue-white structures	☐
Total score	**1**

Fig. 7 Seborrheic keratosis.

This seborrheic keratosis demonstrates a great deal of asymmetry of color and structure, but the other two criteria needed to diagnose melanoma are absent. If the multiple milia-like cysts (*white arrows*) and the numerous follicular openings (*black arrows*) diagnostic of seborrheic keratosis cannot be recognized, excise the lesion.

Checklist	
Asymmetry	☑
Atypical network	☐
Blue-white structures	☐
Total score	**1**

Fig. 8 Nevus.

Some melanomas are featureless, so beware! The color and structure in the left upper quarter of the lesion is not a mirror image in any other quarter of the lesion. The presence of an irregular black blotch in the left upper quarter (*circle*) adds to the asymmetry. An atypical pigment network and blue-white structures are not seen. In our estimation this is a nevus warranting careful consideration for its management.

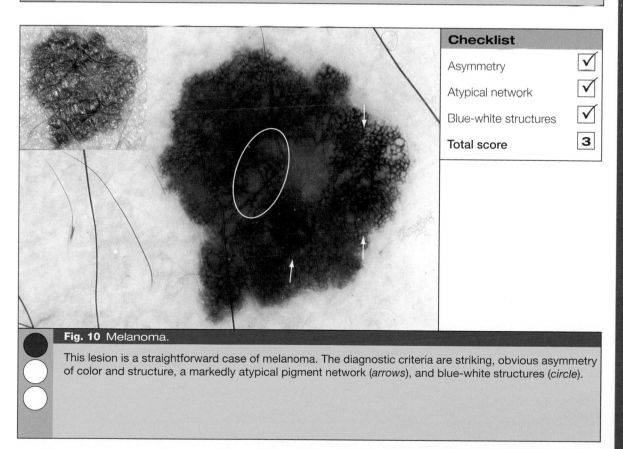

Checklist	
Asymmetry	☐
Atypical network	☐
Blue-white structures	☐
Total score	**0**

Fig. 9 Nevus.

If in doubt, cut it out! With practice, fewer lesions that look like this will be excised. This is rather symmetrical, and there is a great example of a regular pigment network in the periphery of this banal nevus. Do not be fooled by the dark central color—it is not always a sign of malignancy. No blue-white structures are seen.

Checklist	
Asymmetry	☑
Atypical network	☑
Blue-white structures	☑
Total score	**3**

Fig. 10 Melanoma.

This lesion is a straightforward case of melanoma. The diagnostic criteria are striking, obvious asymmetry of color and structure, a markedly atypical pigment network (*arrows*), and blue-white structures (*circle*).

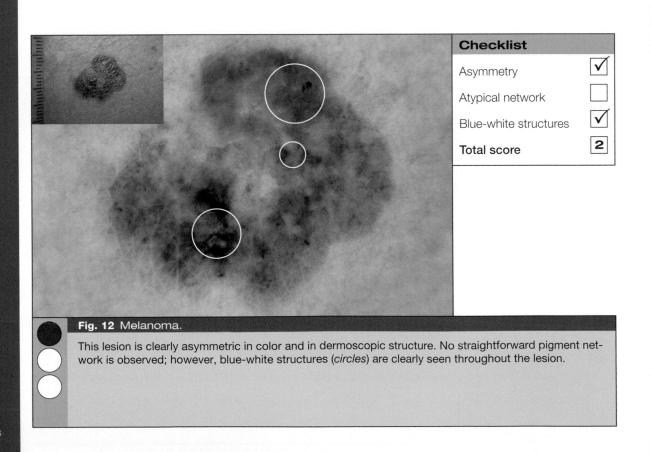

Checklist

Asymmetry	☑
Atypical network	☐
Blue-white structures	☐
Total score	1

Fig. 11 Nevus.

The clinical ABCDs could lead you astray with this banal nevus. There is slight asymmetry, but there is also a typical pigment network fading out at the periphery and blue-white structures are absent.

Checklist

Asymmetry	☑
Atypical network	☐
Blue-white structures	☑
Total score	2

Fig. 12 Melanoma.

This lesion is clearly asymmetric in color and in dermoscopic structure. No straightforward pigment network is observed; however, blue-white structures (*circles*) are clearly seen throughout the lesion.

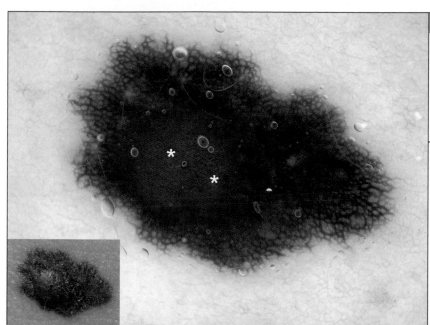

Checklist	
Asymmetry	☑
Atypical network	☑
Blue-white structures	☑
Total score	**3**

Fig. 13 Melanoma.

Clinicians might think that this lesion is nothing to worry about until they examine it with dermoscopy. There is asymmetry of color and structure, an atypical pigment network, and blue-white structures (*asterisks*) cover part of the lesion.

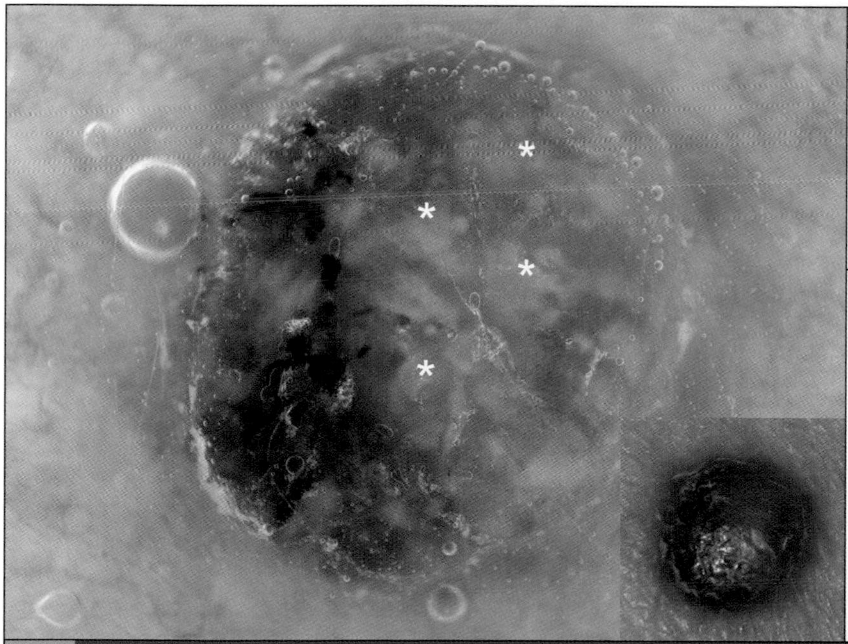

Checklist	
Asymmetry	☑
Atypical network	☐
Blue-white structures	☑
Total score	**2**

Fig. 14 Melanoma.

The extensive blue-white structures (*asterisks*) are the first clue to the seriousness of this lesion. Particularly color is clearly asymmetrical. A pigment network is absent, and there are well-developed blue-white structures.

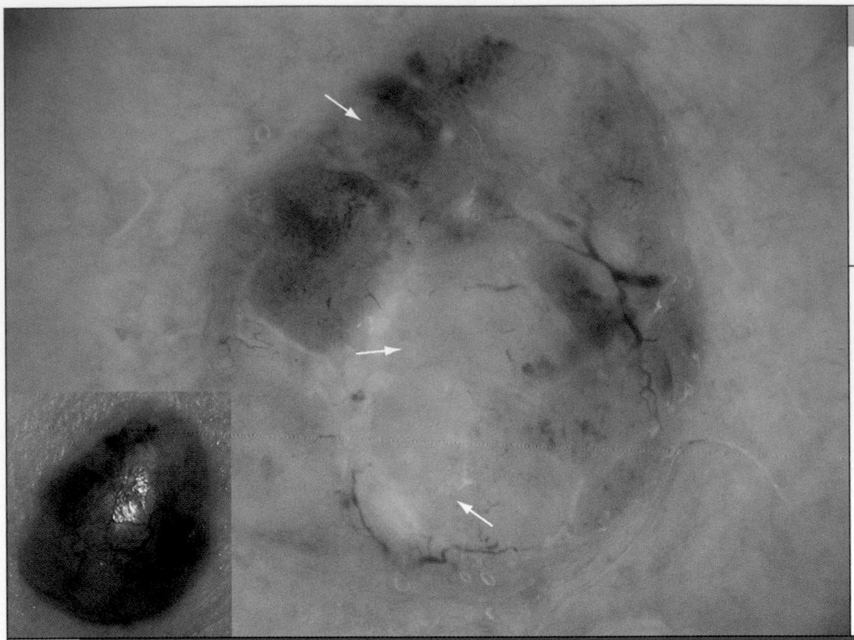

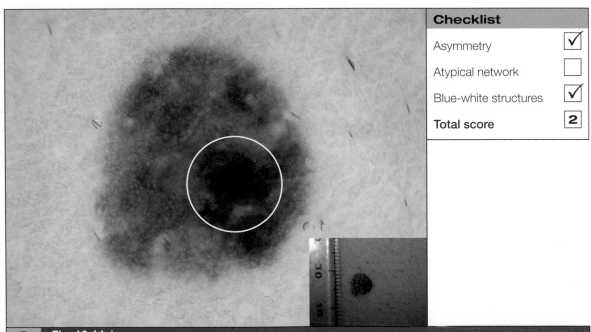

Checklist	
Asymmetry	☑
Atypical network	☐
Blue-white structures	☑
Total score	**2**

Fig. 15 Basal cell carcinoma.

This lesion demonstrates nicely the in-focus arborizing vessels typical for a nodular basal cell carcinoma. Two positive features of the checklist are clearly present—asymmetry and blue-white structures (*arrows*). There is no pigment network.

Checklist	
Asymmetry	☑
Atypical network	☐
Blue-white structures	☑
Total score	**2**

Fig. 16 Melanoma.

Asymmetry is unmistakably present in this lesion, but whether the pigment network is atypical in several foci of this lesion is debatable. Blue-white structures (*circle*) are clearly seen. There is no doubt this lesion needs to be excised.

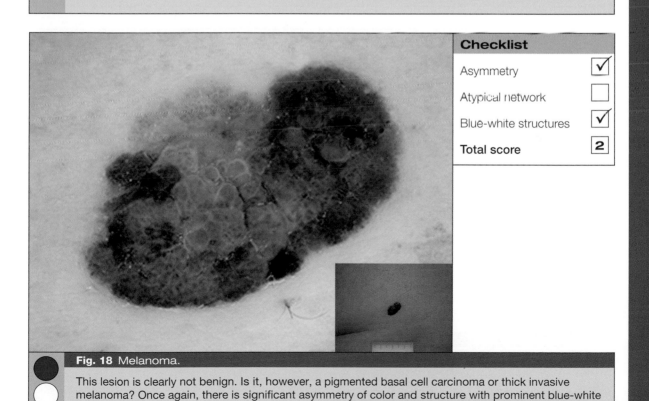

Checklist	
Asymmetry	☑
Atypical network	☐
Blue-white structures	☑
Total score	2

Fig. 17 Basal cell carcinoma.

This lesion is so bizarre looking that you should excise it as soon as possible. There is asymmetry of color and structure, and delicate blue-white structures are found throughout. No pigment network is seen. Because two of the three criteria from the 3-point checklist are present, the lesion should be excised.

Checklist	
Asymmetry	☑
Atypical network	☐
Blue-white structures	☑
Total score	2

Fig. 18 Melanoma.

This lesion is clearly not benign. Is it, however, a pigmented basal cell carcinoma or thick invasive melanoma? Once again, there is significant asymmetry of color and structure with prominent blue-white structures. A pigment network is not present, which is often actually observed in thick melanomas. This lesion needs to be completely excised urgently.

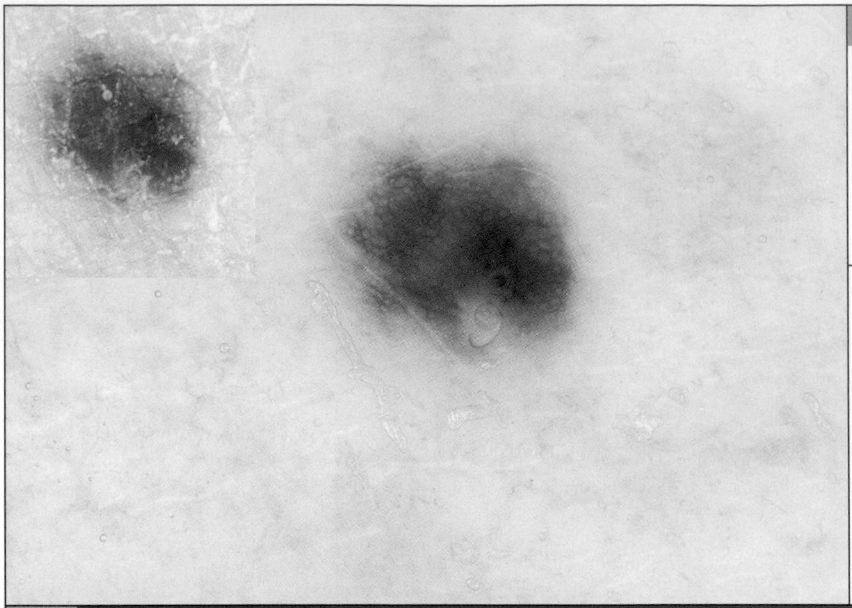

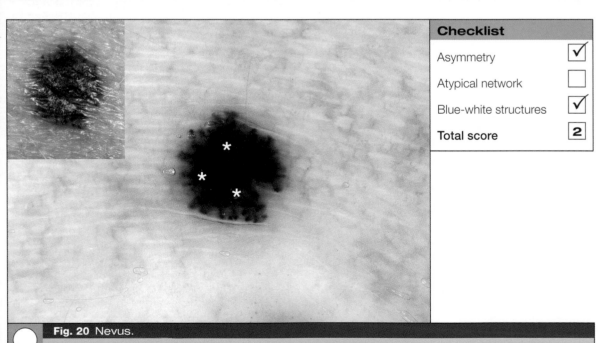

Checklist

Asymmetry	☑
Atypical network	☐
Blue-white structures	☐
Total score	1

Fig. 19 Nevus.

This stereotypical benign nevus is commonly seen when performing dermoscopy. The blotch of dark brown color is not significant. Although there is slight asymmetry of color and structure, the lesion is characterized by a typical pigment network, and no clear-cut blue-white structures are seen.

Checklist

Asymmetry	☑
Atypical network	☐
Blue-white structures	☑
Total score	2

Fig. 20 Nevus.

The pattern of criteria shown here is most often seen with a Spitz nevus, but the differential diagnosis should include Clark (dysplastic) nevus and melanoma. There is slight asymmetry of color and structure. A pigment network is absent, with blue-white structures (*asterisks*). The checklist will not work for all lesions, and it is important to take into account the history and age of the patient when deciding what to do.

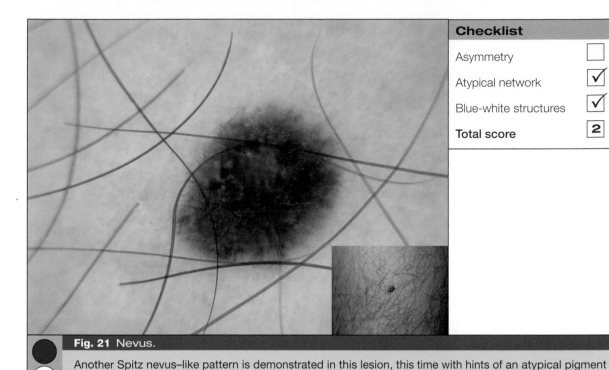

Checklist

Asymmetry	☐
Atypical network	☑
Blue-white structures	☑
Total score	**2**

Fig. 21 Nevus.

Another Spitz nevus–like pattern is demonstrated in this lesion, this time with hints of an atypical pigment network in the left lower corner. Blue-white structures are visible throughout the lesion. A lesion like this one should be excised without hesitation.

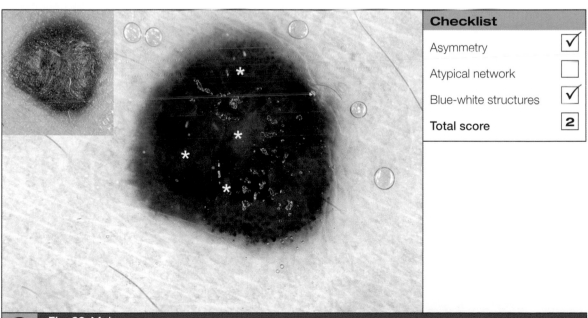

Checklist

Asymmetry	☑
Atypical network	☐
Blue-white structures	☑
Total score	**2**

Fig. 22 Melanoma.

This rather banal-looking clinical lesion has a strikingly worrisome dermoscopic appearance, with asymmetry of color and structure. No pigment network is present, but blue-white structures are seen throughout the lesion (*asterisks*).

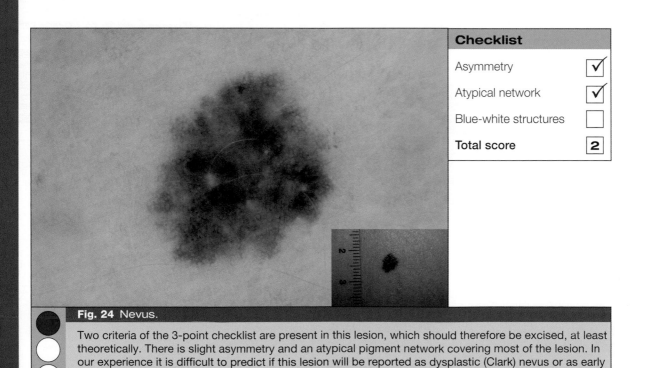

Checklist

Asymmetry	☑
Atypical network	☐
Blue-white structures	☐
Total score	**1**

Fig. 23 Nevus.

This lesion is benign. Compare it with the other lesions shown in this chapter with more obvious asymmetry of color and structure, an atypical pigment network, and blue-white structures. There is slight asymmetry of color and structure, although 100% symmetry is never found in nature. No pigment network or blue-white structures are seen.

Checklist

Asymmetry	☑
Atypical network	☑
Blue-white structures	☐
Total score	**2**

Fig. 24 Nevus.

Two criteria of the 3-point checklist are present in this lesion, which should therefore be excised, at least theoretically. There is slight asymmetry and an atypical pigment network covering most of the lesion. In our experience it is difficult to predict if this lesion will be reported as dysplastic (Clark) nevus or as early in situ melanoma. As our patient had several similar-looking lesions, we opted for close follow-up using sequential dermoscopy imaging.

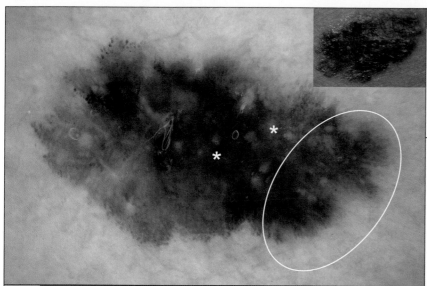

Checklist	
Asymmetry	☑
Atypical network	☑
Blue-white structures	☑
Total score	**3**

Fig. 25 Melanoma.

This is a clear-cut melanoma because of the striking asymmetry of color and structure and the presence of diffuse blue-white structures (*asterisks*). An atypical pigment network can be discerned in the right part of the lesion (*circle*).

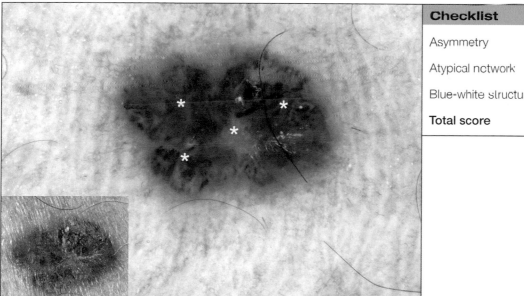

Checklist	
Asymmetry	☑
Atypical network	☐
Blue-white structures	☑
Total score	**2**

Fig. 26 Basal cell carcinoma.

There is no doubt that this pigmented neoplasm displays two criteria of the 3-point checklist. Note the striking asymmetry. No pigment network is seen, but several blue-white structures are present (*asterisks*).

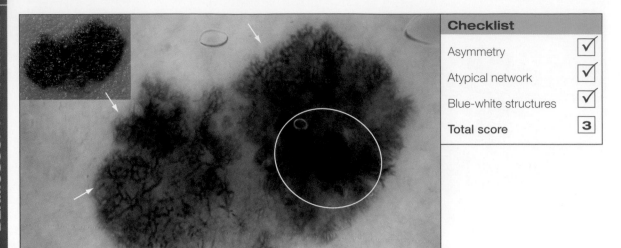

Fig. 27 Melanoma.

All three checklist criteria are seen in this lesion. There is significant asymmetry of color and structure with a well-developed atypical pigment network (*arrows*). In the right lower part of the lesion, a blue-white structure can be discerned (*circle*).

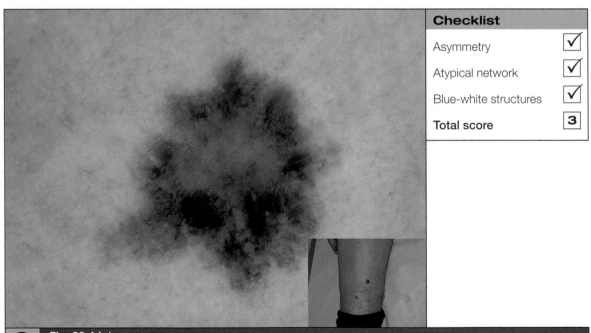

Checklist	
Asymmetry	☑
Atypical network	☑
Blue-white structures	☑
Total score	3

Fig. 28 Melanoma.

Significant asymmetry of color and dermoscopic structure can be easily recognized in this lesion. In addition, there is a paracentrally-located blue-white structure (actually more whitish) and there are also obvious foci of an atypical pigment network. This lesion needs to be excised.

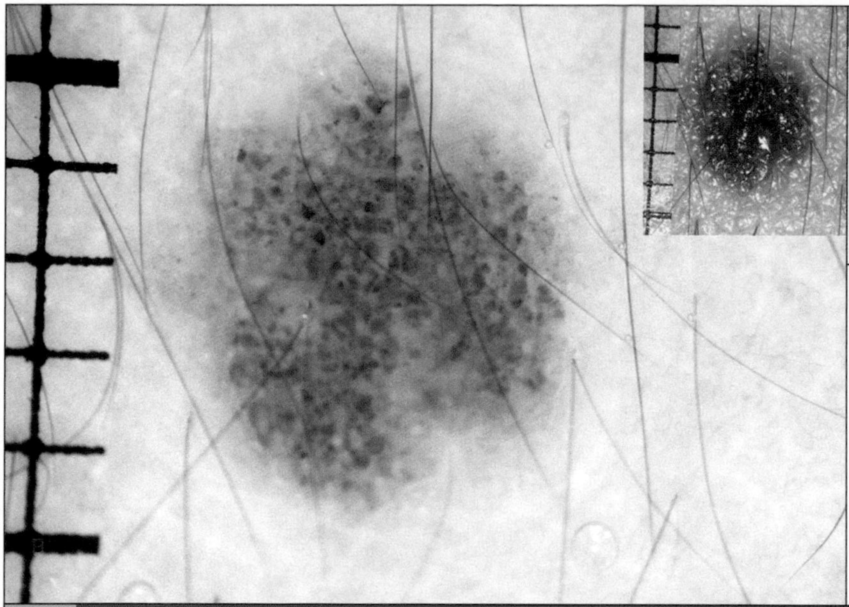

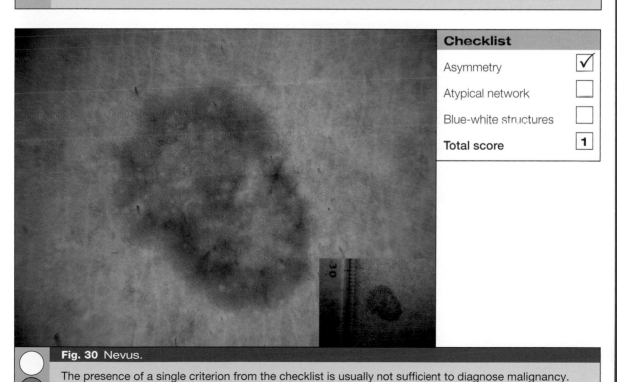

Checklist	
Asymmetry	☑
Atypical network	☐
Blue-white structures	☐
Total score	**1**

Fig. 29 Nevus.

Only one of the checklist criteria is present in this lesion, so this lesion is benign. The lower half of the lesion does not mirror the upper half, thereby displaying subtle asymmetry. No pigment network or blue-white structures are seen.

Checklist	
Asymmetry	☑
Atypical network	☐
Blue-white structures	☐
Total score	**1**

Fig. 30 Nevus.

The presence of a single criterion from the checklist is usually not sufficient to diagnose malignancy. Note the subtle asymmetry of color and structure—the left side of the lesion is not a mirror image of the right side, and the upper side does not mirror the lower side. An atypical pigment network and blue-white structures are absent.

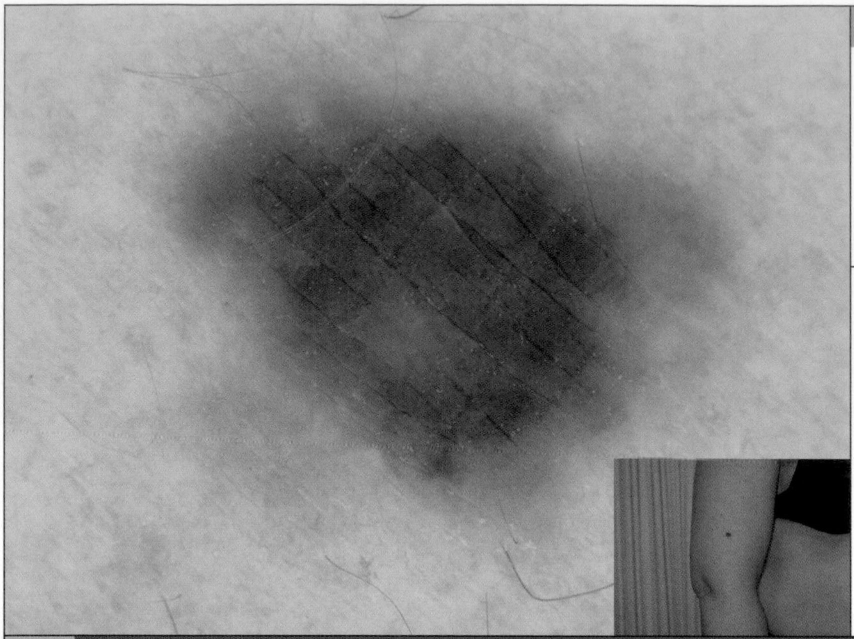

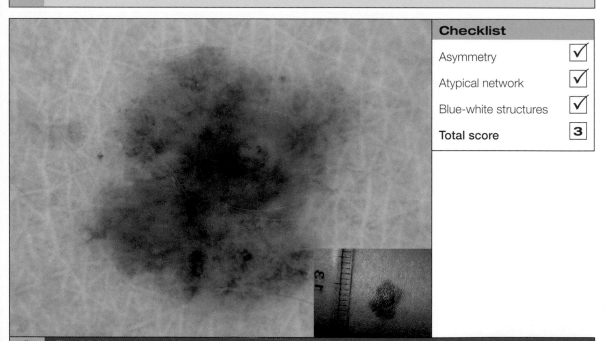

Checklist

Asymmetry	☐
Atypical network	☐
Blue-white structures	☑
Total score	**1**

Fig. 31 Melanoma.

This is a difficult lesion to interpret. Although only one criterion of the 3-point checklist is present, the overall appearance may raise some suspicion that it could be a melanoma. The lesion is rather symmetrical and there is no pigment network. However, blue-white structures are clearly present throughout this quite worrisome-looking lesion.

Checklist

Asymmetry	☑
Atypical network	☑
Blue-white structures	☑
Total score	**3**

Fig. 32 Melanoma.

All criteria of the 3-point checklist are present, underlining the impression that this lesion is a melanoma. Although the contour is symmetrical, there is asymmetry of color and dermoscopic structure within. Tiny loci of subtle thickened pigment network are present at the upper pole of the lesion, with a small focus of blue-white structures in the center of the lesion. This early melanoma might go undiagnosed if dermoscopy is not used.

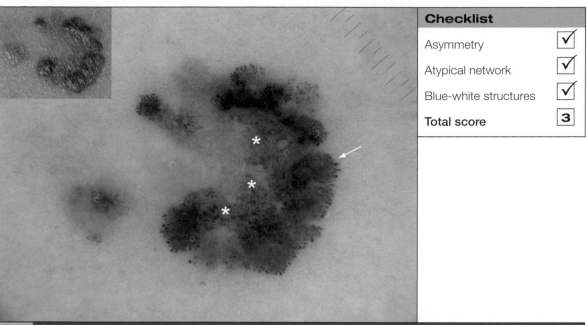

Checklist	
Asymmetry	☑
Atypical network	☑
Blue-white structures	☑
Total score	**3**

Fig. 33 Melanoma.

Once again, all three features of the checklist are clearly present and even a novice dermoscopist should immediately suspect a melanoma. There is striking asymmetry of color and structure with zones displaying an atypical pigment network (*arrow*). There are also clear-cut areas with another variation on the theme of blue-white structures, namely peppering (*asterisks*).

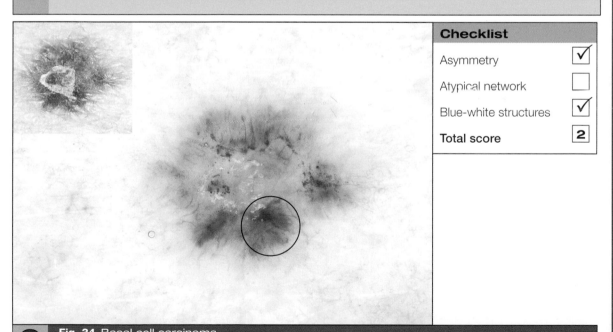

Checklist	
Asymmetry	☑
Atypical network	☐
Blue-white structures	☑
Total score	**2**

Fig. 34 Basal cell carcinoma.

The lower half of this lesion is not a mirror image of the upper half, and the right side is not a mirror image of the left side; therefore, this is an asymmetrical lesion. No pigment network is identified, but there are numerous blue-white structures seen throughout (*circle*). Remember, when two criteria are identified, the lesion should be excised.

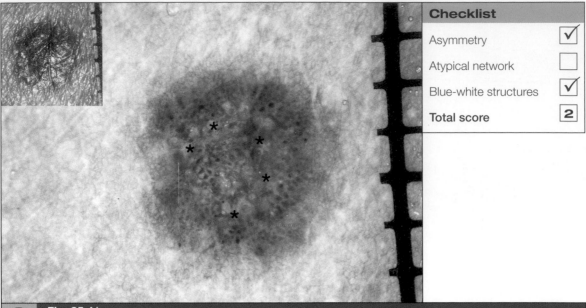

Checklist

Asymmetry	☑
Atypical network	☐
Blue-white structures	☑
Total score	2

Fig. 35 Nevus.

Despite the rather compelling asymmetry of color and structure, this lesion is benign. There is no hint of a pigment network, but numerous blue-white structures are present (*asterisks*). With a score of 2, excise this lesion or show it to a more experienced dermoscopist. Also remember to always compare the dermoscopic features of several nevi of a given patient; every so often blue-white structures are found in several nevi of a patient. Dermoscopic findings always need to be interpreted in the overall clinical context.

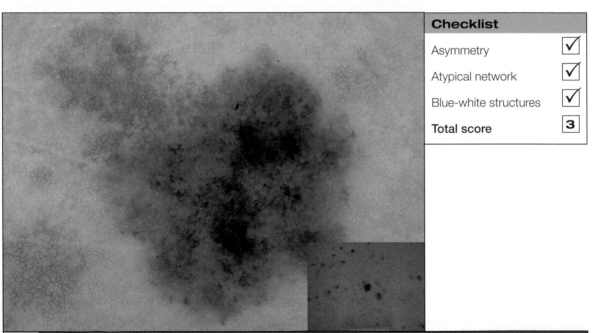

Checklist

Asymmetry	☑
Atypical network	☑
Blue-white structures	☑
Total score	3

Fig. 36 Melanoma.

This is a difficult lesion to diagnose because there is a discrepancy between the clinical and the dermoscopic images. Dermoscopically all three features are present, albeit the atypical pigment network is very subtle if at all present. Asymmetry is obvious, and blue-white structures can be seen clearly in the right part of the lesion. If you have any doubt, the lesion needs to be excised.

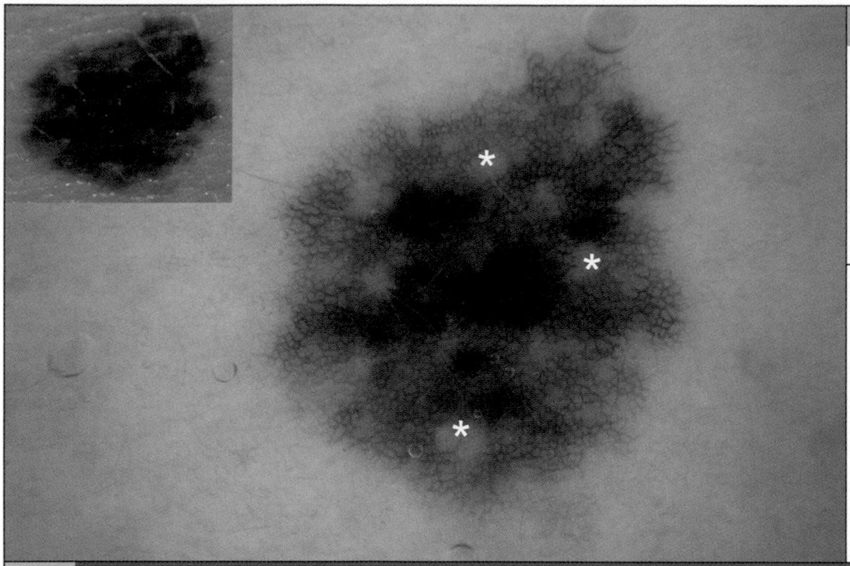

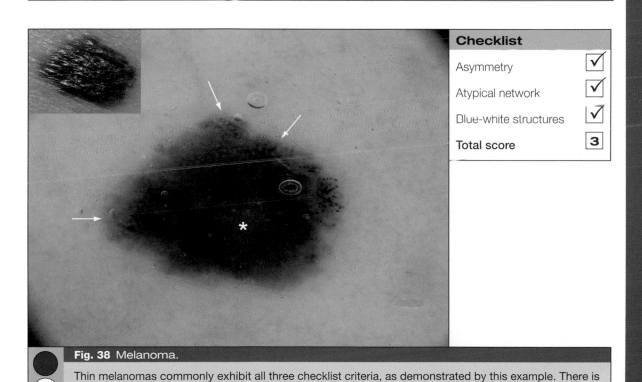

Checklist	
Asymmetry	☑
Atypical network	☐
Blue-white structures	☐
Total score	1

Fig. 37 Nevus.

This is a slightly asymmetrical lesion with a typical pigment network. Do not confuse the multifocal hypo-pigmentation (*asterisks*) with the white color that can be seen in blue-white structures.

Checklist	
Asymmetry	☑
Atypical network	☑
Blue-white structures	☑
Total score	3

Fig. 38 Melanoma.

Thin melanomas commonly exhibit all three checklist criteria, as demonstrated by this example. There is asymmetry of color and structure with a few foci (*arrows*) of an atypical pigment network. In the center, an area of blue-white structures is also seen (*asterisk*). The dermoscopic differential diagnosis includes severely dysplastic nevus and in situ melanoma.

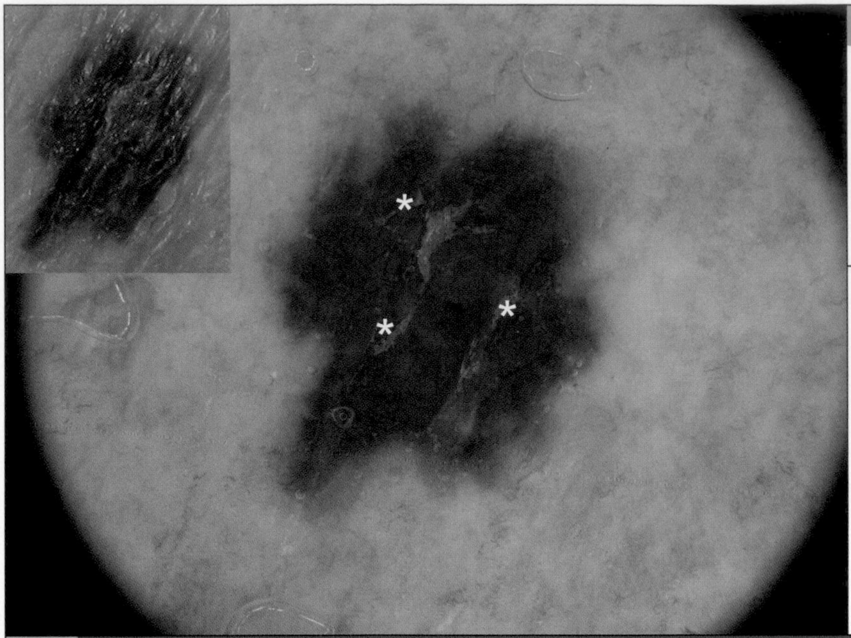

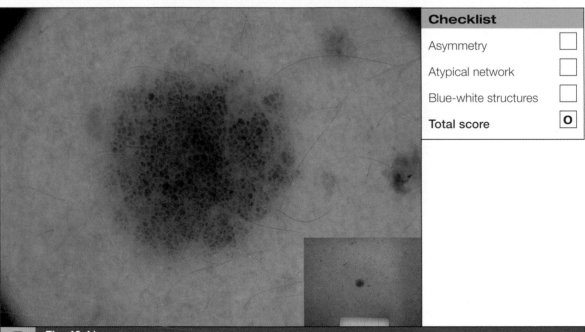

Checklist	
Asymmetry	☑
Atypical network	☐
Blue-white structures	☑
Total score	**2**

Fig. 39 Melanoma.

This dark lesion is a cause for concern. Note the shape asymmetry and multiple anastomosing blue-white structures throughout the lesion (*asterisks*). With two out of three well-developed criteria present, this melanoma will not be misdiagnosed if the 3-point checklist is used.

Checklist	
Asymmetry	☐
Atypical network	☐
Blue-white structures	☐
Total score	**0**

Fig. 40 Nevus.

There is an obvious lack of striking criteria in this lesion compared to the melanomas already seen in this chapter. An atypical pigment network and blue-white structures are not seen in this rather symmetrical lesion.

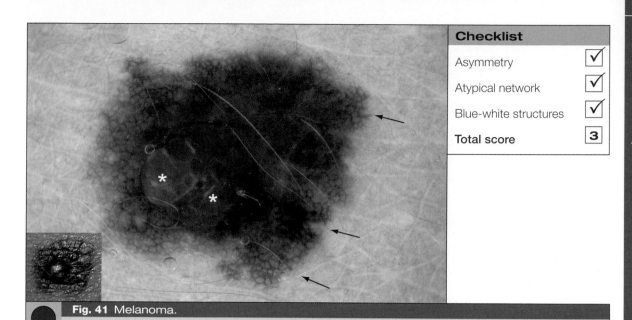

Checklist	
Asymmetry	☑
Atypical network	☑
Blue-white structures	☑
Total score	3

Fig. 41 Melanoma.

This is a clear-cut example of a melanoma with a checklist score of 3. There is striking asymmetry of color and structure. Several zones exhibit variations of the morphology of an atypical pigment network (*arrows*). In paracentral location, blue-white structures can be clearly seen (*asterisks*). Always concentrate and focus attention to identify important criteria that might be present in a lesion.

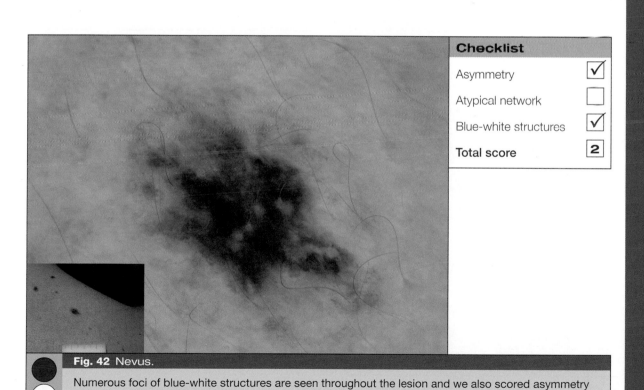

Checklist	
Asymmetry	☑
Atypical network	☐
Blue-white structures	☑
Total score	2

Fig. 42 Nevus.

Numerous foci of blue-white structures are seen throughout the lesion and we also scored asymmetry here. An atypical pigment network is not seen. The dark color and blue-white structures are very worrisome here and therefore we excised this lesion. This turned out to be a high-risk nevus, so it is better to err on the side of safety and remove these borderline lesions.

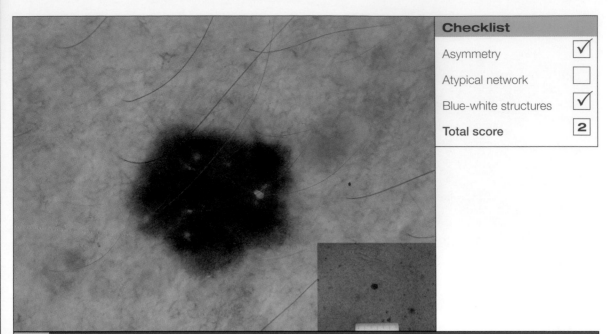

Checklist	
Asymmetry	☑
Atypical network	☐
Blue-white structures	☑
Total score	2

Fig. 43 Nevus.

This lesion is difficult to score and a score of 2 can be achieved for this lesion only if it is considered to be asymmetrical. The pigment network is rather typical and is therefore not scored. There are, however, subtle foci of blue-white structures in the center of the lesion.

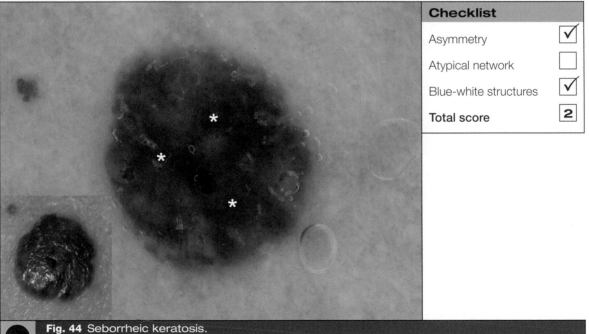

Checklist	
Asymmetry	☑
Atypical network	☐
Blue-white structures	☑
Total score	2

Fig. 44 Seborrheic keratosis.

Strictly following the 3-point checklist gives this lesion a score of 2. There is slight asymmetry of color and structure with a few areas of blue-white structures (*asterisks*). There is no pigment network. With a score of 2, the novice dermoscopist should remove this lesion, though there will always be exceptions to every rule. With experience, clinicians will become confident in diagnosing seborrheic keratosis.

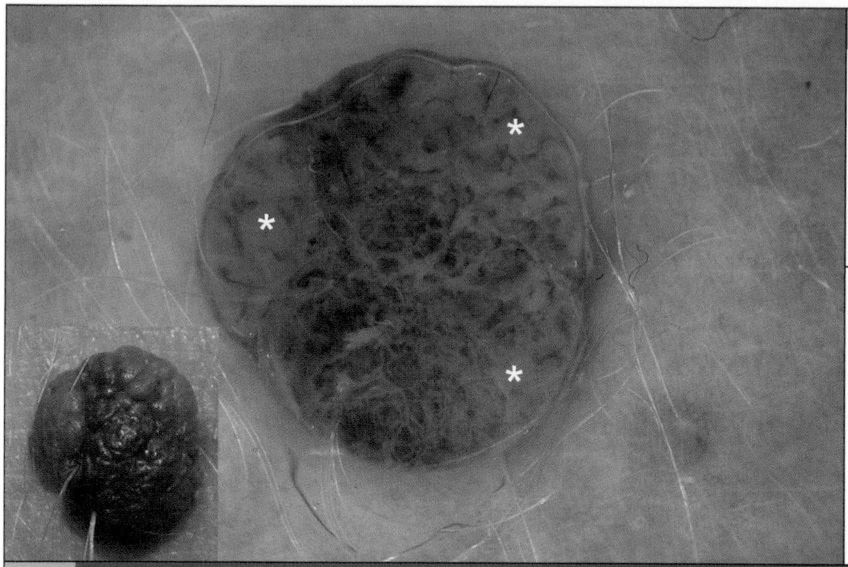

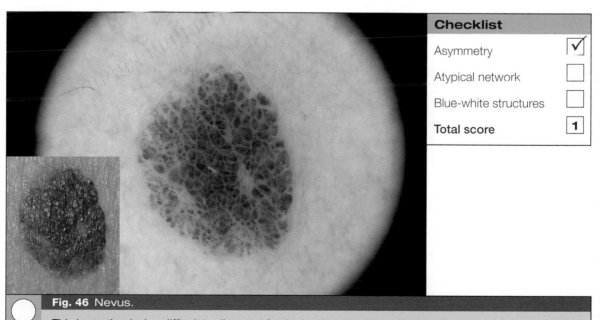

Checklist	
Asymmetry	☐
Atypical network	☐
Blue-white structures	☑
Total score	**1**

Fig. 45 Nevus.

This lesion has a 3-point checklist score of 1. It is relatively symmetrical and there is no pigment network. Blue-white structures (*asterisks*), in this instance only whitish, are clearly visible. This example can be a potential pitfall for the 3-point checklist because nodular basal cell carcinomas can mimic dermal nevi dermoscopically, particularly when the vascular structures are not carefully examined.

Checklist	
Asymmetry	☑
Atypical network	☐
Blue-white structures	☐
Total score	**1**

Fig. 46 Nevus.

This is another lesion difficult to diagnose for the beginner because its checklist score may be 1 or 2. Always remember: if a lesion could be high risk, excise it or follow the patient closely. There is slight asymmetry of dermoscopic structures (globules) but no pigment network. Very subtle whitish areas may be interpreted as blue-white structures.

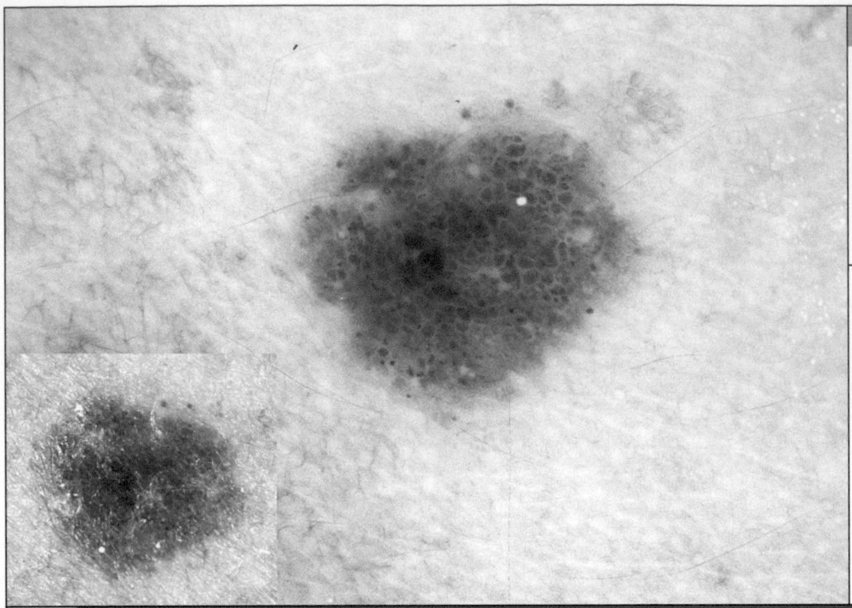

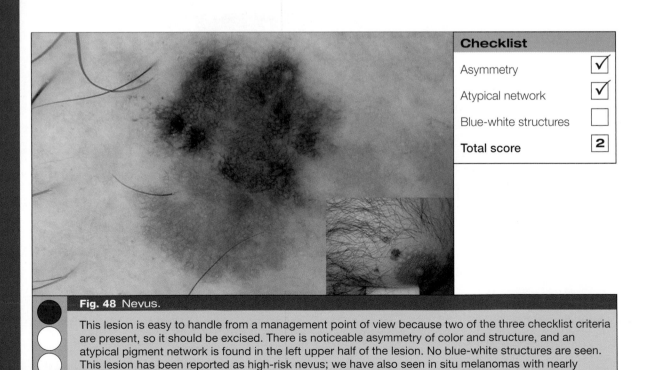

Checklist	
Asymmetry	☑
Atypical network	☐
Blue-white structures	☐
Total score	**1**

Fig. 47 Nevus.

The checklist score for this lesion is only 1, with slight asymmetry of color and structure.

Checklist	
Asymmetry	☑
Atypical network	☑
Blue-white structures	☐
Total score	**2**

Fig. 48 Nevus.

This lesion is easy to handle from a management point of view because two of the three checklist criteria are present, so it should be excised. There is noticeable asymmetry of color and structure, and an atypical pigment network is found in the left upper half of the lesion. No blue-white structures are seen. This lesion has been reported as high-risk nevus; we have also seen in situ melanomas with nearly identical dermoscopic features.

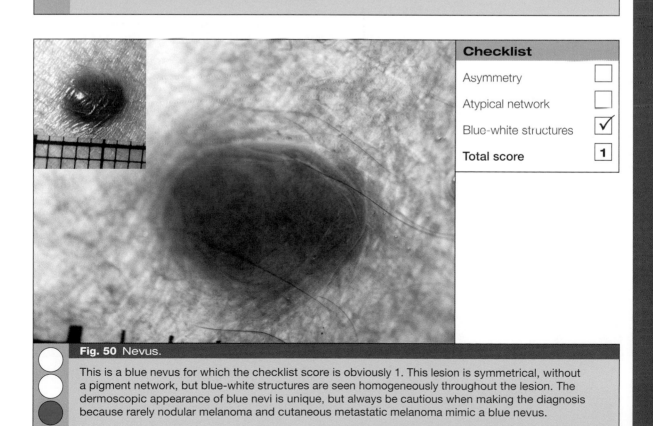

Checklist	
Asymmetry	☑
Atypical network	☑
Blue-white structures	☐
Total score	**2**

Fig. 49 Nevus.

This dermoscopic image is a bit worrisome, showing two of the three checklist criteria. There is asymmetry of color and structure and foci of an atypical thickened and branched pigment network (*circles*). The novice should excise a lesion with this dermoscopic appearance, although the pathology report might not detect any high-risk features.

Checklist	
Asymmetry	☐
Atypical network	☐
Blue-white structures	☑
Total score	**1**

Fig. 50 Nevus.

This is a blue nevus for which the checklist score is obviously 1. This lesion is symmetrical, without a pigment network, but blue-white structures are seen homogeneously throughout the lesion. The dermoscopic appearance of blue nevi is unique, but always be cautious when making the diagnosis because rarely nodular melanoma and cutaneous metastatic melanoma mimic a blue nevus.

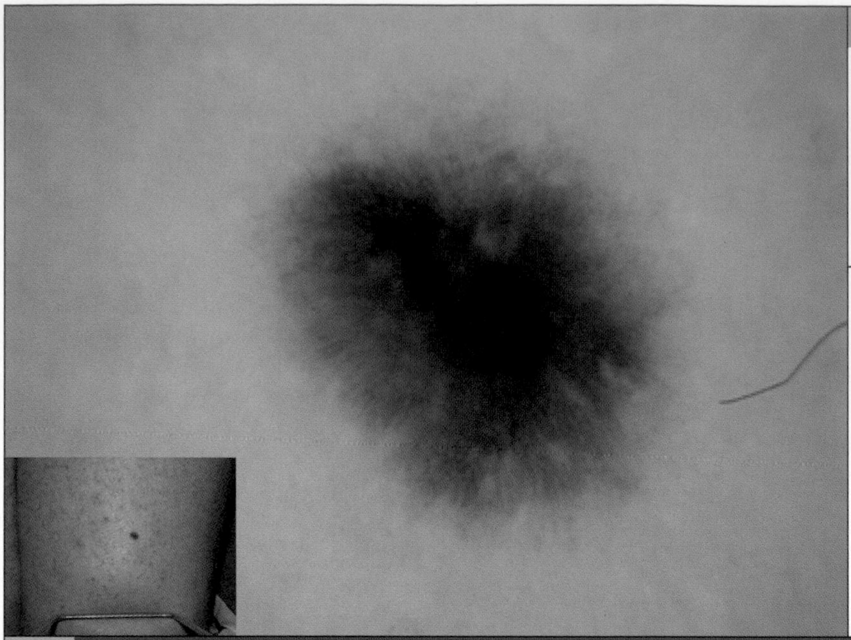

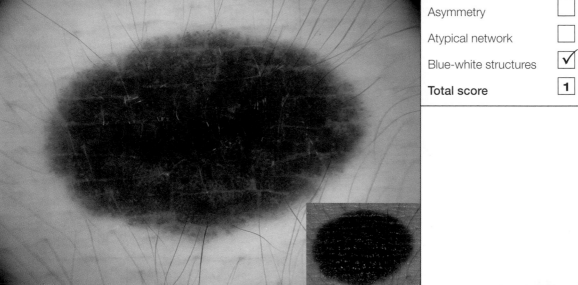

Checklist	
Asymmetry	☑
Atypical network	☑
Blue-white structures	☐
Total score	2

Fig. 51 Nevus.

Again, the management of this lesion after evaluating it with the 3-point checklist is straightforward. With a score of 2, this could be a high-risk lesion. There is asymmetry of shape and structure. An atypical pigment network is observed throughout the periphery of the lesion. No blue-white structures are seen. The discordance between the positive 3-point checklist score and pathology is well known for this type of nevus with prominent central hyperpigmentation.

Checklist	
Asymmetry	☐
Atypical network	☐
Blue-white structures	☑
Total score	1

Fig. 52 Nevus.

In contrast to the lesion above, the checklist score for this nevus is just 1. There is no significant asymmetry of structure with only delicate foci of blue-white structures in the centre of the lesion. No atypical pigment network can be discerned.

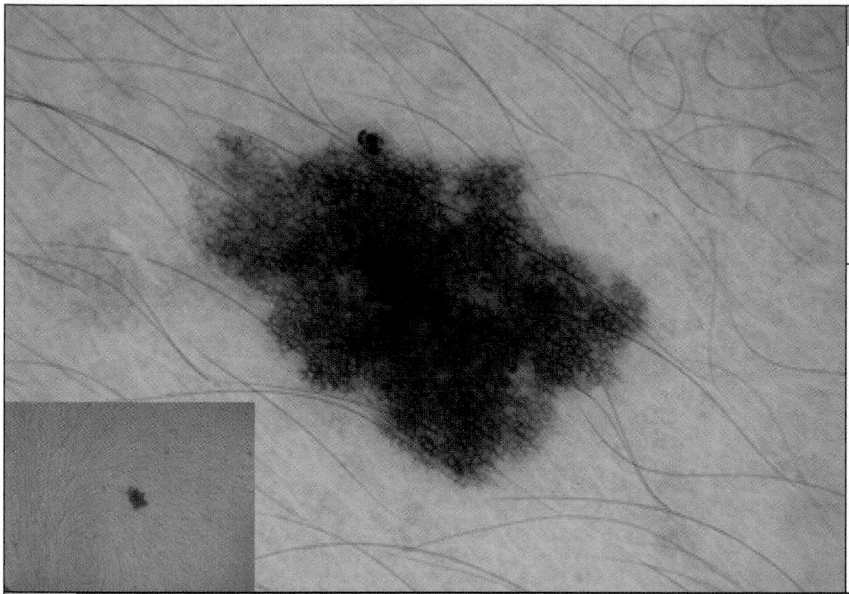

Checklist

Asymmetry	☑
Atypical network	☑
Blue-white structures	☐
Total score	**2**

Fig. 53 Nevus.

This lesion also has a checklist score of 2. This example shows the limitations of the 3-point checklist. There is asymmetry because the lower half does not mirror the upper half. Also note that the pigment network is atypical pretty much throughout the whole lesion. Blue-white structures are not observed. Please remember your final management decision always needs to take into consideration the clinical context including the morphologic features of other nevi in the same patient.

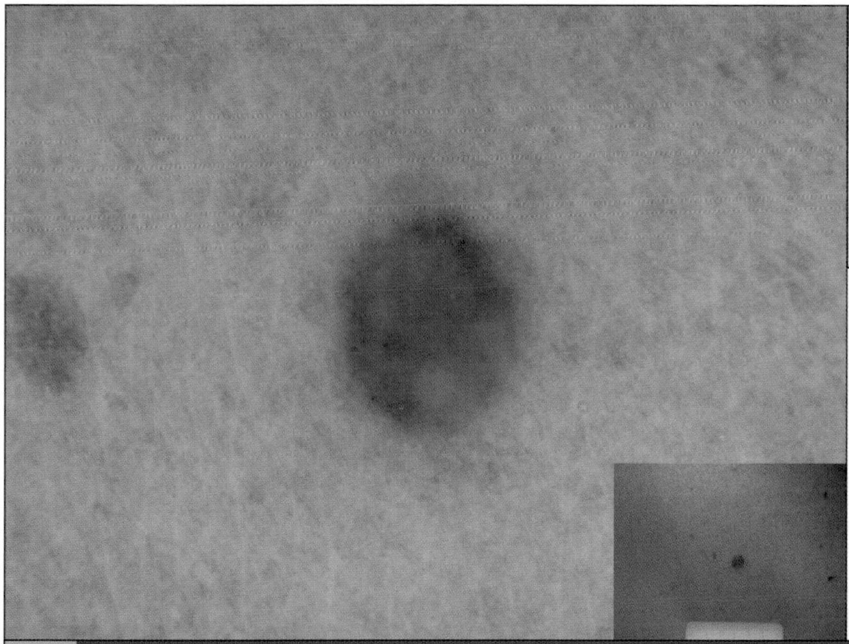

Checklist

Asymmetry	☐
Atypical network	☐
Blue-white structures	☐
Total score	**0**

Fig. 54 Nevus.

This is a rather featureless lesion and we did not score this lesion at all. The slight asymmetry related to the subtle area with a typical pigment network in the right upper corner was deemed not enough to call this lesion asymmetric. And do not confuse the para central delicate hypopigmentation with blue-white structures.

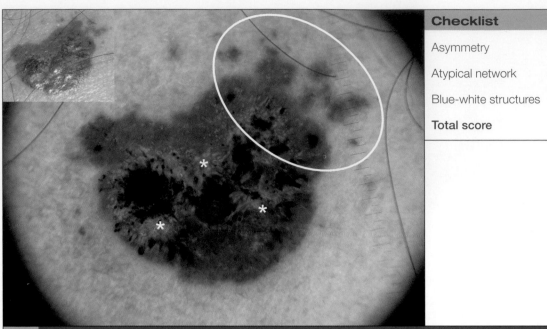

Checklist	
Asymmetry	☑
Atypical network	☐
Blue-white structures	☑
Total score	2

Fig. 55 Melanoma.

There are two strikingly positive features present here—asymmetry and blue-white structures. Because there are also a few satellite lesions (*circle*), it should be excised with high priority. Clear-cut asymmetry of shape and structure and conspicuous blue-white structures (*asterisks*) are seen throughout the lesion. No pigment network is seen, not even at the periphery.

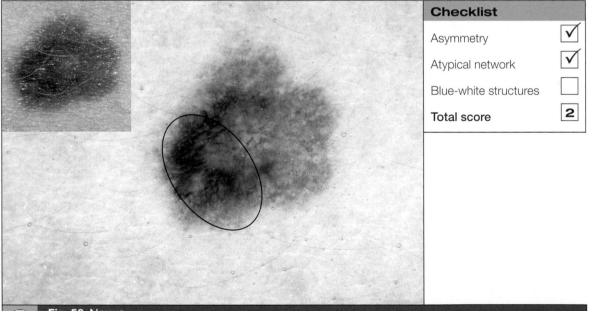

Checklist	
Asymmetry	☑
Atypical network	☑
Blue-white structures	☐
Total score	2

Fig. 56 Nevus.

The atypical pigment network (*circle*) in this asymmetrical lesion is worrisome, and the lesion should be excised. No blue-white structures are seen. Although the histology was benign, this dermoscopic picture might also be seen in in situ melanoma.

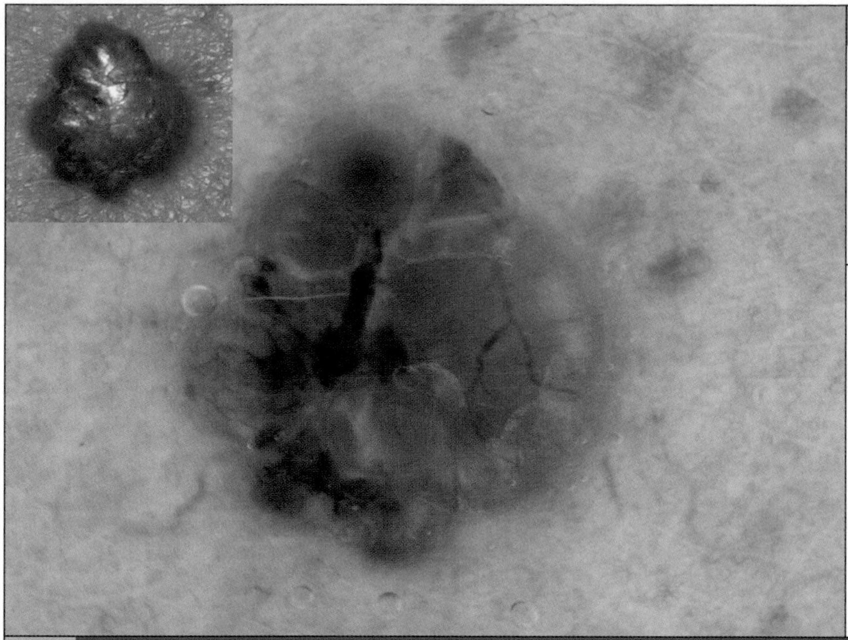

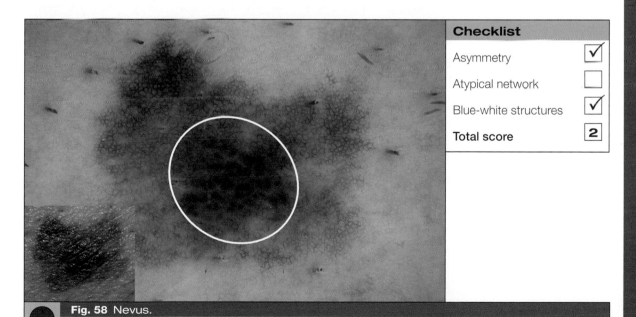

Checklist

Asymmetry	☑
Atypical network	☐
Blue-white structures	☑
Total score	**2**

Fig. 57 Basal cell carcinoma.

The checklist score for this lesion is 2; because it is nodular, excision is recommended. Note the asymmetry of color and structure and numerous blue-white structures throughout the lesion. No pigment network can be identified.

Checklist

Asymmetry	☑
Atypical network	☐
Blue-white structures	☑
Total score	**2**

Fig. 58 Nevus.

Two of the 3-point checklist criteria are present. Asymmetry of color and shape is evident, and centrally located blue-white structures (*circle*) are seen. Because of a 3-point checklist score of 2, excision of this lesion is recommended.

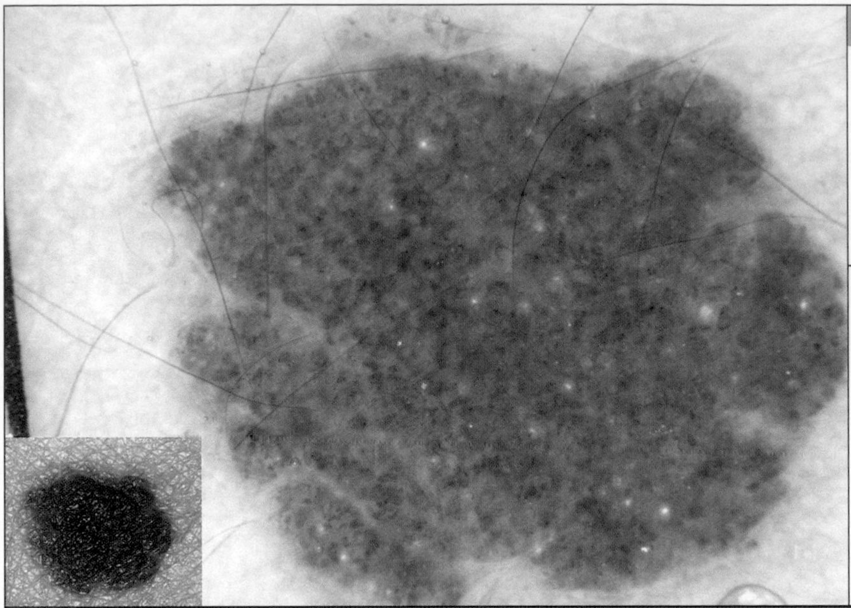

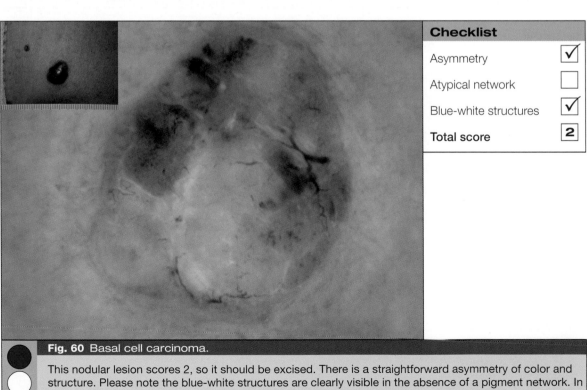

Checklist

Asymmetry	☐
Atypical network	☐
Blue-white structures	☐
Total score	**0**

Fig. 59 Nevus.

The checklist score for this lesion is zero.

Checklist

Asymmetry	☑
Atypical network	☐
Blue-white structures	☑
Total score	**2**

Fig. 60 Basal cell carcinoma.

This nodular lesion scores 2, so it should be excised. There is a straightforward asymmetry of color and structure. Please note the blue-white structures are clearly visible in the absence of a pigment network. In addition, the typical arborizing vessels of basal cell carcinoma are present.

Pattern analysis

Dermoscopic criteria for specific diagnoses

Dermoscopic analysis of pigmented skin lesions is based on four algorithms:

- pattern analysis;
- the ABCD rule;
- Menzies' 11-point checklist; and
- the 7-point checklist.

The common denominator of all these diagnostic algorithms is the identification and analysis of dermoscopic criteria found in the lesions. The majority of the dermatologists who participated in the second consensus meeting were proponents of pattern analysis. The basic principle is that pigmented skin lesions are characterized by global patterns and combinations of local criteria.

Four global dermoscopic patterns for melanocytic nevi

Reticular pattern

The reticular pattern is the most common global pattern in melanocytic lesions. It is characterized by a pigment network covering most parts of a lesion. The pigment network appears as a grid of line segments (honeycomb-like) in different shades of black, brown, or gray. Modifications of the pigment network vary with changes in the biologic behavior of melanocytic skin lesions, and these variations therefore merit special attention.

Globular pattern

Variously sized, round to oval brown structures fill these melanocytic lesions. This pattern can be found in congenital and acquired melanocytic and Clark (dysplastic) nevi.

Homogeneous pattern

This pattern is characterized by a diffuse, uniform, structureless color filling most of the lesion. Colors include black, brown, gray, blue, white, or red. A predominantly bluish color is the morphologic hallmark of blue nevi.

Starburst pattern

The starburst pattern is characterized by the presence of pigmented streaks and/or dots and globules in a radial arrangement at the periphery of a melanocytic lesion. This pattern is the stereotypical morphology in Spitz nevi.

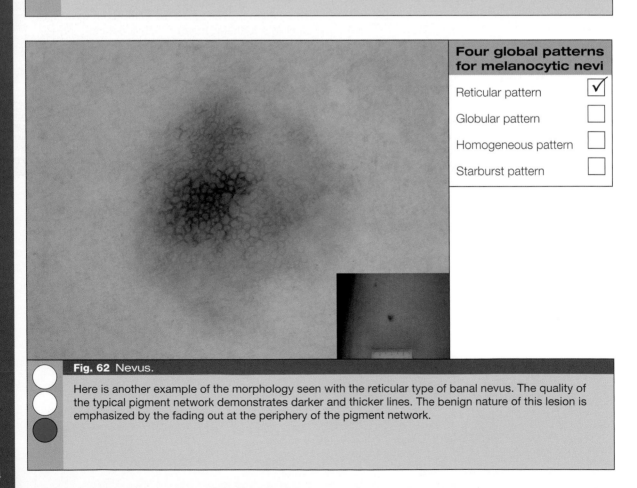

Four global patterns for melanocytic nevi

Reticular pattern ☑
Globular pattern ☐
Homogeneous pattern ☐
Starburst pattern ☐

Fig. 61 Nevus.

The reticular type is probably the most common dermoscopic feature of a flat acquired melanocytic nevus. It is characterized by a typical pigment network that fades out at the periphery. There are also a few small islands of hypopigmentation—a common finding in benign nevi. The histopathologic distinction between a junctional nevus and a compound nevus is commonly given, but the distinction cannot always be made dermoscopically. Moreover, it is clinically irrelevant.

Four global patterns for melanocytic nevi

Reticular pattern ☑
Globular pattern ☐
Homogeneous pattern ☐
Starburst pattern ☐

Fig. 62 Nevus.

Here is another example of the morphology seen with the reticular type of banal nevus. The quality of the typical pigment network demonstrates darker and thicker lines. The benign nature of this lesion is emphasized by the fading out at the periphery of the pigment network.

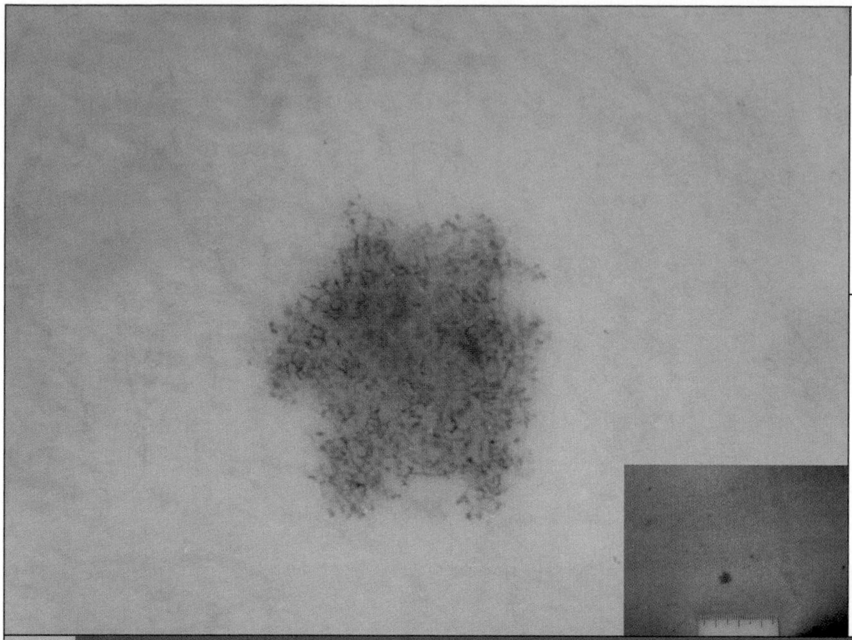

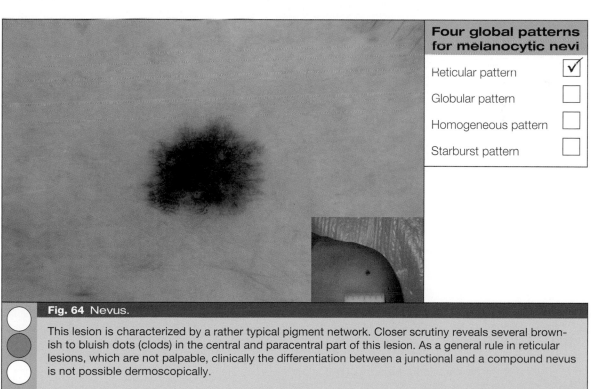

Four global patterns for melanocytic nevi

Reticular pattern	☑
Globular pattern	☐
Homogeneous pattern	☐
Starburst pattern	☐

Fig. 63 Nevus.

This is a reticular-type lesion with a few dots. Please note in the center of the lesion, the pigment network is lacking. In addition, there are a few brown dots (also called clods) at the periphery; an indication that this nevus is still growing. This lesion can also be called a Clark, dysplastic, or atypical nevus; it is not a melanoma.

Four global patterns for melanocytic nevi

Reticular pattern	☑
Globular pattern	☐
Homogeneous pattern	☐
Starburst pattern	☐

Fig. 64 Nevus.

This lesion is characterized by a rather typical pigment network. Closer scrutiny reveals several brownish to bluish dots (clods) in the central and paracentral part of this lesion. As a general rule in reticular lesions, which are not palpable, clinically the differentiation between a junctional and a compound nevus is not possible dermoscopically.

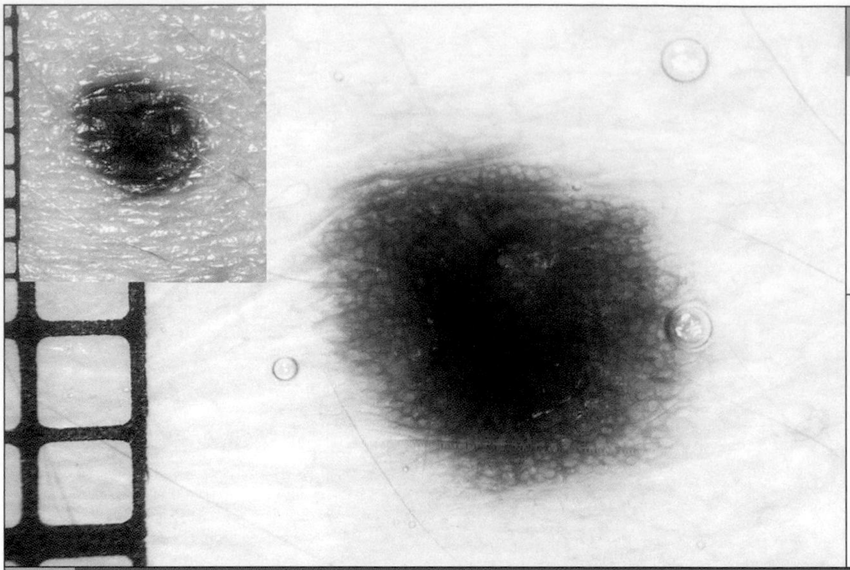

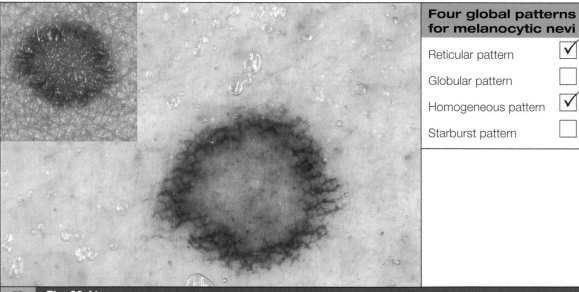

Four global patterns for melanocytic nevi

Reticular pattern	☑
Globular pattern	☐
Homogeneous pattern	☑
Starburst pattern	☐

Fig. 65 Nevus.

A reticular-homogeneous pattern, as seen here, can be seen in banal nevi. In the center, there is homogeneous black pigmentation (black lamella), and at the periphery there is an annular distribution of a typical pigment network. Once again, the pigment network fades at the periphery—a sign of a benign nature. If this was a solitary lesion, in situ melanoma would be the differential diagnosis. Most people with this dermoscopic appearance have multiple similar-appearing nevi, favoring low-risk pathology. Tape stripping can peel away the black lamella and allows one to see whether there are any underlying typical or atypical structures.

Four global patterns for melanocytic nevi

Reticular pattern	☑
Globular pattern	☐
Homogeneous pattern	☑
Starburst pattern	☐

Fig. 66 Nevus.

The unusual type of reticular-homogeneous pattern seen here is more often found in younger pediatric patients. In the center of the lesion, there is homogeneous hypopigmentation (not to be confused with the bony-milky white color of regression), and this is surrounded by a small rim of pigment network. The lines of the pigment network are thickened and the meshes are slightly irregular. The overall architecture of the network, however, is symmetrical and regular.

2 Pattern analysis

Four global patterns for melanocytic nevi

Reticular pattern	☑
Globular pattern	☐
Homogeneous pattern	☑
Starburst pattern	☐

Fig. 67 Nevus.

A stereotypical reticular pattern is seen here. The pigment network is typical, but unevenly distributed and fades out at the periphery. In addition, there are hypopigmented areas throughout the lesion (*arrows*). This nevus does not reveal criteria used to diagnose melanoma (melanoma-specific criteria). Because of the uneven distribution of the pigment network and variations in the shades of brown, the novice dermoscopist should consider excision or close dermoscopic and clinical follow-up.

Four global patterns for melanocytic nevi

Reticular pattern	☑
Globular pattern	☐
Homogeneous pattern	☐
Starburst pattern	☐

Fig. 68 Nevus.

The patchy reticular pattern shown here is associated with an uneven distribution of a typical pigment network. The intensity of pigmentation of the lines alternates, giving this pigment network a patchy appearance. The general principle to remember is that any unevenness of a relatively regular-appearing pigment network is a minor cause for concern. Please note the whitish halo around a hair at the lower left pole of the lesion. This is a rather common finding in reticular nevi.

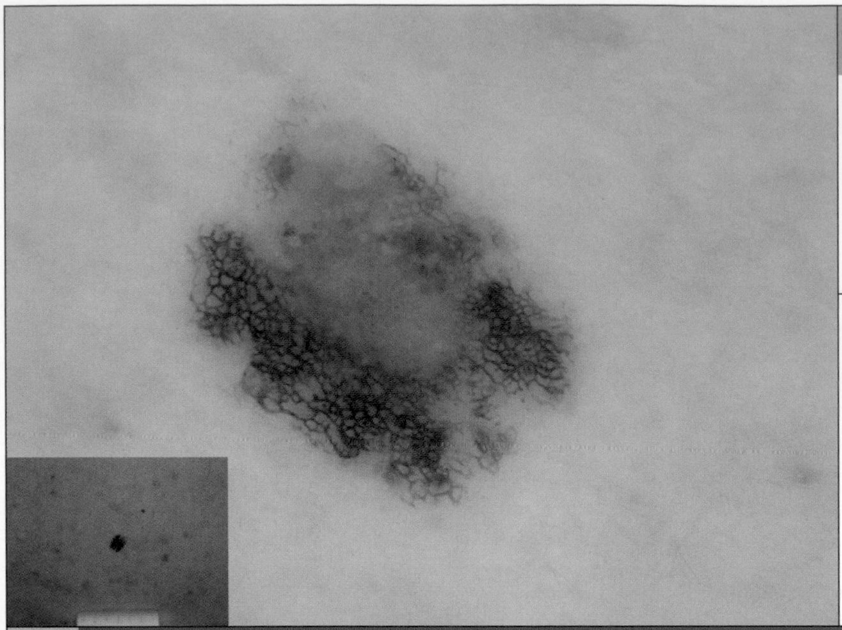

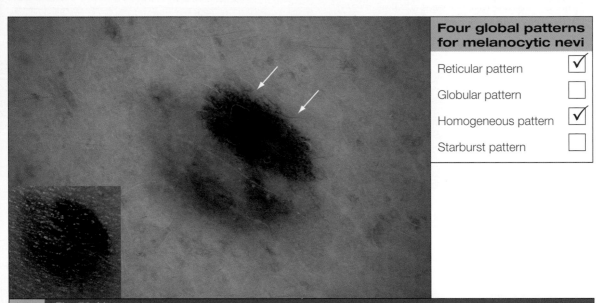

Four global patterns for melanocytic nevi

Reticular pattern	☑
Globular pattern	☐
Homogeneous pattern	☑
Starburst pattern	☐

Fig. 69 Nevus.

This nevus shows a variation of reticular-pattern morphology. Note the zone of homogeneous hypopigmentation in upper half of the lesion. This is not an area of regression that would be seen in melanoma. Still, this lesion is clearly asymmetric in shape and dermoscopic structure and therefore this lesion was excised and called a high-risk nevus. Always remember: when in doubt cut it out.

Four global patterns for melanocytic nevi

Reticular pattern	☑
Globular pattern	☐
Homogeneous pattern	☑
Starburst pattern	☐

Fig. 70 Nevus.

This dermoscopic picture is very worrying. The reticular pattern with eccentric hyperpigmentation dermoscopically simulates in situ melanoma arising in a pre-existing nevus. The upper right half of this lesion is characterized by a slightly atypical pigment network (*arrows*). On the left lower side, there is an area of homogeneous hypopigmentation with a few foci of delicate pigmentation commonly seen in benign nevi. Do not hesitate to excise a lesion that looks like this as soon as possible. The final histopathologic diagnosis is in situ melanoma within a pre-existing nevus in 10% of similar-appearing lesions. In this case, the diagnosis was Clark (dysplastic) nevus, compound type.

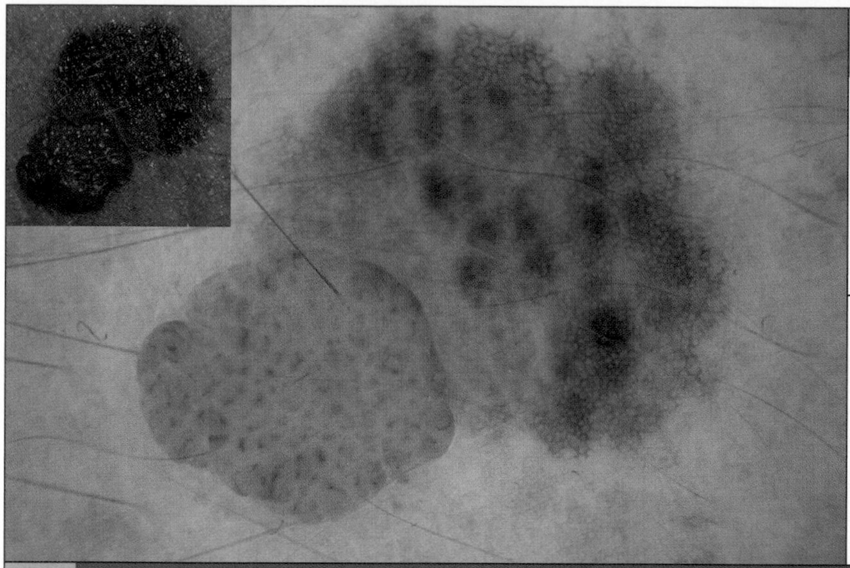

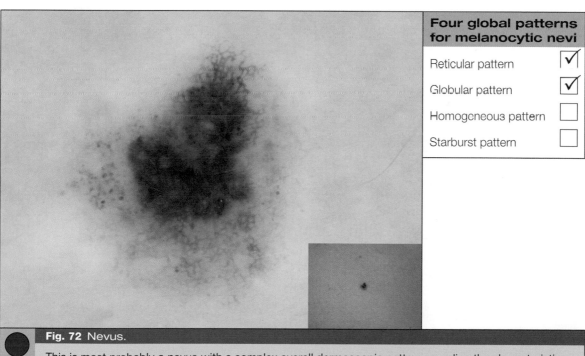

Four global patterns for melanocytic nevi	
Reticular pattern	☑
Globular pattern	☑
Homogeneous pattern	☐
Starburst pattern	☐

Fig. 71 Nevus.

This is a rather unusual combined nevus, with a dome-shaped globular nevus on the lower left site and a variation on the theme of a flat reticular nevus on the upper right site. This lesion should undoubtedly be excised because the differential diagnosis represents a hypomelanotic nodular melanoma arising within a superficial melanoma or a pre-existing dysplastic (Clark) nevus. However, this lesion turned out to be a dysplastic (Clark) nevus adjacent to a benign dermal nevus.

Four global patterns for melanocytic nevi	
Reticular pattern	☑
Globular pattern	☑
Homogeneous pattern	☐
Starburst pattern	☐

Fig. 72 Nevus.

This is most probably a nevus with a complex overall dermoscopic pattern revealing the characteristics of a reticular and a globular nevus (left pole). This lesion displays several unusual dermoscopic aspects with prominent blue-white structures (more bluish-black) in the center. Always excise a lesion like this one. The histopathology diagnosis here was a dysplastic (Clark) nevus, compound type.

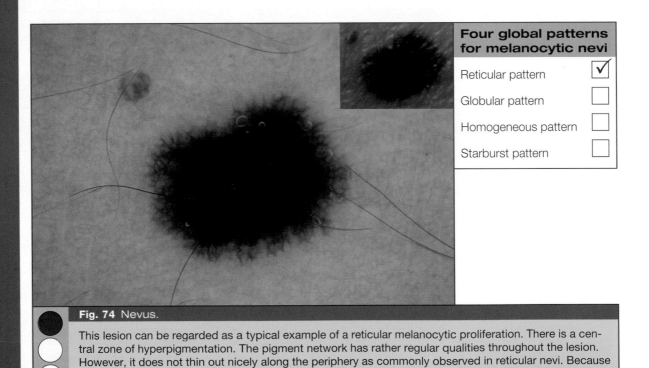

Four global patterns for melanocytic nevi

Reticular pattern	☑
Globular pattern	☐
Homogeneous pattern	☑
Starburst pattern	☐

Fig. 73 Nevus.

This light-brown pinkish lesion reveals a central hypopigmented homogeneous area surrounded by a subtle, not very pronounced pigment network in a ring-like fashion. The unusual aspect of this lesion is its pinkish color, and in the absence of any history of growth, annual follow-up is the management approach we choose for this patient.

Four global patterns for melanocytic nevi

Reticular pattern	☑
Globular pattern	☐
Homogeneous pattern	☐
Starburst pattern	☐

Fig. 74 Nevus.

This lesion can be regarded as a typical example of a reticular melanocytic proliferation. There is a central zone of hyperpigmentation. The pigment network has rather regular qualities throughout the lesion. However, it does not thin out nicely along the periphery as commonly observed in reticular nevi. Because of this dermoscopic finding and heavy pigmentation, this is potentially a high-risk lesion. Histopathologically, this was diagnosed as a junctional type of dysplastic (Clark) nevus. Novice dermoscopists should not hesitate to excise lesions that look like this.

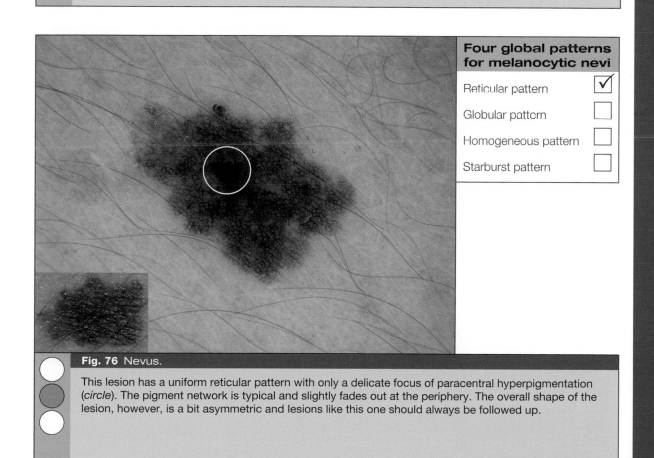

Four global patterns for melanocytic nevi

Reticular pattern	☑
Globular pattern	☐
Homogeneous pattern	☑
Starburst pattern	☐

Fig. 75 Nevus.

This is another example of a reticular-homogeneous nevus with an annular reticular pattern in the periphery and large central homogeneous hypopigmented area. The color of the hypopigmented area is not bony-white as observed in regressive melanoma, and because of the overall symmetry of this lesion, annual follow-up can be advised confidently by the novice dermoscopist.

Four global patterns for melanocytic nevi

Reticular pattern	☑
Globular pattern	☐
Homogeneous pattern	☐
Starburst pattern	☐

Fig. 76 Nevus.

This lesion has a uniform reticular pattern with only a delicate focus of paracentral hyperpigmentation (*circle*). The pigment network is typical and slightly fades out at the periphery. The overall shape of the lesion, however, is a bit asymmetric and lesions like this one should always be followed up.

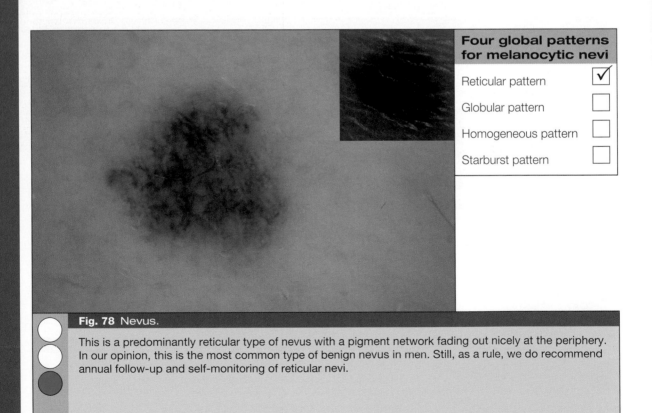

Four global patterns for melanocytic nevi

Reticular pattern	☑
Globular pattern	☐
Homogeneous pattern	☐
Starburst pattern	☐

Fig. 77 Nevus.

This is another example of the protean variation of morphology within melanocytic proliferations exhibiting the reticular pattern. In contrast to Fig. 76, the pigment network here is mostly atypical with a tendency to stop abruptly at the periphery. This high-risk nevus cannot be distinguished dermoscopically from a superficial melanoma (or an in situ melanoma) and needs to be excised.

Four global patterns for melanocytic nevi

Reticular pattern	☑
Globular pattern	☐
Homogeneous pattern	☐
Starburst pattern	☐

Fig. 78 Nevus.

This is a predominantly reticular type of nevus with a pigment network fading out nicely at the periphery. In our opinion, this is the most common type of benign nevus in men. Still, as a rule, we do recommend annual follow-up and self-monitoring of reticular nevi.

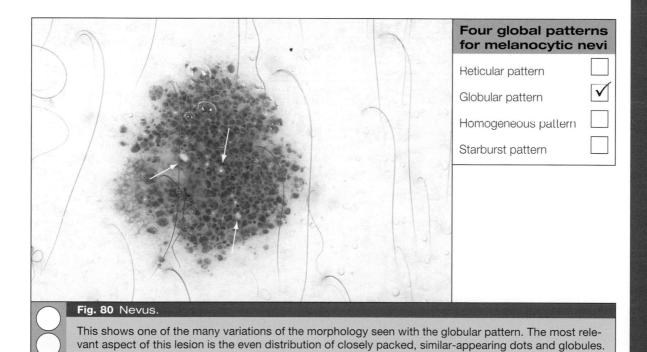

Four global patterns for melanocytic nevi

Reticular pattern	☐
Globular pattern	☑
Homogeneous pattern	☐
Starburst pattern	☐

Fig. 79 Nevus.

This shows a stereotypical globular pattern of a benign nevus. There are numerous dots and globules of similar shape and varying size throughout the lesion. No melanoma-specific dermoscopic criteria are seen. This pattern is most commonly seen in adolescents but can also be found in adults. The histopathology could show a junctional or compound nevus.

Four global patterns for melanocytic nevi

Reticular pattern	☐
Globular pattern	☑
Homogeneous pattern	☐
Starburst pattern	☐

Fig. 80 Nevus.

This shows one of the many variations of the morphology seen with the globular pattern. The most relevant aspect of this lesion is the even distribution of closely packed, similar-appearing dots and globules. In addition, there are a few milia-like cysts in the center of the lesion (*arrows*). Milia-like cysts are not seen only in seborrheic keratosis.

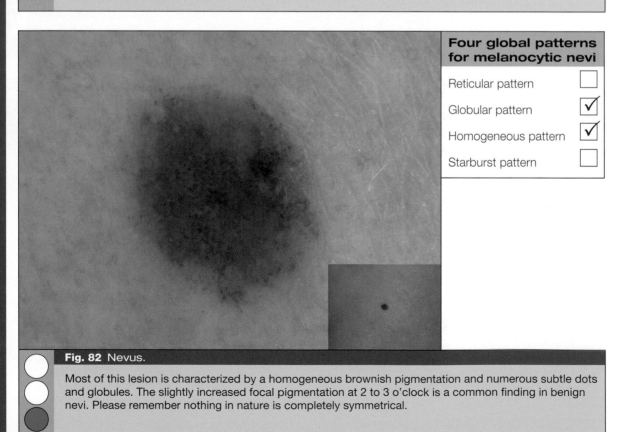

Four global patterns for melanocytic nevi

Reticular pattern ☐
Globular pattern ☑
Homogeneous pattern ☐
Starburst pattern ☐

Fig. 81 Nevus.

This globular pattern shows dots and globules that are not closely packed together, are similar in size and shape, and have a slightly uneven distribution. Please note an increase of globules at the periphery of the lesion (peripheral rim of globules). This specific pattern is commonly observed in symmetrically growing nevi. No melanoma-specific criteria are seen in this otherwise banal lesion.

Four global patterns for melanocytic nevi

Reticular pattern ☐
Globular pattern ☑
Homogeneous pattern ☑
Starburst pattern ☐

Fig. 82 Nevus.

Most of this lesion is characterized by a homogeneous brownish pigmentation and numerous subtle dots and globules. The slightly increased focal pigmentation at 2 to 3 o'clock is a common finding in benign nevi. Please remember nothing in nature is completely symmetrical.

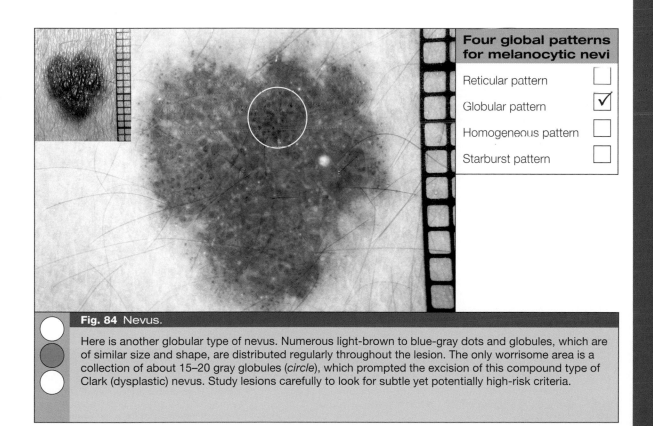

Four global patterns for melanocytic nevi	
Reticular pattern	☐
Globular pattern	☑
Homogeneous pattern	☐
Starburst pattern	☐

Fig. 83 Nevus.

This image shows a more worrisome variation of the globular pattern. Numerous dots and globules are unevenly distributed throughout the lesion (*circle*) and vary in size and shape.

Four global patterns for melanocytic nevi	
Reticular pattern	☐
Globular pattern	☑
Homogeneous pattern	☐
Starburst pattern	☐

Fig. 84 Nevus.

Here is another globular type of nevus. Numerous light-brown to blue-gray dots and globules, which are of similar size and shape, are distributed regularly throughout the lesion. The only worrisome area is a collection of about 15–20 gray globules (*circle*), which prompted the excision of this compound type of Clark (dysplastic) nevus. Study lesions carefully to look for subtle yet potentially high-risk criteria.

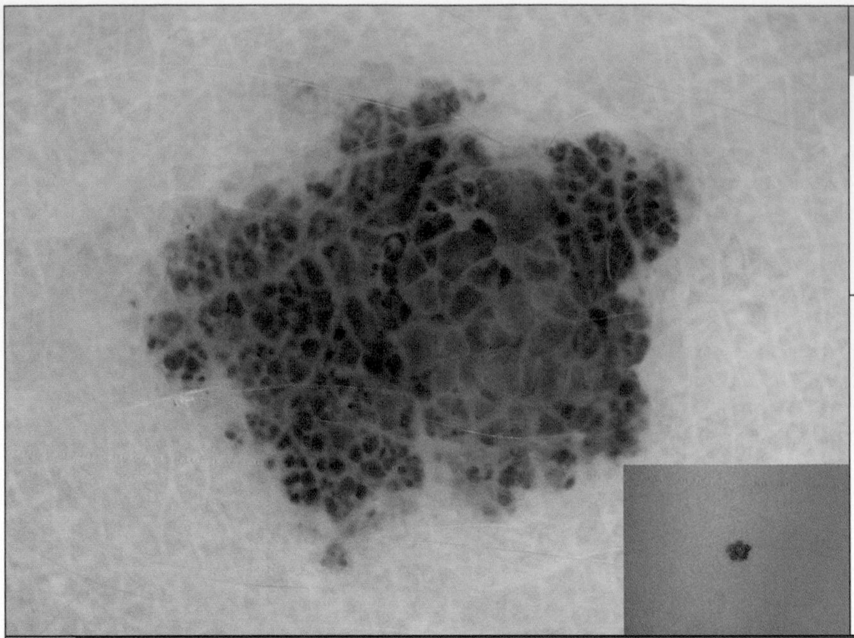

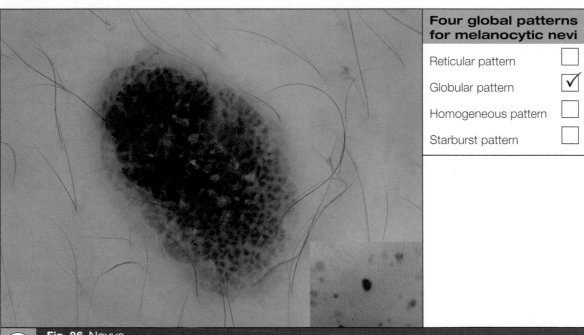

Four global patterns for melanocytic nevi

Reticular pattern ☐
Globular pattern ☑
Homogeneous pattern ☐
Starburst pattern ☐

Fig. 85 Nevus.

This is another stereotypical example of the globular pattern of nevus, in which the globules are very easy to see. Throughout this lesion several dark-brown dots and globules display a rectangular shape (cobblestone-like). This morphologic phenomenon is often found in congenital or congenital-like nevi. Dermoscopically, this lesion gives the impression of a papillomatous or raised character. Histopathologic examination revealed a predominantly dermal compound nevus.

Four global patterns for melanocytic nevi

Reticular pattern ☐
Globular pattern ☑
Homogeneous pattern ☐
Starburst pattern ☐

Fig. 86 Nevus.

The globular pattern seen here is very similar to that in Fig. 85. The lesion is composed of closely packed dots and globules characterized by various shades of brown. In addition, there are several whitish dots and globules representing keratin accumulation. The variation of the color might alarm the inexperienced dermoscopist. Remember, if in doubt, cut it out. This was a benign, mostly dermal nevus. After seeing and excising a few lesions with this dermoscopic appearance, the dermoscopist will feel more comfortable about not excising lesions that look like this.

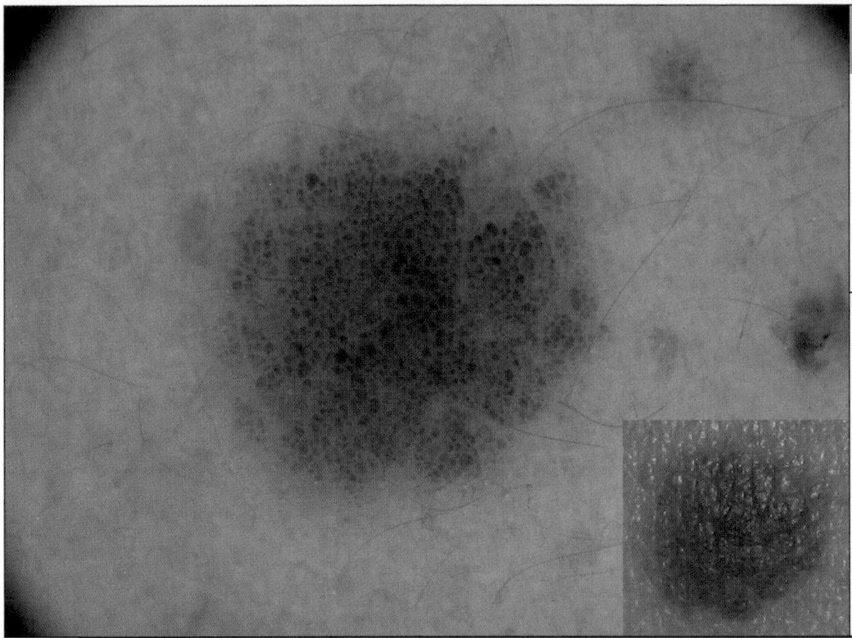

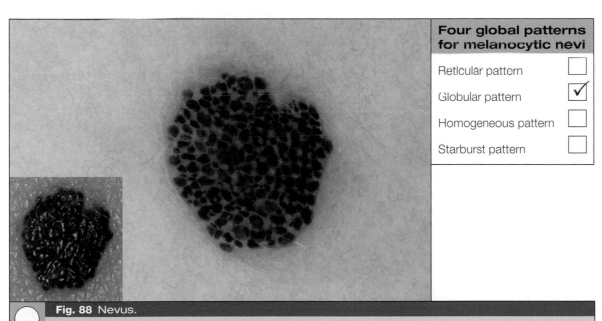

Four global patterns for melanocytic nevi	
Reticular pattern	☐
Globular pattern	☑
Homogeneous pattern	☐
Starburst pattern	☐

Fig. 87 Nevus.

This lesion shows again a globular pattern. It contains numerous brown to gray globules, which are evenly distributed throughout the lesion. The gray globules are situated predominantly in the center of the lesion and correspond to nests of pigmented nevus cells in the papillary dermis. Remarkably, globular nevi represent the stereotypical nevus subtype among children and teenagers.

Four global patterns for melanocytic nevi	
Reticular pattern	☐
Globular pattern	☑
Homogeneous pattern	☐
Starburst pattern	☐

Fig. 88 Nevus.

It is amazing to see the many different variations on the theme of globular nevi. In the previous pages, we have seen quite a few benign globular nevi, but all are morphologically different and unique. The striking aspect of this uniformly pigmented globular nevus is its dark brown pigmentation. We are happy to follow this nevus and recommend self-monitoring.

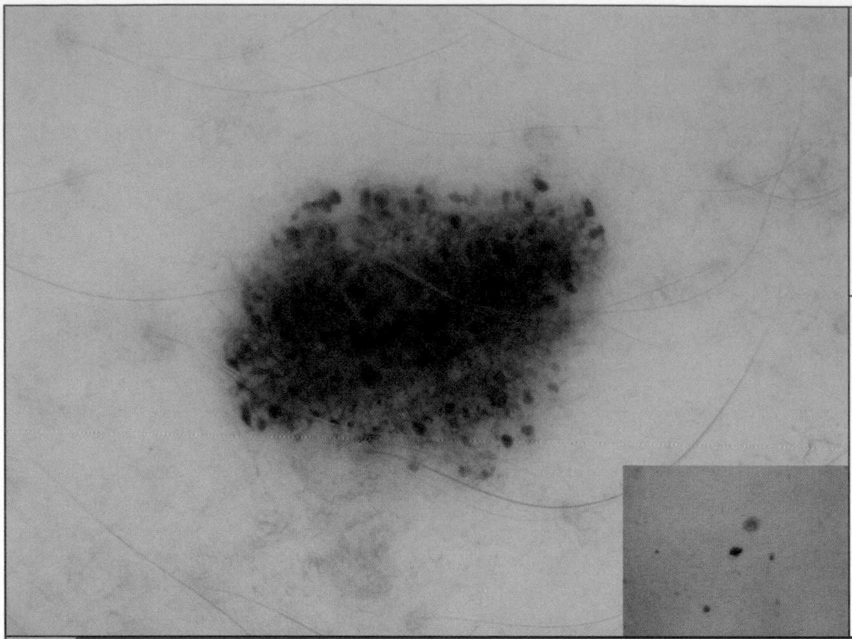

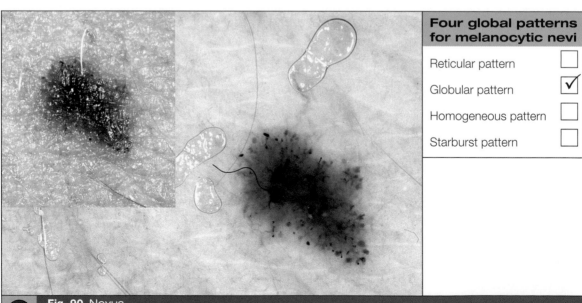

Four global patterns for melanocytic nevi

Reticular pattern	☐
Globular pattern	☑
Homogeneous pattern	☐
Starburst pattern	☐

Fig. 89 Nevus.

This globular nevus raises at least the orange flag because the globules composing this lesion vary slightly in size, shape, and color and are also slightly unevenly distributed throughout the lesion. In addition, this lesion has an incomplete rim of peripheral globules, indicating that this lesion will continue to grow. Because the patient was concerned about this lesion, a deep shave biopsy was performed. The final histopathologic diagnosis was a compound type of dysplastic (Clark) nevus.

Four global patterns for melanocytic nevi

Reticular pattern	☐
Globular pattern	☑
Homogeneous pattern	☐
Starburst pattern	☐

Fig. 90 Nevus.

Numerous irregularly sized brownish dots and globules are seen throughout this lesion. Although it is rather small, the dermoscopic asymmetry is striking. The pinkish color is an important clue that this could be a high-risk lesion. Because of its high-risk appearance, a lesion like this one warrants a second histopathologic opinion if it is signed out as a benign nevus as was the case here.

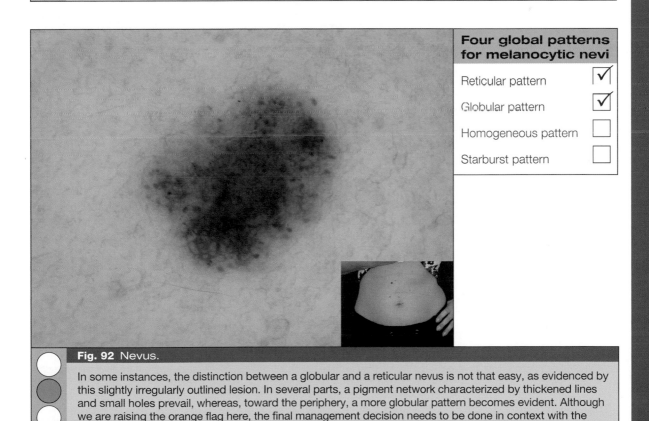

Four global patterns for melanocytic nevi

Reticular pattern	☐
Globular pattern	☑
Homogeneous pattern	☐
Starburst pattern	☐

Fig. 91 Nevus.

One has to look carefully to recognize that this heavily pigmented nevus reveals a globular and not a homogeneous pattern in its central part. The lighter pigmented peripheral ring displays a pattern reminiscent of globules and reticulated lines telling us that in morphology there is always an overlap of features. We were confident that this lesion was a variation on the theme of a benign globular nevus and recommended annual follow-up and self-monitoring.

Four global patterns for melanocytic nevi

Reticular pattern	☑
Globular pattern	☑
Homogeneous pattern	☐
Starburst pattern	☐

Fig. 92 Nevus.

In some instances, the distinction between a globular and a reticular nevus is not that easy, as evidenced by this slightly irregularly outlined lesion. In several parts, a pigment network characterized by thickened lines and small holes prevail, whereas, toward the periphery, a more globular pattern becomes evident. Although we are raising the orange flag here, the final management decision needs to be done in context with the clinical setting. We have excised this lesion and the histopathology has ruled out a melanoma.

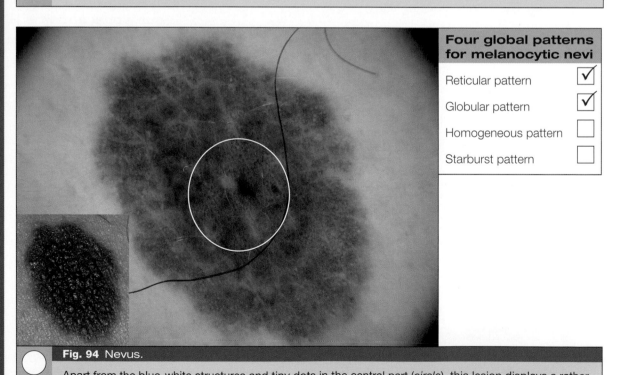

Four global patterns for melanocytic nevi

Reticular pattern	☐
Globular pattern	☐
Homogeneous pattern	☑
Starburst pattern	☐

Fig. 93 Nevus.

This lesion is characterized by diffuse homogeneous pigmentation. There is a subtle rim of radially oriented line segments at the periphery at 9 o'clock and subtle blue-white structures in the center. The dermoscopic differential diagnosis includes Clark (dysplastic) nevus and Spitz nevus. We raised the orange flag and excised this lesion. The lesion was reported as a compound type of Clark (dysplastic) nevus with so-called spitzoid features.

Four global patterns for melanocytic nevi

Reticular pattern	☑
Globular pattern	☑
Homogeneous pattern	☐
Starburst pattern	☐

Fig. 94 Nevus.

Apart from the blue-white structures and tiny dots in the central part (*circle*), this lesion displays a rather uniform subtle reticular pattern, which made us comfortable to follow up this lesion. We are well aware that some colleagues would prefer to excise a lesion like this one for peace of mind. Also the clinical image was reassuring for us that we were dealing with a nevus.

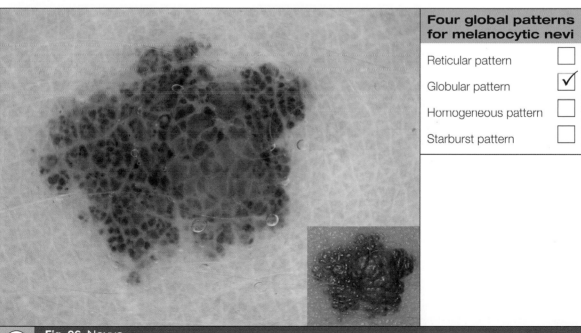

Four global patterns for melanocytic nevi	
Reticular pattern	☑
Globular pattern	☐
Homogeneous pattern	☑
Starburst pattern	☐

Fig. 95 Nevus.

This lesion is characterized by a reticular-homogeneous pattern. Please note the focus of atypical pigment network (*circle*). In addition, the left lower part of the lesion exhibits blue-white structures, and these two signs are sufficient to warrant excision. In the realm of dysplastic (Clark) nevus, it is difficult to determine whether a lesion is low or high-risk dermoscopically; therefore, the novice is best advised to excise gray-zone lesions as this one.

Four global patterns for melanocytic nevi	
Reticular pattern	☐
Globular pattern	☑
Homogeneous pattern	☐
Starburst pattern	☐

Fig. 96 Nevus.

This is another example of a benign globular nevus with globules slightly varying in size, shape, and coloration. Despite the irregular outline of this lesion, no action but follow-up has to be undertaken.

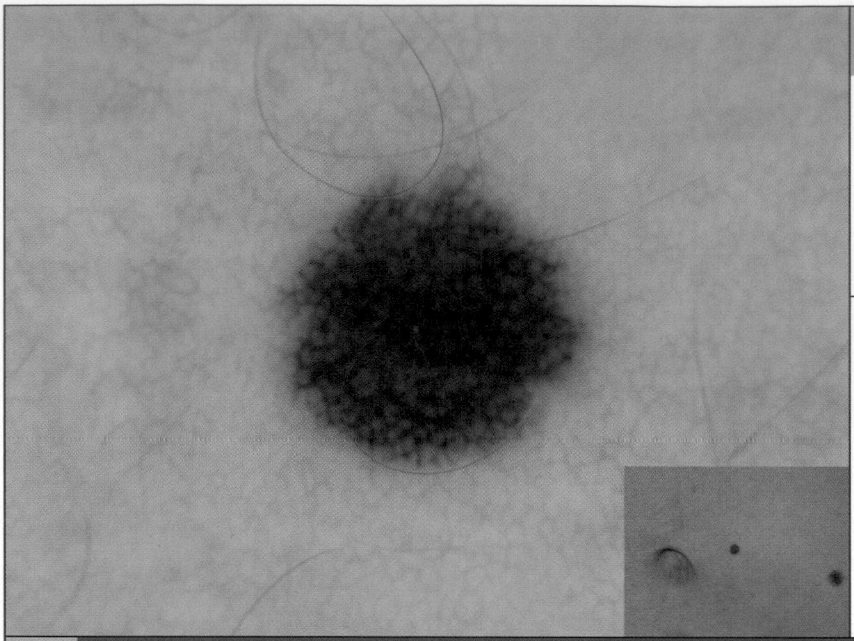

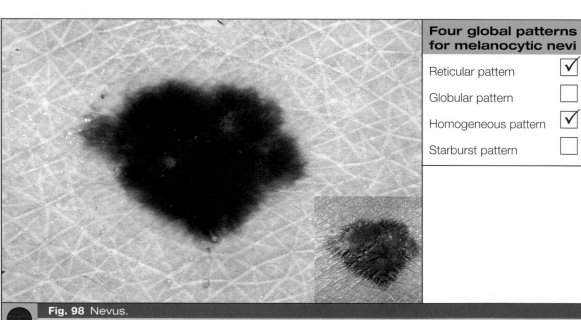

Four global patterns for melanocytic nevi

Reticular pattern	☑
Globular pattern	☐
Homogeneous pattern	☐
Starburst pattern	☐

Fig. 97 Nevus.

This is a rather commonly observed variation on the theme of a reticular type of nevus. These lesions are frequently found in adults. We judge this pigment network as somewhat atypical and despite rather uniformly distributed in this roundish lesion, we raise the orange flag. It is also not really fading out at the periphery, which is rather infrequently seen in reticular nevi. Without any specific history of growth by the patient, we were happy with short-term follow-up of this nevus and, in addition, recommended self-monitoring.

Four global patterns for melanocytic nevi

Reticular pattern	☑
Globular pattern	☐
Homogeneous pattern	☑
Starburst pattern	☐

Fig. 98 Nevus.

This lesion is a variation of the homogeneous-reticular type of nevus reminiscent of a so-called black nevus. Multiple jet-black homogeneous zones are seen at the periphery. Use tape stripping for this black lesion mimicking in situ melanoma.

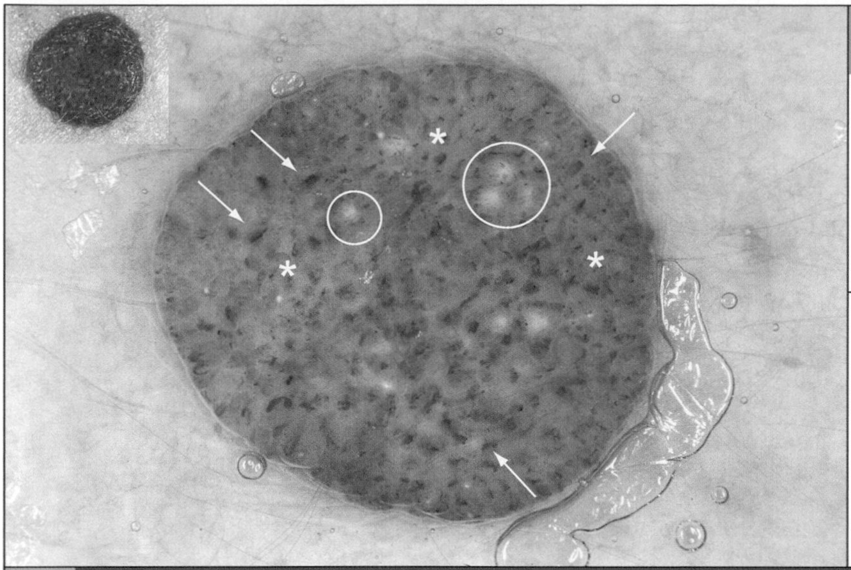

Four global patterns for melanocytic nevi

Reticular pattern	☐
Globular pattern	☑
Homogeneous pattern	☐
Starburst pattern	☐

Fig. 99 Nevus.

This is a dome-shaped melanocytic nevus that reveals a subtle globular pattern with numerous light-brown dots and globules throughout. Multiple blood vessels with dotted (*asterisks*) and comma-like appearances (*arrows*) are seen. There are also a few milia-like cysts (*circles*), but this is not a seborrheic keratosis. Clinically this lesion could be confused with a basal cell carcinoma, but the vessels in a basal cell carcinoma are thick and branched (arborizing) and there would be no yellow color.

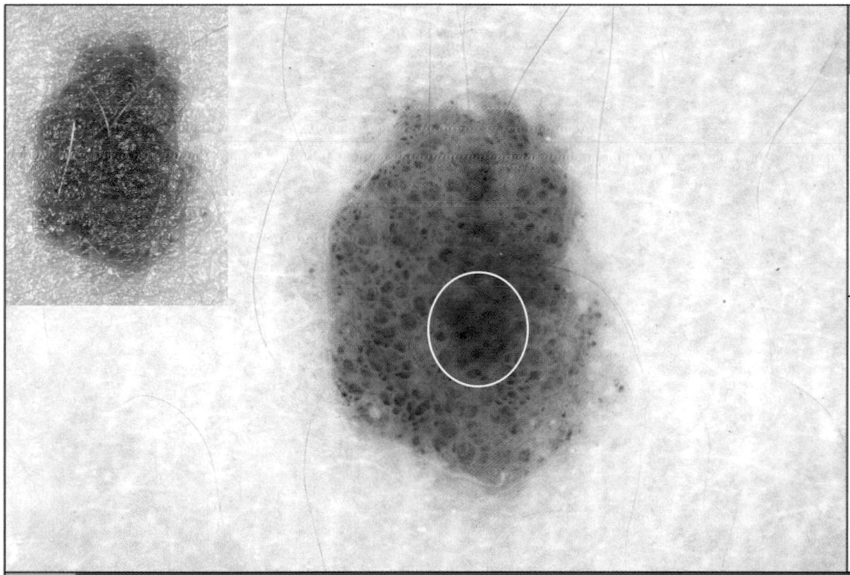

Four global patterns for melanocytic nevi

Reticular pattern	☐
Globular pattern	☑
Homogeneous pattern	☐
Starburst pattern	☐

Fig. 100 Nevus.

This lesion has a globular pattern containing numerous brownish-blue dots and globules, which vary in size and shape, and a central irregular brownish blotch (*circle*).

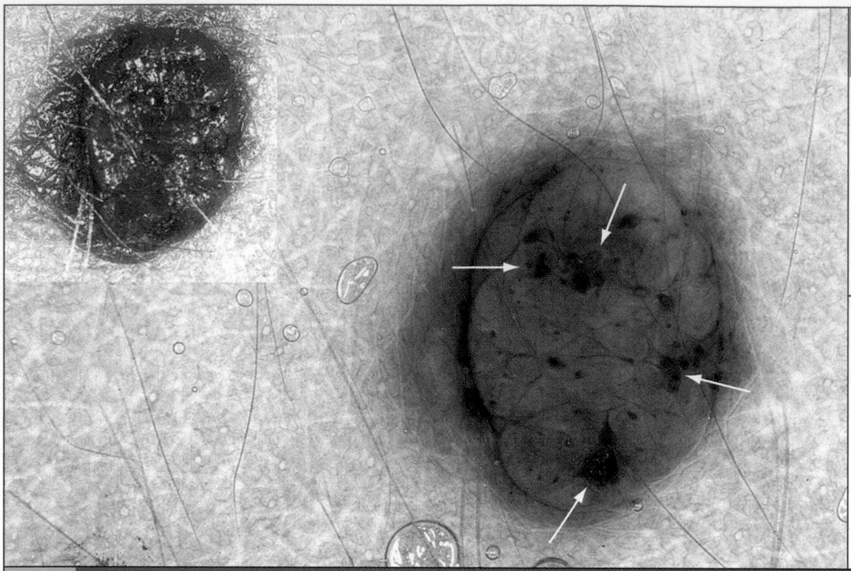

Four global patterns for melanocytic nevi

Reticular pattern	☐
Globular pattern	☑
Homogeneous pattern	☐
Starburst pattern	☐

Fig. 101 Nevus.

This clinically broad sessile nodule has a papillomatous surface and a few irregularly shaped comedo-like openings (*arrows*). Sometimes it is not possible to differentiate the comedo-like openings from globules. The thin pigmented lines are not pigment network but pigmentation in the furrows of the lesion. The soft, compressible nature points to it being low risk. Palpate suspicious lesions, but if in doubt, cut them out.

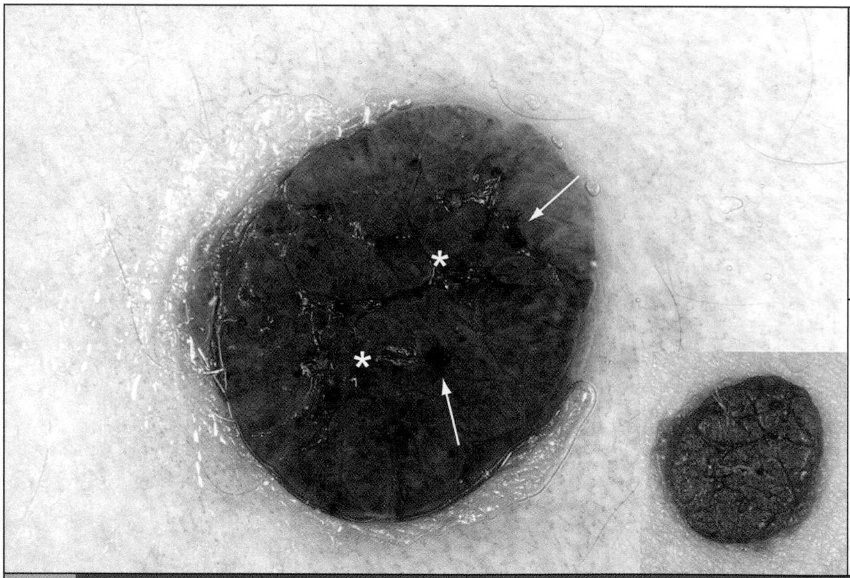

Four global patterns for melanocytic nevi

Reticular pattern	☐
Globular pattern	☑
Homogeneous pattern	☐
Starburst pattern	☐

Fig. 102 Nevus.

This is another broad, sessile nodule characterized by a papillomatous surface. There are some comedo-like openings (*arrows*) and a few bluish dots and globules (*asterisks*). These can be confused with blue-white structures.

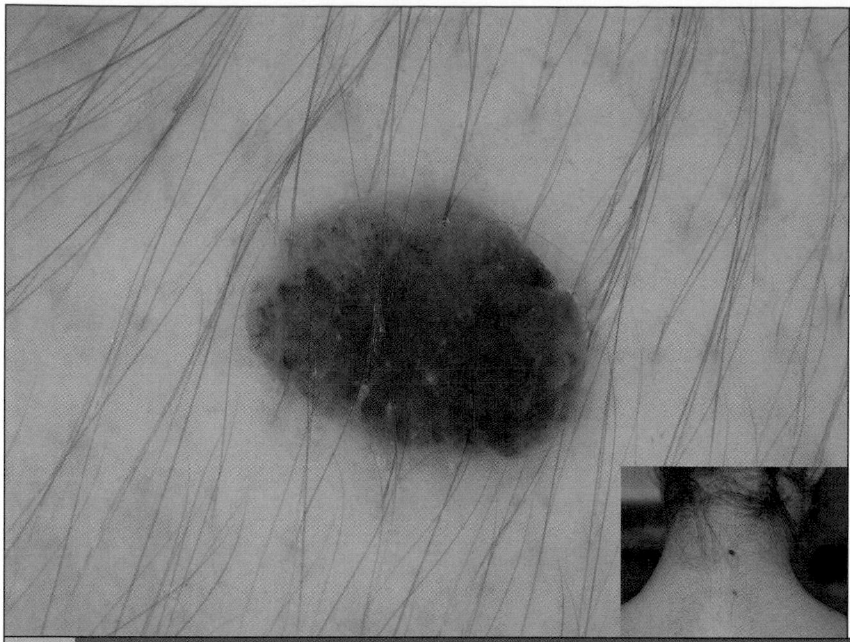

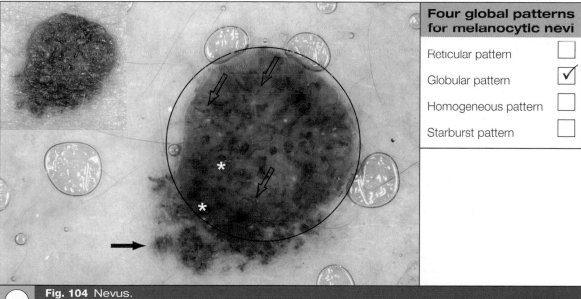

Four global patterns for melanocytic nevi

Reticular pattern	☐
Globular pattern	☐
Homogeneous pattern	☑
Starburst pattern	☐

Fig. 103 Nevus.

Here is another papillomatous dermal nevus. Please note the subtle variation of gray and brown colors throughout this slightly papillomatous nodule. Also, the presence of numerous terminal hairs within this nevus is rather typical for a benign lesion. This is another lesion to palpate. Compressibility and easy movement from side to side are good clinical signs in favor of its benign nature.

Four global patterns for melanocytic nevi

Reticular pattern	☐
Globular pattern	☑
Homogeneous pattern	☐
Starburst pattern	☐

Fig. 104 Nevus.

It is common to see a papillomatous nevus (*circle*) in transition with a flat melanocytic nevus (*solid arrow*). The flat component can give a worrisome clinical appearance, which in most cases is not high risk when viewed with dermoscopy. The dome-shaped nodule is characterized by numerous comedo-like openings (*asterisks*). In addition, there are comma-like vessels (*open arrows*) throughout the lesion. Comma-shaped vessels are not characteristically seen in melanomas. At the lower margin, there is a flat brownish area with regular dots and globules.

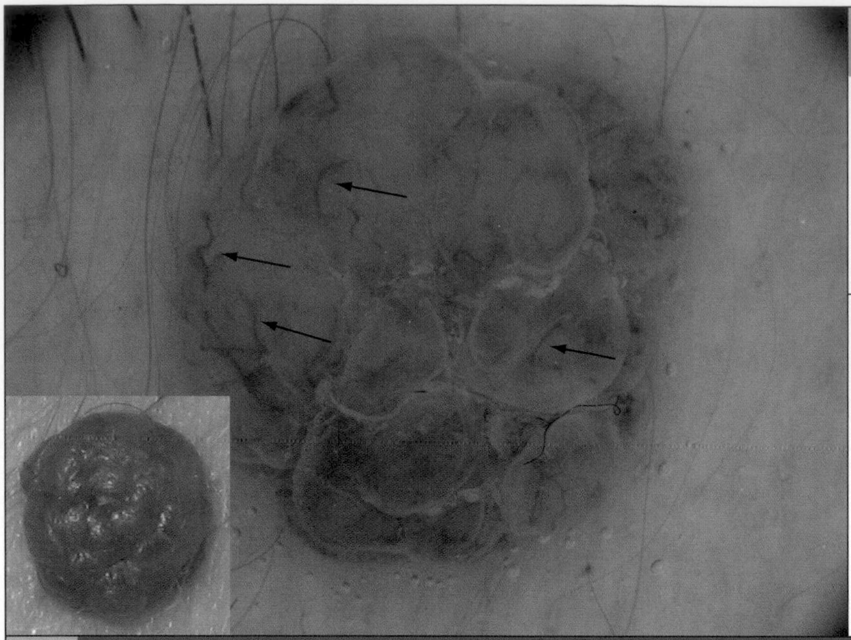

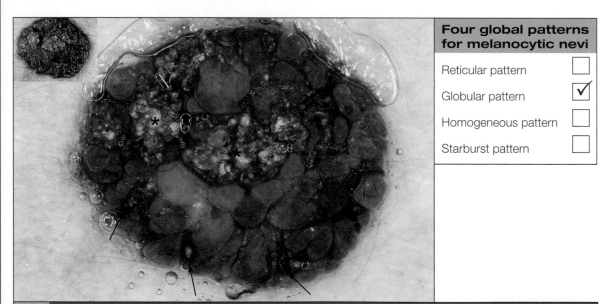

Four global patterns for melanocytic nevi	
Reticular pattern	☐
Globular pattern	☐
Homogeneous pattern	☑
Starburst pattern	☐

Fig. 105 Nevus.

This papillomatous dermal nevus is relatively featureless, but the blood vessels (*arrows*) might make one consider basal cell carcinoma in the differential diagnosis. The vessels of basal cell carcinoma, however, are linear, sharp in focus, and branched (arborizing). This elevated papillomatous nodule reveals a homogeneous pattern and has a light-brown color. Commonly these nevi are irritated due to incidental traumas.

Four global patterns for melanocytic nevi	
Reticular pattern	☐
Globular pattern	☑
Homogeneous pattern	☐
Starburst pattern	☐

Fig. 106 Nevus.

In this bizarre dermoscopic picture, there are several densely aggregated exophytic papillary structures and ridges, which look like globules. There are also a few irregular crypts and furrows (*arrows*), which represent a variation of the morphology seen with comedo-like openings. In the center, there is an accumulation of yellowish-white keratotic material (*asterisks*). Palpate this lesion and it will be soft, which will be one criterion in favor of it being a banal nevus.

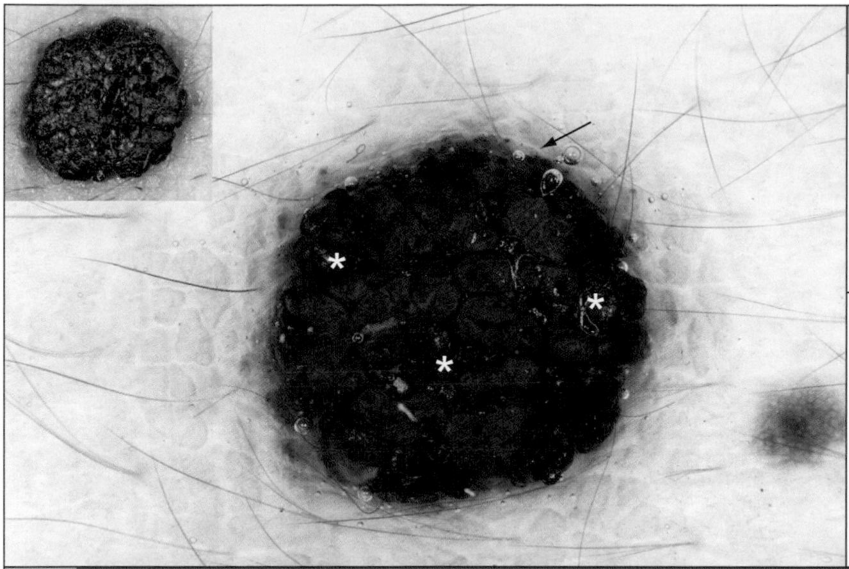

Four global patterns for melanocytic nevi	
Reticular pattern	☐
Globular pattern	☑
Homogeneous pattern	☐
Starburst pattern	☐

Fig. 107 Nevus.

This lesion is similar to that in Fig. 106 and is composed of densely aggregated exophytic papillary structures intermingled with furrows (*asterisks*). In addition, there are a few regular brown dots and globules (*arrow*) and blue-white structures. A small banal reticular-type nevus is seen in the right lower corner.

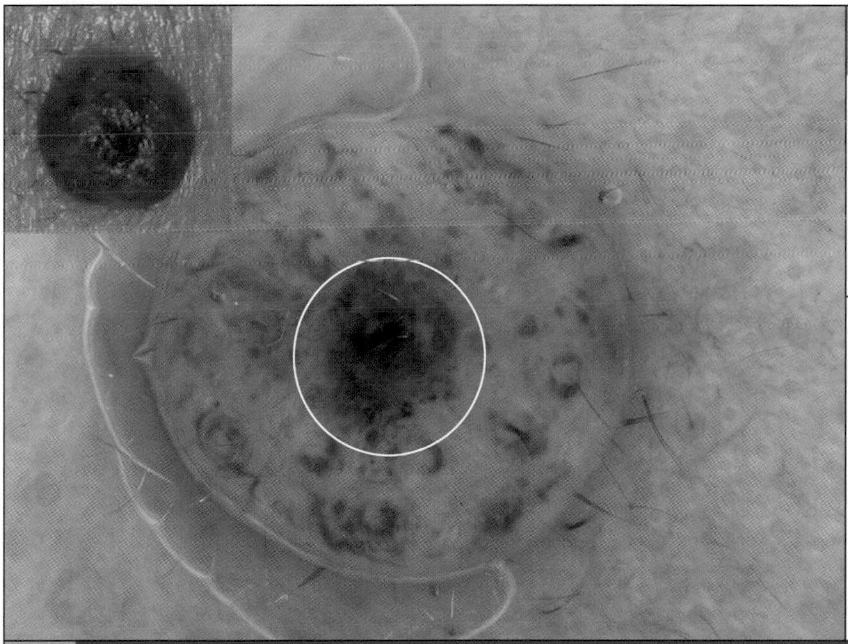

Four global patterns for melanocytic nevi	
Reticular pattern	☐
Globular pattern	☑
Homogeneous pattern	☑
Starburst pattern	☐

Fig. 108 Nevus.

This elevated nevus on the forehead is characterized by some light- to dark-brown dots and globules, particularly in the center of the lesion (*circle*). Please note the presence of roundish holes representing hair follicles. Closer scrutiny shows hairs in the center of a few follicles. These nevi are so often inflamed due to ingrown hairs and ruptured hair follicles. Because of the relatively pronounced pigmentation, we raised the orange flag. This benign nevus was excised as requested by the patient.

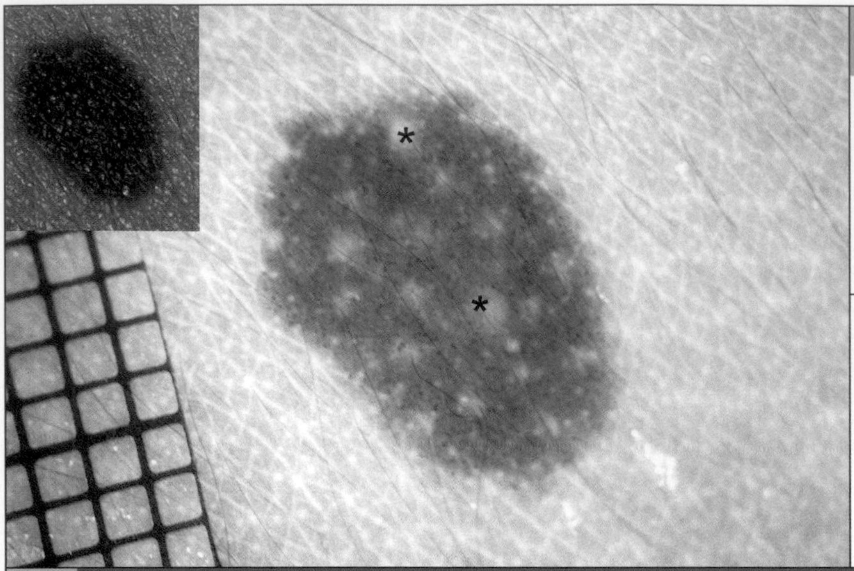

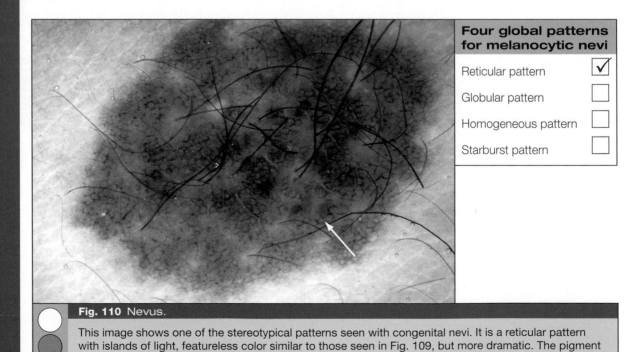

Four global patterns for melanocytic nevi

Reticular pattern	☐
Globular pattern	☑
Homogeneous pattern	☐
Starburst pattern	☐

Fig. 109 Nevus.

Here is a very subtle type of globular pattern in a flat melanocytic nevus with numerous tiny dots and multifocal hypopigmentation (*asterisks*). This pattern can be seen with congenital or Clark (dysplastic) nevi.

Four global patterns for melanocytic nevi

Reticular pattern	☑
Globular pattern	☐
Homogeneous pattern	☐
Starburst pattern	☐

Fig. 110 Nevus.

This image shows one of the stereotypical patterns seen with congenital nevi. It is a reticular pattern with islands of light, featureless color similar to those seen in Fig. 109, but more dramatic. The pigment network in the central portion is more heavily pigmented and the lines are thickened when compared to those at the periphery. There is also a focus of blue-white structures (*arrow*). Commonly, congenital nevi look worrisome with dermoscopy but not histologically. Islands of normal skin + islands of criteria = congenital melanocytic nevus.

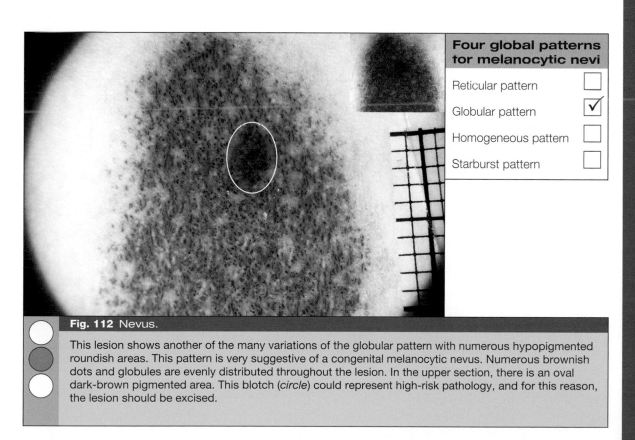

Four global patterns for melanocytic nevi

Reticular pattern	☐
Globular pattern	☑
Homogeneous pattern	☐
Starburst pattern	☐

Fig. 111 Nevus.

The globular pattern seen here is intermingled with roundish white holes and is characterized by numerous tiny bluish dots and globules (*circle*) situated predominantly in the center of the lesion, and many light-brownish globules peripherally. The overall dermoscopic architecture of this lesion is symmetrical and regular, and excision is not indicated.

Four global patterns tor melanocytic nevi

Reticular pattern	☐
Globular pattern	☑
Homogeneous pattern	☐
Starburst pattern	☐

Fig. 112 Nevus.

This lesion shows another of the many variations of the globular pattern with numerous hypopigmented roundish areas. This pattern is very suggestive of a congenital melanocytic nevus. Numerous brownish dots and globules are evenly distributed throughout the lesion. In the upper section, there is an oval dark-brown pigmented area. This blotch (*circle*) could represent high-risk pathology, and for this reason, the lesion should be excised.

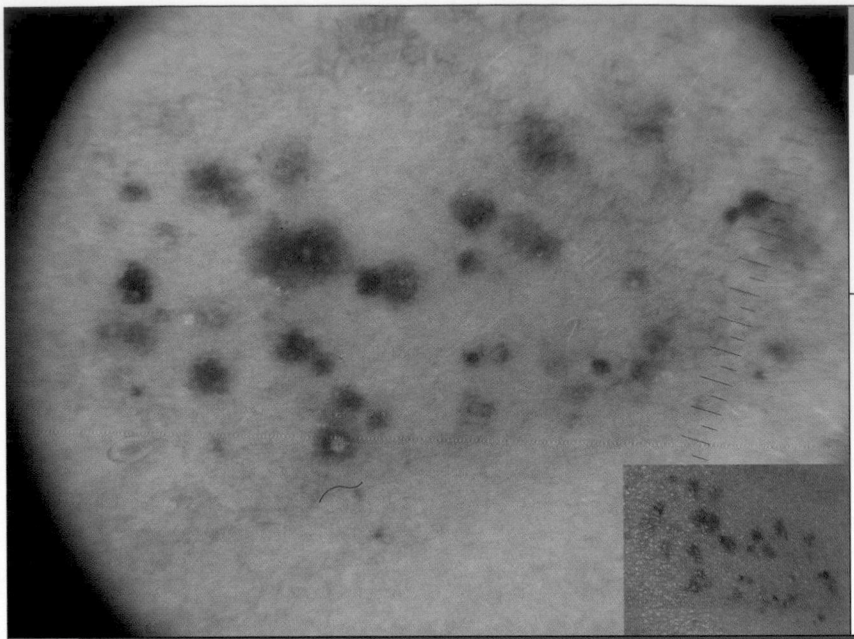

Four global patterns for melanocytic nevi

Reticular pattern ☐
Globular pattern ☑
Homogeneous pattern ☑
Starburst pattern ☐

Fig. 113 Nevus.

This lesion with a particular homogeneous pattern is a congenital speckled nevus, also called nevus spilus. There is a rather characteristic pattern of several brownish homogeneous dots and clods on a homogeneous light brown to skin-colored background. The novice may be confounded by this lesion and consider an unusual melanoma in the differential diagnosis. We felt confident to recommend follow-up and self-monitoring of this special type of congenital nevus.

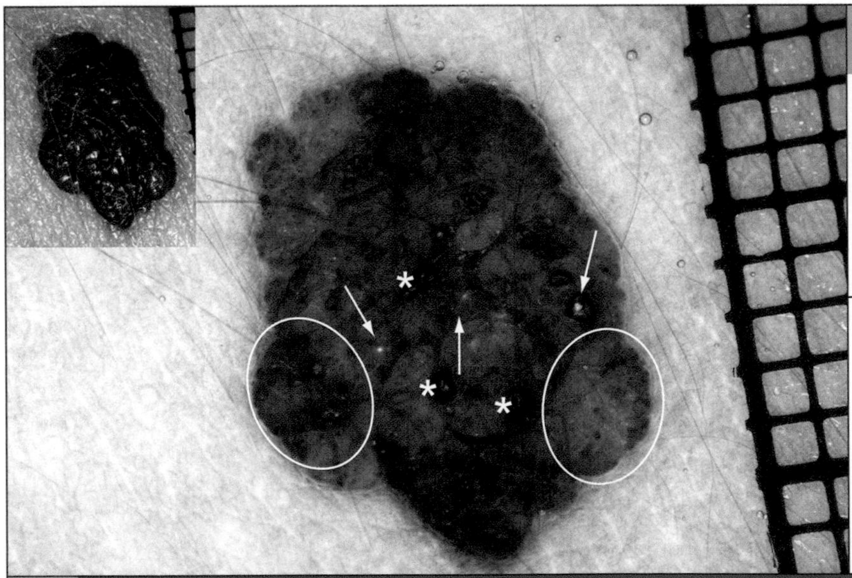

Four global patterns for melanocytic nevi

Reticular pattern ☐
Globular pattern ☑
Homogeneous pattern ☐
Starburst pattern ☐

Fig. 114 Nevus.

This papillomatous nevus is composed of a few exophytic papillary structures (*circles*) and some comedo-like openings (*asterisks*). In addition, there are a few milia-like cysts (*arrows*) and blue-white structures. If a worrisome-looking lesion like this is palpated, it should be soft and compressible—this sign indicates that it is benign.

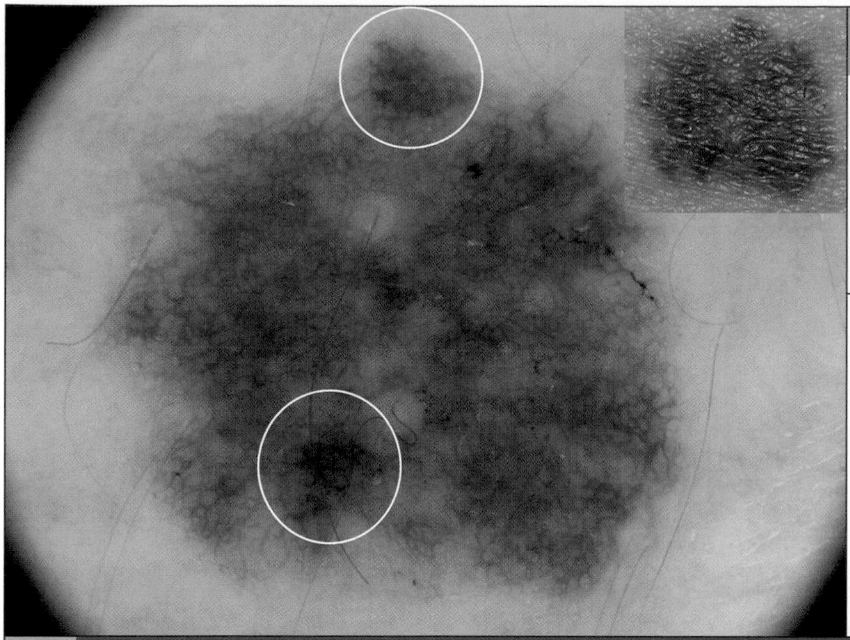

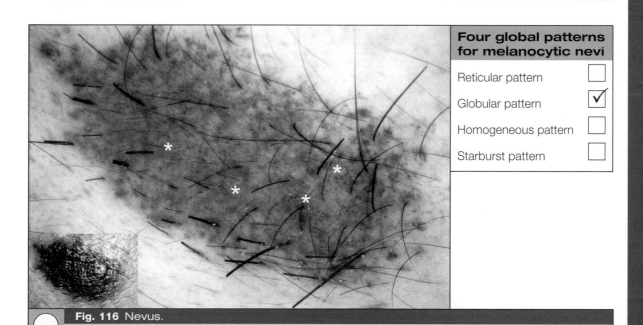

Four global patterns for melanocytic nevi

Reticular pattern	☑
Globular pattern	☐
Homogeneous pattern	☐
Starburst pattern	☐

Fig. 115 Nevus.

This reticular nevus is characterized by a pigment network pattern that immediately raises our suspicion. There are certainly areas with a thickened and branched pigment network (*circles*) and also the other parts of the pigment network reveal some features of irregularity. This dysplastic (Clark) nevus simulates in situ melanoma and should be excised.

Four global patterns for melanocytic nevi

Reticular pattern	☐
Globular pattern	☑
Homogeneous pattern	☐
Starburst pattern	☐

Fig. 116 Nevus.

This nevus is characterized by the presence of numerous hairs, which is diagnostic of a congenital melanocytic nevus. There are also brownish globules throughout the lesion intermingled with numerous small blue dots (*asterisks*), which represent collections of melanophages in the papillary dermis and raise the suspicion of a regressing melanoma. Against the dermoscopic diagnosis of melanoma are the presence of multiple hairs and symmetry of color and structure.

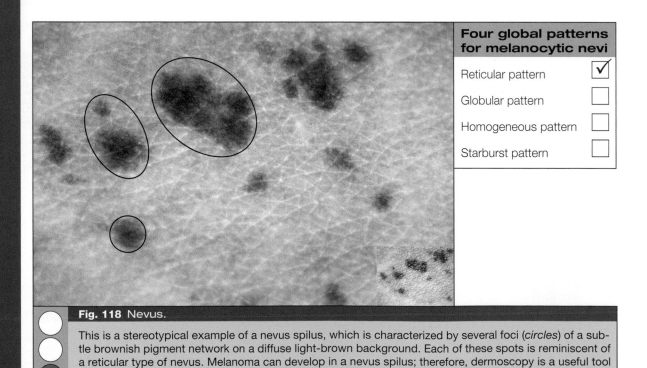

Four global patterns for melanocytic nevi

Reticular pattern	✓
Globular pattern	☐
Homogeneous pattern	☐
Starburst pattern	☐

Fig. 117 Nevus.

Here is another example of a nevus with dark hairs, which might be best interpreted as a small congenital melanocytic nevus on the face. The dermoscopic hallmark of this lesion is a regular pseudopigment network formed by numerous round areas, which represent follicular openings. This criterion is site specific. Because of the dermoscopic symmetry of color and structure, a melanoma can be ruled out with certainty. Pigment network is not the same as pseudopigment network.

Four global patterns for melanocytic nevi

Reticular pattern	✓
Globular pattern	☐
Homogeneous pattern	☐
Starburst pattern	☐

Fig. 118 Nevus.

This is a stereotypical example of a nevus spilus, which is characterized by several foci (*circles*) of a subtle brownish pigment network on a diffuse light-brown background. Each of these spots is reminiscent of a reticular type of nevus. Melanoma can develop in a nevus spilus; therefore, dermoscopy is a useful tool for examining these lesions. Look for the same high-risk criteria as for other types of melanocytic nevi.

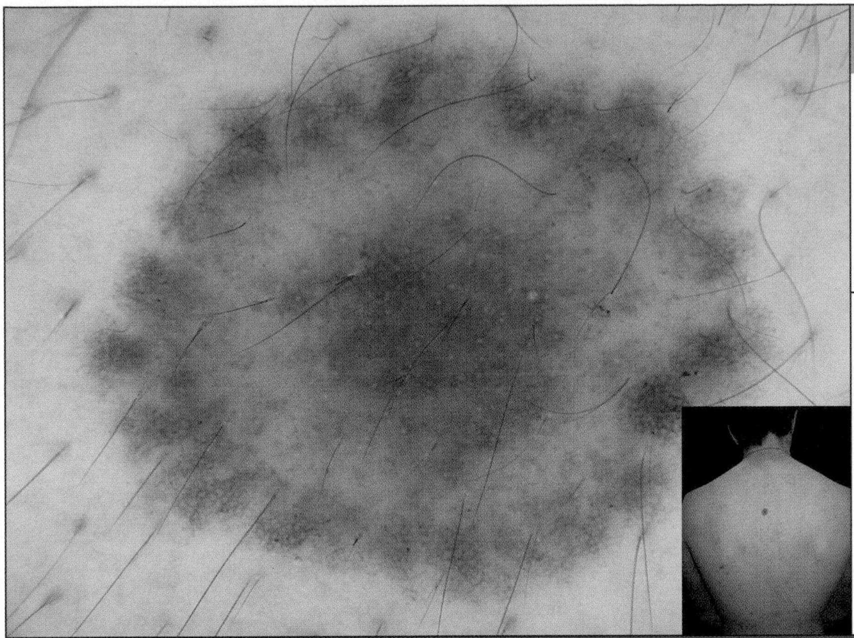

Four global patterns for melanocytic nevi

Reticular pattern	☑
Globular pattern	☐
Homogeneous pattern	☑
Starburst pattern	☐

Fig. 119 Nevus.

This nevus exhibits a reticular-homogeneous pattern, with the homogenous zone in the center of the lesion. The periphery is characterized by a regular patchy distribution of small foci of typical pigment network arranged in an annular pattern. This lesion reveals a very distinct "Gestalt" called a cockade and is nowadays commonly termed targetoid or cockade nevus (nevus en cocarde). Because of the overall symmetrical aspect of this lesion, we are raising the green flag. Of course, monitoring of this lesion and annual follow-up is recommended.

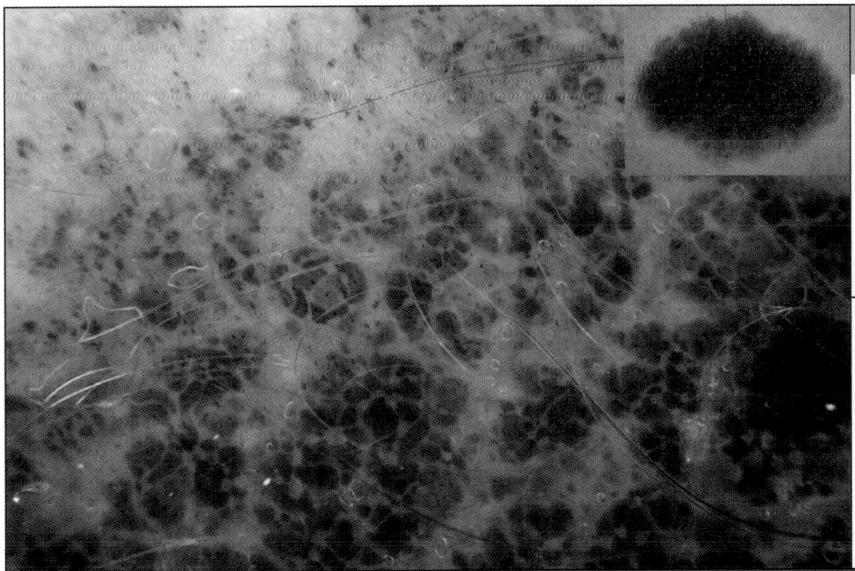

Four global patterns for melanocytic nevi

Reticular pattern	☐
Globular pattern	☑
Homogeneous pattern	☐
Starburst pattern	☐

Fig. 120 Nevus.

At higher magnification, this congenital nevus has a very worrisome appearance dermoscopically because there is asymmetry of color and also of structure. However, in melanocytic lesions larger than 1 cm in diameter, we have always taken into consideration the clinical appearance. It is well known that dermoscopy of congenital nevi may be confounding and lead us astray. Putting together the clinical and the dermoscopic features of this lesion, we are confident to follow up this congenital nevus.

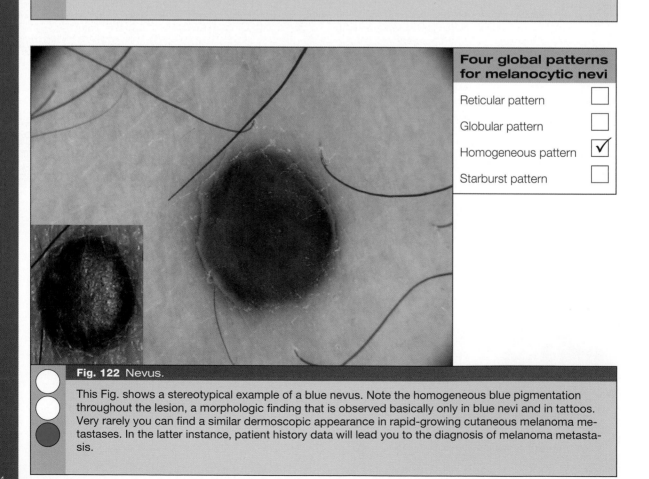

Four global patterns for melanocytic nevi

Reticular pattern ☐

Globular pattern ☐

Homogeneous pattern ☑

Starburst pattern ☐

Fig. 121 Nevus.

This is a stereotypical example of a blue nevus characterized by diffuse homogeneous pigmentation. There is also a small rim of brownish pigmentation. The differential diagnosis of this blue nevus is a hemangioma and nodular or cutaneous metastatic melanoma. The history of the lesion is vital to make the correct dermoscopic diagnosis.

Four global patterns for melanocytic nevi

Reticular pattern ☐

Globular pattern ☐

Homogeneous pattern ☑

Starburst pattern ☐

Fig. 122 Nevus.

This Fig. shows a stereotypical example of a blue nevus. Note the homogeneous blue pigmentation throughout the lesion, a morphologic finding that is observed basically only in blue nevi and in tattoos. Very rarely you can find a similar dermoscopic appearance in rapid-growing cutaneous melanoma metastases. In the latter instance, patient history data will lead you to the diagnosis of melanoma metastasis.

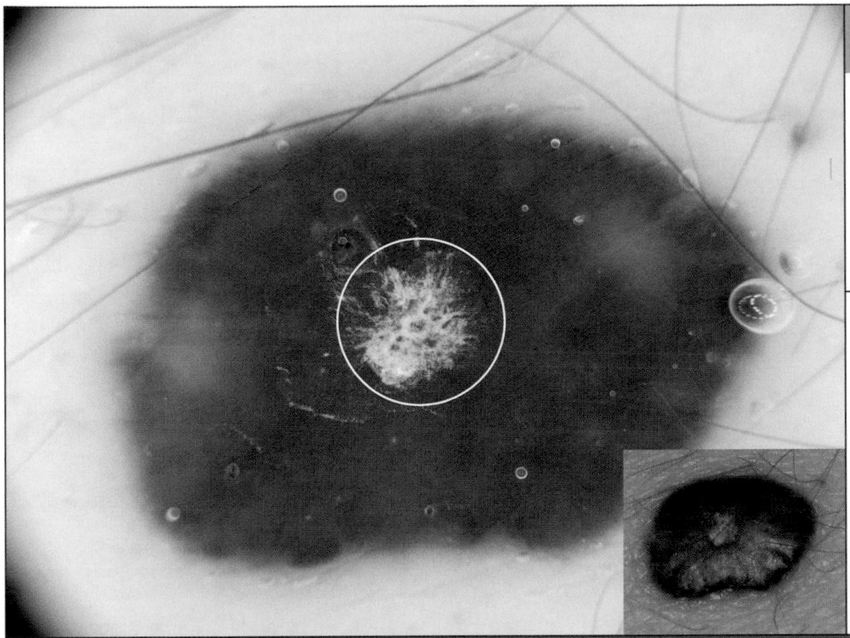

Four global patterns for melanocytic nevi

Reticular pattern	☐
Globular pattern	☐
Homogeneous pattern	☑
Starburst pattern	☐

Fig. 123 Nevus.

This image shows another example of a typical blue nevus. The whitish area in the center of the lesion (*circle*) is just a scale. If there is no history of growth, we can confidently raise the green flag here.

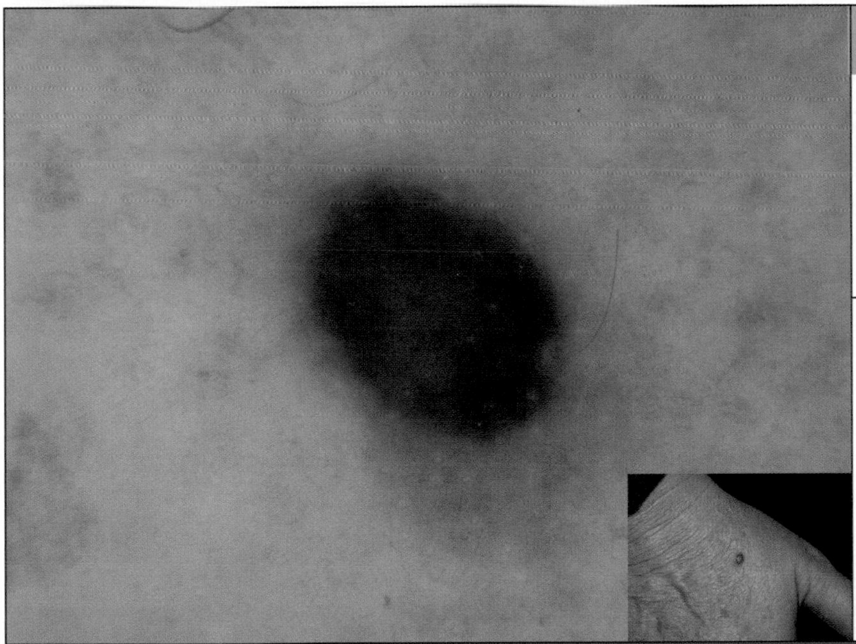

Four global patterns for melanocytic nevi

Reticular pattern	☐
Globular pattern	☐
Homogeneous pattern	☑
Starburst pattern	☐

Fig. 124 Nevus.

This is a blue nevus with a central whitish zone simulating a regressive Clark (dysplastic) nevus or even a regressing melanoma. There is also an off-center light brown homogenous zone. The brown zone, set asymmetrically to the main body of the lesion, may concern dermoscopists. Remember, if in doubt, cut it out, and this is particularly relevant for nodular lesions. We decided to completely excise this lesion, and the histopathologic diagnosis here was a cellular blue nevus.

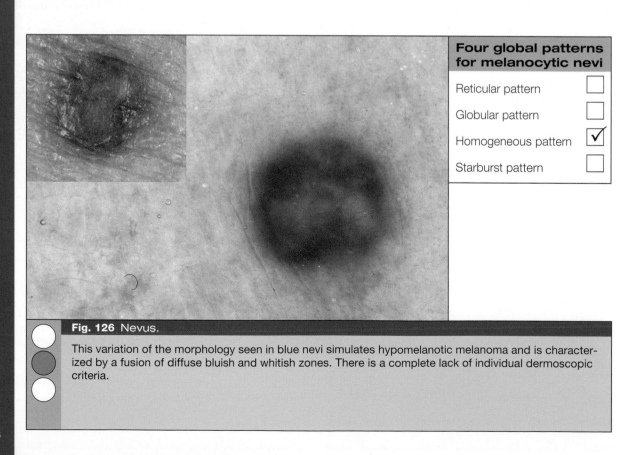

Four global patterns for melanocytic nevi

Reticular pattern ☐
Globular pattern ☐
Homogeneous pattern ☑
Starburst pattern ☐

Fig. 125 Nevus.

This blue nevus is a predominantly firm nodule with a smooth surface. The clinical differential diagnosis includes hypomelanotic melanoma, dermatofibroma, or dermal nevus. The nevus has a diffuse light-brownish color bordered by small zones of darker pigmentation and blue-white structures (*asterisks*). No other dermoscopic criteria are seen. Because a hypomelanotic melanoma cannot be ruled out with certainty, a lesion with this dermoscopic picture should be excised.

Four global patterns for melanocytic nevi

Reticular pattern ☐
Globular pattern ☐
Homogeneous pattern ☑
Starburst pattern ☐

Fig. 126 Nevus.

This variation of the morphology seen in blue nevi simulates hypomelanotic melanoma and is characterized by a fusion of diffuse bluish and whitish zones. There is a complete lack of individual dermoscopic criteria.

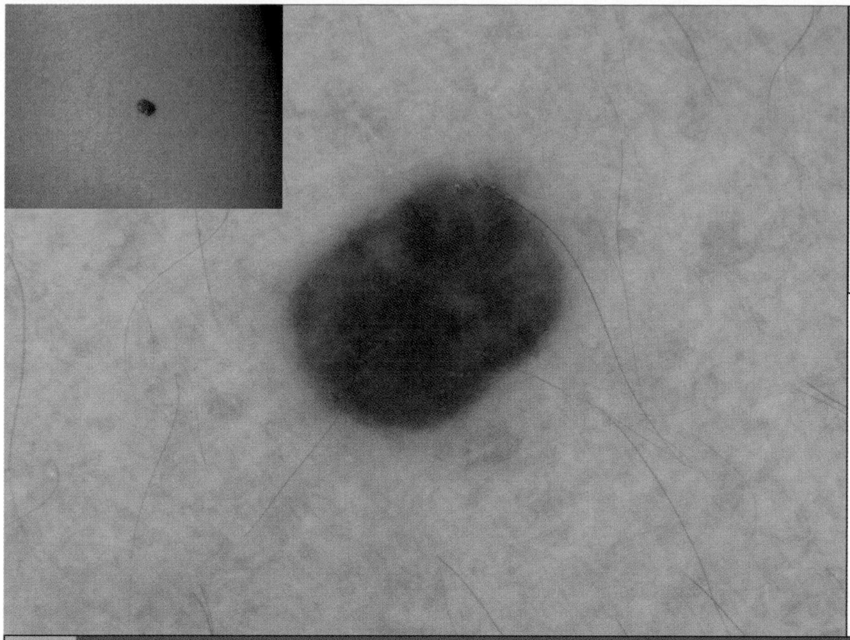

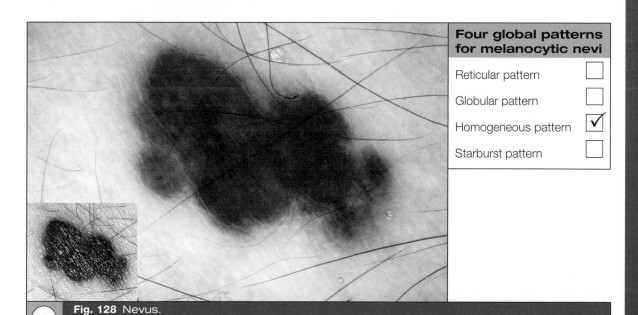

Four global patterns for melanocytic nevi

Reticular pattern ☐

Globular pattern ☐

Homogeneous pattern ☑

Starburst pattern ☐

Fig. 127 Nevus.

This is an example of an unusual blue nevus with asymmetric zones of bluish-brown pigmentation and whitish zones. A lesion like this one raises important differential diagnostic considerations, such as Spitz nevus and nodular melanoma. Although there is a small probability that this is indeed a nodular melanoma, we are raising the red flag here.

Four global patterns for melanocytic nevi

Reticular pattern ☐

Globular pattern ☐

Homogeneous pattern ☑

Starburst pattern ☐

Fig. 128 Nevus.

This lesion is a variation of a blue nevus. Dermoscopically, it is characterized by homogeneous blue and gray color surrounded by a faint ring of lighter blue color. There are no hints of local dermoscopic features, particularly melanoma-specific criteria. Nevertheless, because of the lesion's asymmetry of contour and color, excision is justified to rule out a melanoma. The history is also an important factor in this case.

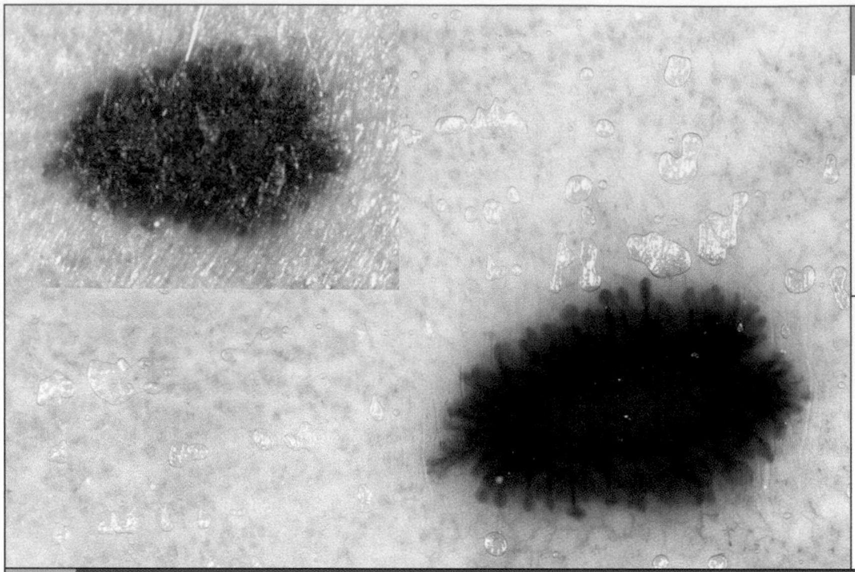

Four global patterns for melanocytic nevi	
Reticular pattern	☐
Globular pattern	☐
Homogeneous pattern	☐
Starburst pattern	☑

Fig. 129 Nevus.

This is a stereotypical example of a Spitz nevus with a starburst pattern. There is a symmetrical ring of streaks around the entire lesion and a central blue-white structure. Both these dermoscopic features are commonly found in Spitz nevi. If the streaks are not at all areas of the periphery, it could be the dermoscopic picture of a melanoma. A starburst pattern should immediately make one think of Spitz nevus.

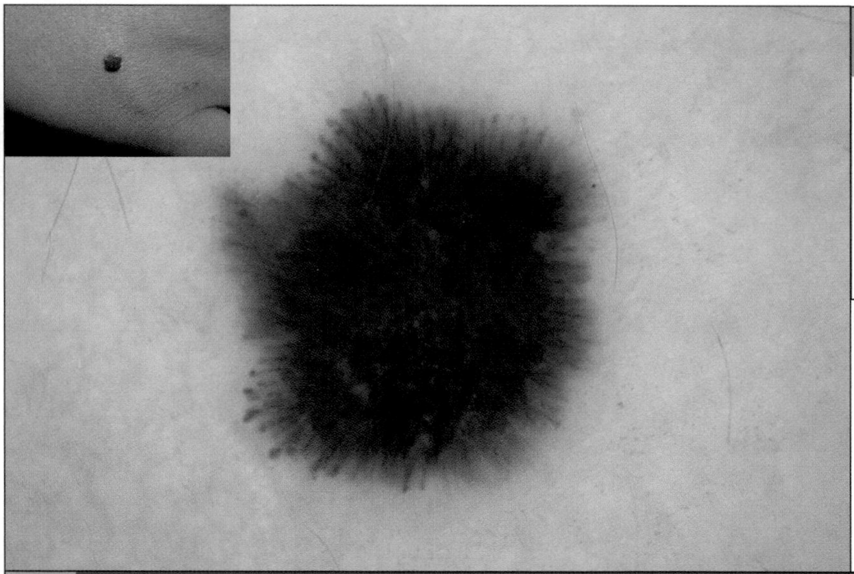

Four global patterns for melanocytic nevi	
Reticular pattern	☐
Globular pattern	☐
Homogeneous pattern	☐
Starburst pattern	☑

Fig. 130 Nevus.

This lesion is also reminiscent of a Spitz/Reed nevus and is similar to that in Fig. 129, but with asymmetrically distributed pseudopods at the periphery. It also has the starburst pattern with a central blue-white structure. As a rule, excision of a lesion with this dermoscopic appearance is recommended, particularly if the individual is over 14 years of age.

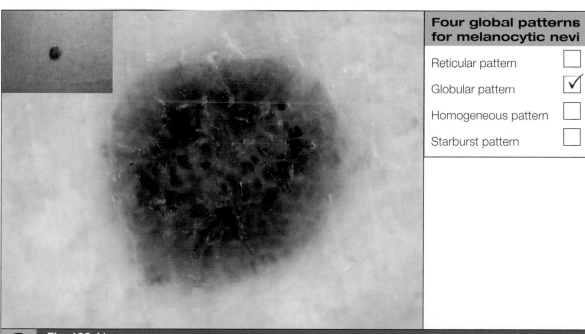

Four global patterns for melanocytic nevi

Reticular pattern	☐
Globular pattern	☑
Homogeneous pattern	☐
Starburst pattern	☐

Fig. 131 Nevus.

This is predominantly a globular type of Spitz nevus, which dermoscopically raises a suspicion of melanoma. It is a relatively symmetrical lesion characterized by numerous brown to bluish globules rather evenly distributed throughout the lesion. In the left lower corner of the lesion, there are several dotted vessels (*circle*). The decision about whether to closely follow or excise a lesion that looks like this depends on the clinical setting.

Four global patterns for melanocytic nevi

Reticular pattern	☐
Globular pattern	☑
Homogeneous pattern	☐
Starburst pattern	☐

Fig. 132 Nevus.

This lesion is similar to the one before, but the dots and globules are more prominent. This globular pattern can be seen in banal, dysplastic (Clark), and Spitz nevi as well as rarely in melanomas. In addition, there are hints of streaks in the periphery (1–2 o'clock) and a so-called negative pigment network in the central parts of the lesion, both features suggestive of a Spitz nevus. There are also several black dots throughout the lesion, making this lesion quite suspicious for melanoma. Because of the equivocal dermoscopic appearance, this lesion was excised and diagnosed histopathologically as a Spitz nevus.

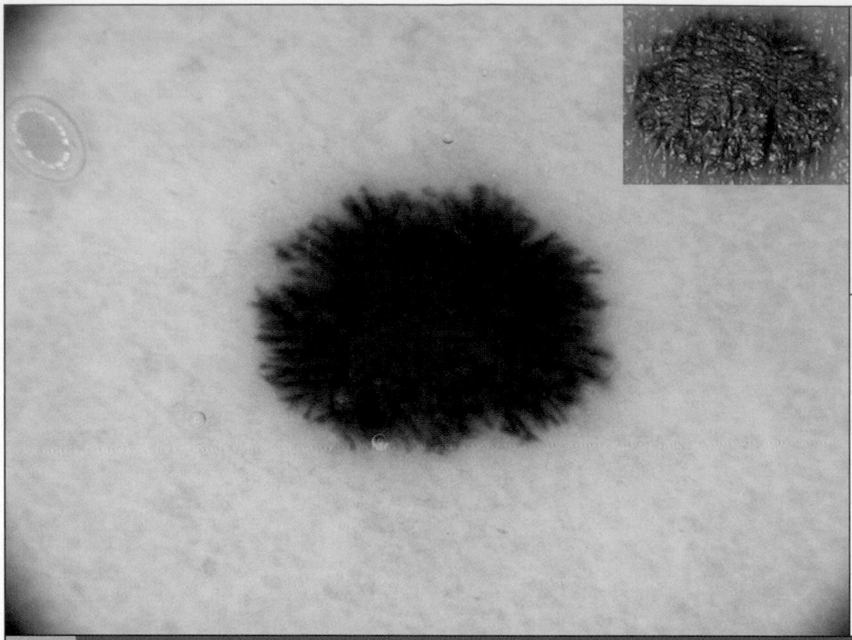

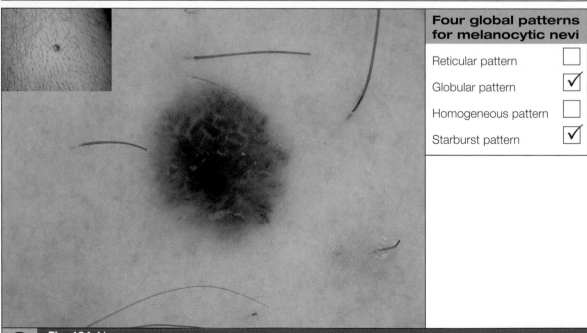

Four global patterns for melanocytic nevi	
Reticular pattern	☑
Globular pattern	☐
Homogeneous pattern	☐
Starburst pattern	☑

Fig. 133 Nevus.

This is a small pigmented Spitz nevus (commonly referred to as pigmented spindle cell nevus or Reed nevus) with a rather typical starburst pattern. In addition, there is a thickened and branched superficial black pigment network throughout the lesion with an accentuation at the periphery. The differential diagnosis includes an in situ melanoma, and therefore the lesion should be excised. Small lesions can be high risk.

Four global patterns for melanocytic nevi	
Reticular pattern	☐
Globular pattern	☑
Homogeneous pattern	☐
Starburst pattern	☑

Fig. 134 Nevus.

This lesion shows another variation of the morphology seen in Spitz nevi. There is dermoscopic symmetry, a relatively large blue-white structure in the center, negative pigment network around large brown globules and streaks with a subtle starburst pattern at the periphery. Grey pseudopods at the periphery (5 o'clock) are a concerning feature. Because a melanoma cannot be ruled out with certainty, this lesion should be excised. The diagnosis here was a Spitz nevus.

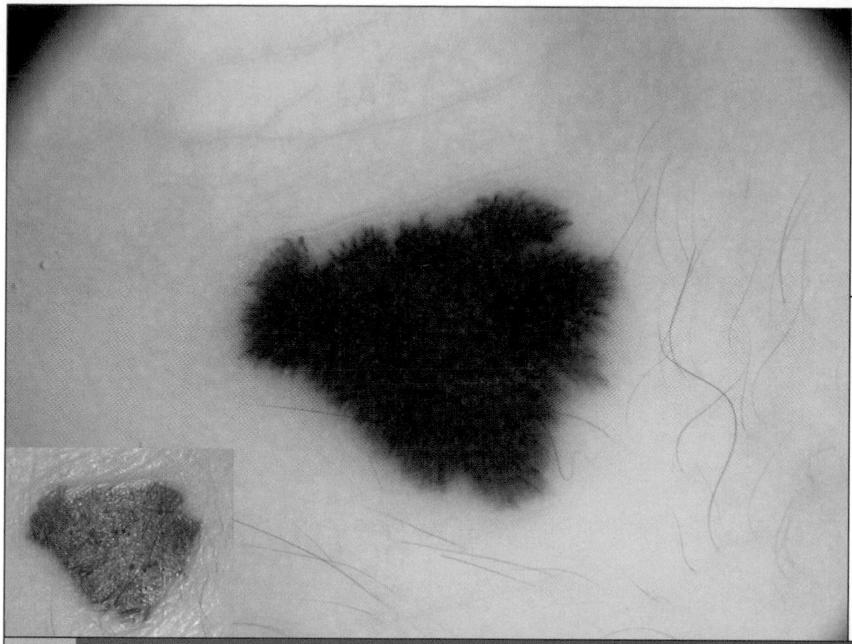

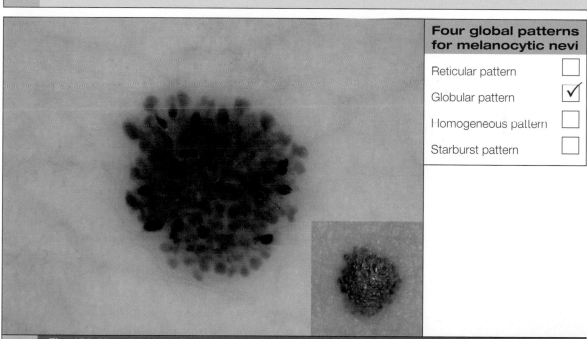

Four global patterns for melanocytic nevi

Reticular pattern	☐
Globular pattern	☐
Homogeneous pattern	☐
Starburst pattern	☑

Fig. 135 Nevus.

The starburst pattern of a Reed (pigmented Spitz) nevus should by now be recognizable. Please note the many streaks at the periphery of this lesion. The numerous tiny white punctate areas are not the milia-like cysts of a seborrheic keratosis but eccrine duct openings. The differential diagnosis of this lesion would be a Clark (dysplastic) nevus or a melanoma; therefore it should be excised.

Four global patterns for melanocytic nevi

Reticular pattern	☐
Globular pattern	☑
Homogeneous pattern	☐
Starburst pattern	☐

Fig. 136 Nevus.

This lesion shows another variation on the morphology observed in Spitz (Reed) nevi and is characterized by numerous globules distributed evenly, varying in color from light brown, dark brown, blue to black. The life cycle of a Spitz (Reed) nevus starts with a globular pattern, followed by the starburst pattern and finally the homogeneous pattern before the lesion starts to involute. Based on the clinical constellation, however, we are raising here the red flag.

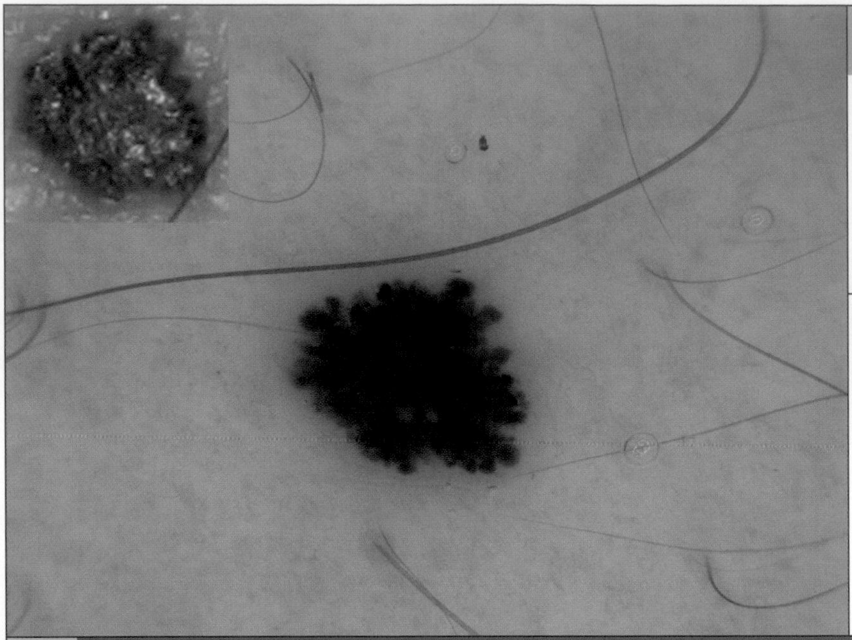

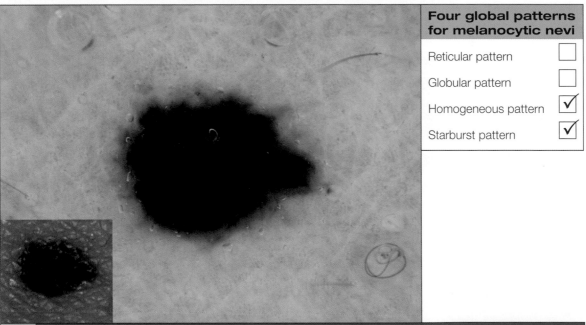

Four global patterns for melanocytic nevi

Reticular pattern ☐
Globular pattern ☐
Homogeneous pattern ☐
Starburst pattern ☑

Fig. 137 Nevus.

It is impossible to see too many variations of Spitz (Reed) nevi, so here is another classic one! The most remarkable aspect of this lesion is a superficial black pigment network forming streaks that create a starburst pattern that is a highly specific sign for Spitz (Reed) nevi. Still, your management decision should always be based on the clinical constellation and never on the dermoscopic findings alone. If this lesion, for example, occurs on the lower leg of a middle-aged woman, raise the red flag.

Four global patterns for melanocytic nevi

Reticular pattern ☐
Globular pattern ☐
Homogeneous pattern ☑
Starburst pattern ☑

Fig. 138 Nevus.

This jet-black Spitz (Reed) nevus is not as easy to diagnose as that in Fig. 137. Although a rather typical starburst pattern can be observed, there is a striking asymmetry at least in one axis and therefore a melanoma should be ruled out, particularly in adults.

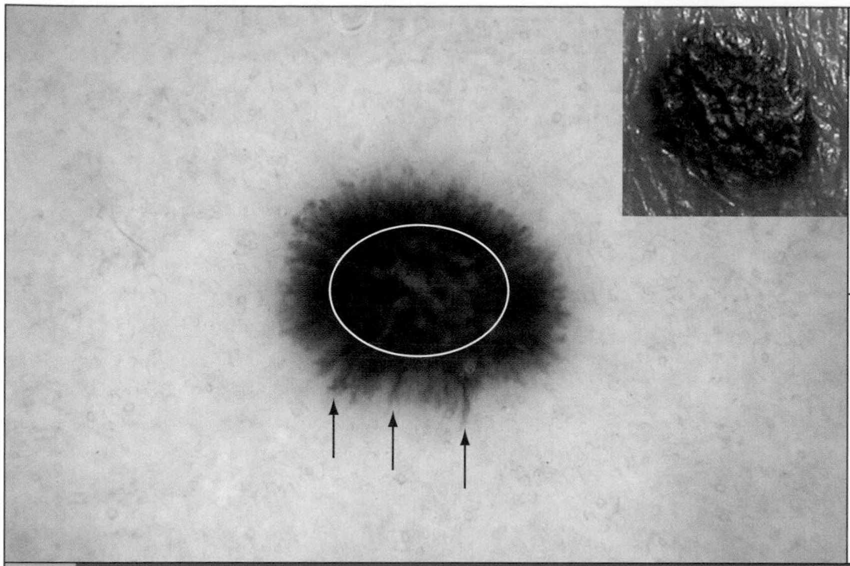

Four global patterns for melanocytic nevi

Reticular pattern	☐
Globular pattern	☑
Homogeneous pattern	☐
Starburst pattern	☑

Fig. 139 Nevus.

Spitz nevi have many faces! This one is harder to diagnose because the dermoscopic features are not distinctive. It has a central diffuse blue-white structure and also a few black dots and globules (*circle*). Please note streaks (*arrows*) arranged radially along the periphery of the lesion suggestive of a starburst pattern. The dermoscopic differential diagnosis includes a dysplastic (Clark) nevus, a Spitz nevus, and an in situ melanoma, so it should be excised.

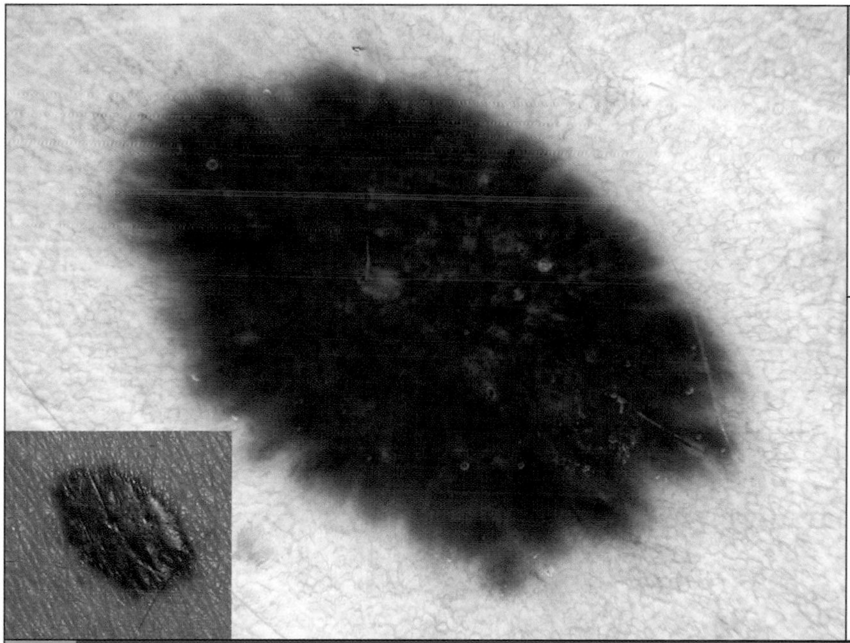

Four global patterns for melanocytic nevi

Reticular pattern	☐
Globular pattern	☐
Homogeneous pattern	☑
Starburst pattern	☑

Fig. 140 Nevus.

This almost structureless lesion has multiple colors—a diffuse black to blue-white coloration in the center and shades of brown in the periphery. There is no clear-cut pigment network visible, but one can recognize a hint of a starburst pattern. If a lesion cannot be categorized with certainty, then it should be excised to rule out melanoma. The large blue-white structure and the starburst pattern favor a pigmented Spitz (Reed) nevus.

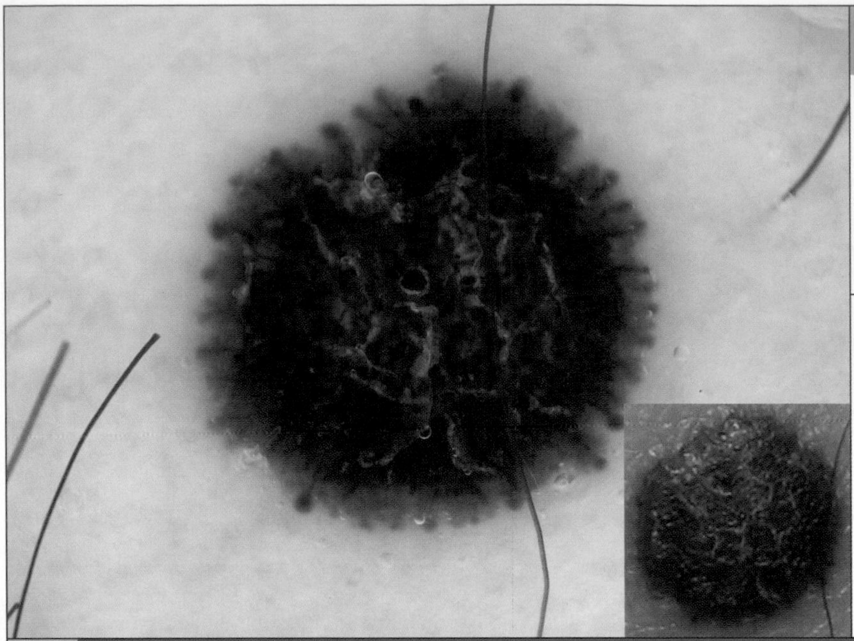

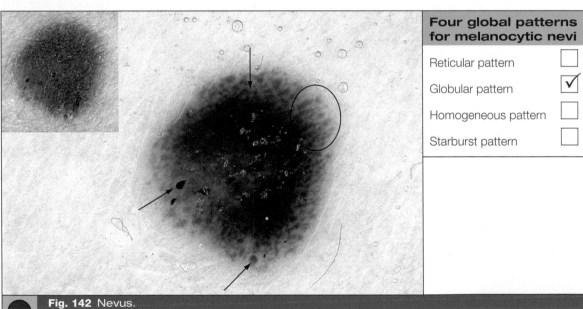

Four global patterns for melanocytic nevi

Reticular pattern	☐
Globular pattern	☐
Homogeneous pattern	☐
Starburst pattern	☑

Fig. 141 Nevus.

This pigmented Spitz nevus (or Reed nevus) clinically strongly mimics a melanoma. However, dermoscopically a classic starburst pattern can be recognized easily and therefore the diagnosis of a pigmented spindle cell (Reed) nevus (also called pigmented Spitz nevus) can be made with confidence. Particularly in children under age 12, this lesion can be followed up and every so often will involute within a few years. In elder children and in younger adults, a lesion like this one always should be removed. Most probably you will not see a similar lesion in adults older than 40 years.

Four global patterns for melanocytic nevi

Reticular pattern	☐
Globular pattern	☑
Homogeneous pattern	☐
Starburst pattern	☐

Fig. 142 Nevus.

This lesion can be categorized as a globular type of Spitz nevus. Because of the asymmetry and multiple colors, it is another lesion that simulates a melanoma. Remember that dermoscopy is not 100% diagnostic of any single lesion. There are numerous asymmetrically located dots and globules (arrows), irregular brown streaks (*circle*), and blue-white structures.

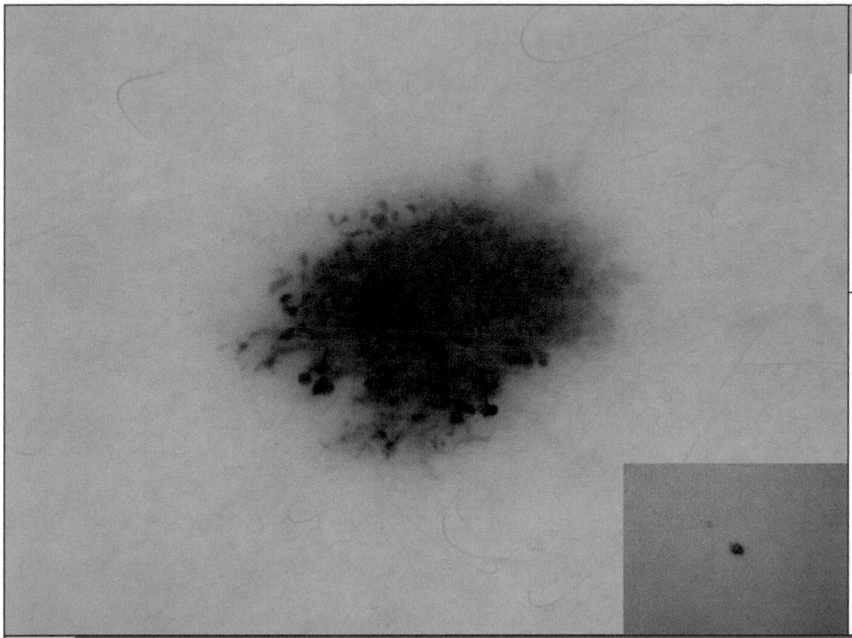

**Four global patterns
for melanocytic nevi**

Reticular pattern ☐

Globular pattern ☑

Homogeneous pattern ☐

Starburst pattern ☐

Fig. 143 Nevus.

This pigmented Spitz nevus is characterized by a sort of globular pattern and again mimics melanoma. There is a central blue-white structure and several irregular black dots and globules, mostly at the periphery of the lesion, and pseudopods distributed unevenly around the lesion, creating structural asymmetry. No pigment network can be identified. Despite this lesion being present in a young adult, an excisional biopsy was performed immediately. Fortunately, the final histopathologic diagnosis was a pigmented Spitz/Reed nevus.

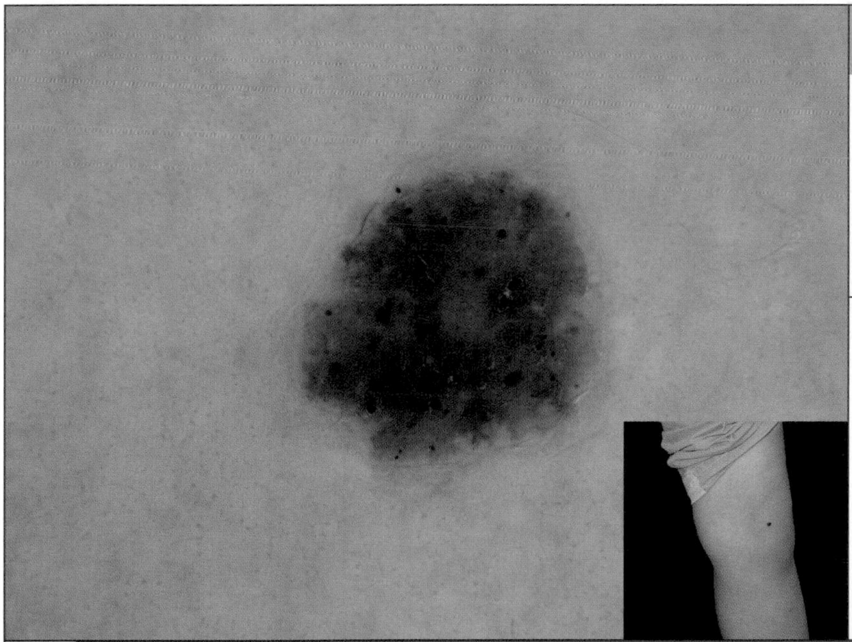

**Four global patterns
for melanocytic nevi**

Reticular pattern ☐

Globular pattern ☑

Homogeneous pattern ☐

Starburst pattern ☐

Fig. 144 Nevus.

On initial impression, this lesion appears high risk because it is so dark already clinically. Remember that black color is not always an ominous sign. This is another variation on the theme of a globular Spitz nevus. Dermoscopically, it is a rather symmetrical lesion characterized by a small homogeneous central zone of blue-white pigmentation surrounded by unevenly distributed black and dark brown dots and globules on a dark background, which is itself surrounded by a pink rim with brown and blue-white structures. Melanoma cannot be ruled out here with certainty; therefore, this lesion should be excised.

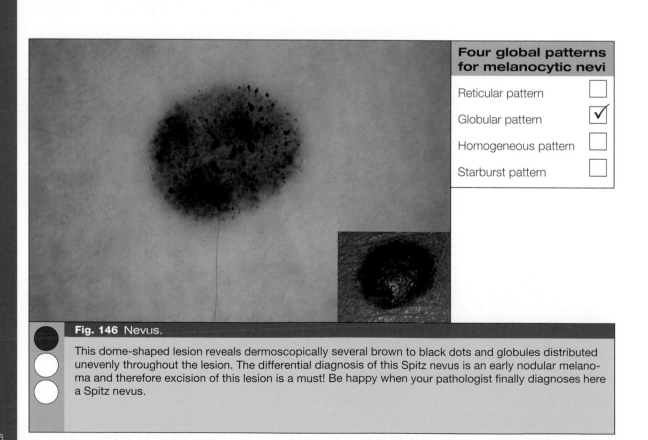

Four global patterns for melanocytic nevi

Reticular pattern	☑
Globular pattern	☐
Homogeneous pattern	☐
Starburst pattern	☑

Fig. 145 Nevus.

A very experienced dermoscopist might recognize this as a pigmented Spitz nevus (Reed nevus). There is a superficial black pigment network and a quite typical starburst pattern with numerous streaks (*arrows*) aligned along the circumference of the lesion. Still, we do recommend excision of this clinically and also dermoscopically rather worrisome lesion. Don't be a "hero" and excise any pigmented lesion when you are not absolutely confident. Keep in mind that about 20% of Spitz nevi can mimic melanoma clinically and dermoscopically.

Four global patterns for melanocytic nevi

Reticular pattern	☐
Globular pattern	☑
Homogeneous pattern	☐
Starburst pattern	☐

Fig. 146 Nevus.

This dome-shaped lesion reveals dermoscopically several brown to black dots and globules distributed unevenly throughout the lesion. The differential diagnosis of this Spitz nevus is an early nodular melanoma and therefore excision of this lesion is a must! Be happy when your pathologist finally diagnoses here a Spitz nevus.

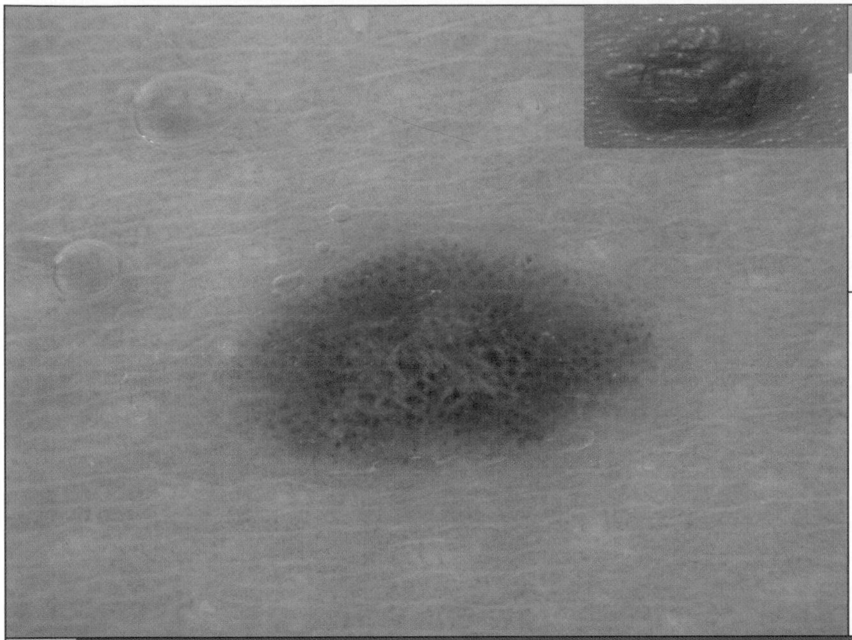

Four global patterns for melanocytic nevi

Reticular pattern	☐
Globular pattern	☑
Homogeneous pattern	☑
Starburst pattern	☐

Fig. 147 Nevus.

This pink homogeneous-globular lesion looks not particularly worrisome but is a Spitz nevus simulating amelanotic melanoma. The most remarkable aspect of this lesion is a central negative pigment network, also called reticular depigmentation. There is a pinkish, rather homogeneous pigmentation throughout. There are also numerous light-brown to pinkish dots throughout the lesion, but one has to look hard to find them. Relatively featureless pinkish lesions should be excised because occasionally they are melanomas. Pink color beware!

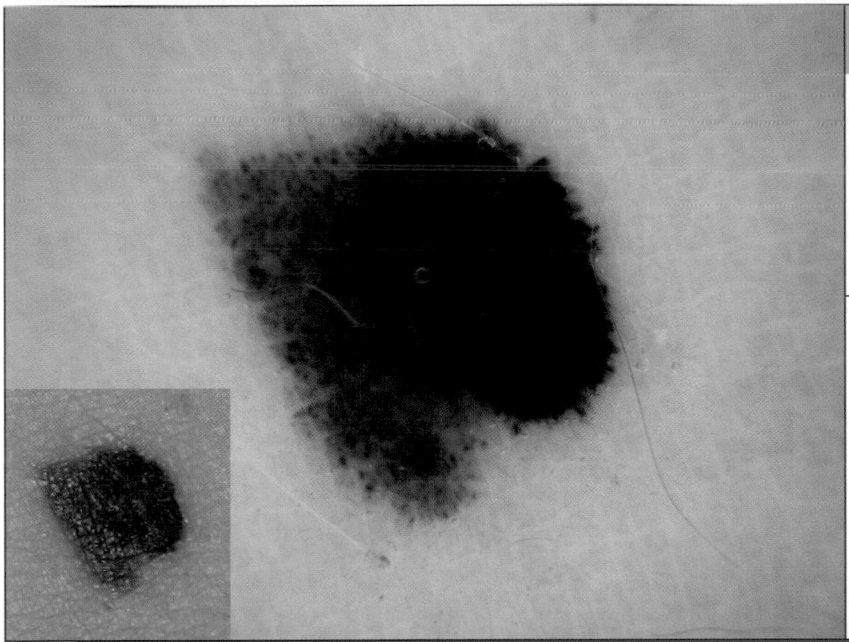

Four global patterns for melanocytic nevi

Reticular pattern	☑
Globular pattern	☑
Homogeneous pattern	☐
Starburst pattern	☑

Fig. 148 Nevus.

Hard to believe that this is not a melanoma—this is a combined nevus composed of a pigmented spindle cell (Reed) nevus (pigmented Spitz nevus) with a rather stereotypical starburst pattern on the right side and an unusual globular-reticular type of dysplastic (Clark) nevus on the left side. There is no doubt a lesion that displays this degree of asymmetry in color, shape, and structure needs to be excised. And even when your pathologist diagnoses this lesion as a benign nevus, we would recommend discussion of this lesion with him or her to make sure that a melanoma has not been missed.

Diagnosis of melanoma using five melanoma-specific criteria

Melanoma is most often characterized by a multicomponent global appearance. The multicomponent pattern is defined as the presence of three or more distinct dermoscopic areas within a given lesion. For example, it might be made up of separate zones of pigment network, clusters of dots and globules, and areas of diffuse hyper- or hypopigmentation. Many combinations of criteria can be seen with this high-risk global pattern. It is highly suggestive of melanoma but can also be found in basal cell carcinoma. Rarely, it is seen in acquired and congenital nevi and in non-melanocytic lesions, such as seborrheic keratoses or angiokeratomas.

To diagnose melanoma, look for the melanoma-specific criteria in a lesion. Melanoma-specific criteria can be seen in benign and malignant lesions but are more specific for melanomas. Finding one or two is enough to warrant a histopathologic diagnosis.

Atypical pigment network

A low-risk pigment network can appear as a delicate thin grid or a honeycomb-like pattern of brownish lines over a diffuse light-brown background. Histopathologically, the lines of the pigment network represent elongated and hyperpigmented rete ridges, whereas the lighter areas between the lines are dermal papillae. This criterion represents the dermoscopic hallmark of melanocytic lesions. Alterations are helpful to differentiate between benign and malignant melanocytic proliferations.

An atypical pigment network is characterized by black, brown, or gray, thickened and branched line segments, distributed irregularly throughout the lesion. A sharp cutoff of an atypical pigment network at the periphery of a lesion is even more suggestive of melanoma.

Irregular streaks

Streaks are dark linear structures of variable thickness found at the periphery of a lesion. The term "streaks" includes radial streaming and pseudopods, which are variations of the same criterion. Streaks represent discrete, linear, heavily pigmented, junctional nests of atypical melanocytes. Although streaks can be found in benign and malignant melanocytic lesions, they are more specific for melanoma, especially when they are unevenly distributed in a lesion. A symmetrical arrangement of streaks around an entire lesion is most often found in Spitz nevi, but this pattern can also be seen in melanomas.

Irregular dots and globules

Dots and globules are sharply circumscribed, round to oval, variously sized, black, brown, or gray structures that can be subdivided as regular or irregular based on their size, shape, and distribution in a lesion. Irregular dots and globules have different sizes and shapes and are unevenly distributed throughout a lesion. Histopathologically dots and globules may represent aggregations of pigmented melanocytes, melanophages, or even clumps of melanin. Dots and globules can be found in benign and malignant melanocytic lesions and are usually irregular in melanomas.

Irregular blotches

Blotches refer to various shades of diffuse hyperpigmentation that obscure the recognition of other dermoscopic features such as pigment network, dots, and globules. Irregular blotches vary in size and shape with irregular borders. A well-demarcated blotch at the periphery is very suggestive of melanoma. Histopathologically blotches represent histopathologic structures that share pronounced melanin pigmentation throughout the epidermis and upper dermis. Localized or diffuse regular blotches are suggestive of benign lesions, whereas localized or diffuse irregular blotches favor malignancy.

Blue-white structures

Blue-white structures can appear as white scar-like depigmented areas (bony-milky white color) or bluish structureless areas, or combinations of both colors. Do not confuse white scar-like areas with hypopigmentation commonly seen in benign lesions. Blue-white structures represent an acanthotic epidermis with compact orthokeratosis and pronounced hypergranulosis overlying a large melanin-containing area such as confluent nests of heavily pigmented melanocytes or melanophages in the upper dermis with variable amounts of fibrosis. Whatever color variations are seen, blue-white structures are a high-risk criterion most often found in melanomas. Blue-white structures can also be seen in Spitz and Clark (dysplastic) nevi.

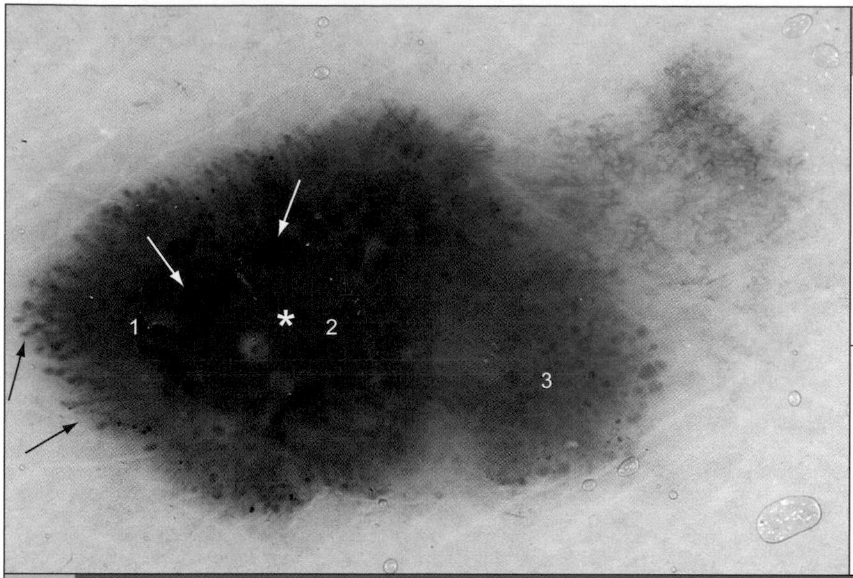

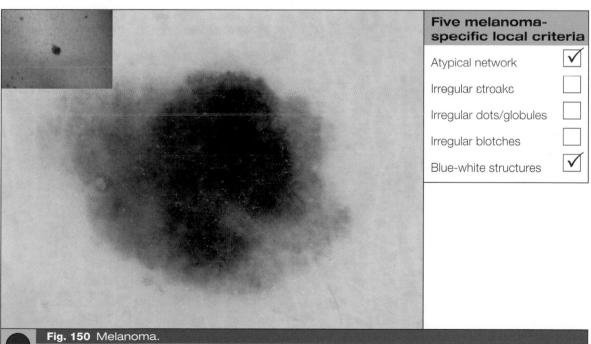

Five melanoma-specific local criteria	
Atypical network	☐
Irregular streaks	☑
Irregular dots/globules	☑
Irregular blotches	☐
Blue-white structures	☑

Fig. 149 Melanoma.

This melanoma demonstrates significant asymmetry of color and structure, multiple vivid colors, and a multicomponent global pattern (*1, 2, 3*). The melanoma-specific criteria are more than sufficient to make the dermoscopic diagnosis, with asymmetrically located irregular streaks (*black arrows*), irregular dots and globules (*white arrows*), and blue structures (*asterisk*).

Five melanoma-specific local criteria	
Atypical network	☑
Irregular streaks	☐
Irregular dots/globules	☐
Irregular blotches	☐
Blue-white structures	☑

Fig. 150 Melanoma.

Remarkably, this dermoscopically straightforward melanoma shows asymmetry of color and structure, although these are not clearly evident clinically. The melanoma-specific criteria found in this lesion include an atypical pigment network, especially at 9 to 11 o'clock, and a slightly off-center area covered by blue-white structures.

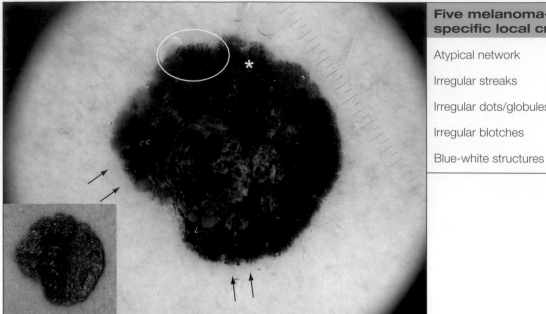

Five melanoma-specific local criteria

Atypical network	☑
Irregular streaks	☑
Irregular dots/globules	☑
Irregular blotches	☐
Blue-white structures	☑

Fig. 151 Melanoma.

This dark black, rather sharply circumscribed lesion displays asymmetry in color, shape, and structure. In addition to a large blue-white structure, there are at least three relevant melanoma-specific criteria present, albeit not very prominent. Remnants of an atypical pigment network are visible at 11 o'clock (circle), few atypical dots/globules are present adjacent to it (*above asterisk*), and variations on the theme of irregular streaks are noted along the periphery of the lesion (*arrows*). Such a constellation of dermoscopic findings allows diagnosing a melanoma with a very high level of confidence.

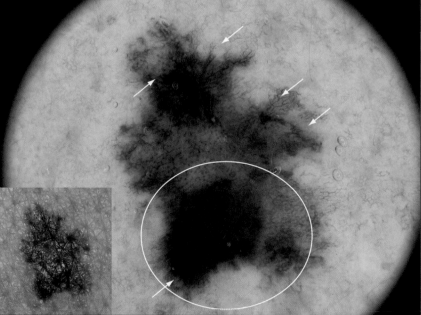

Five melanoma-specific local criteria

Atypical network	☑
Irregular streaks	☑
Irregular dots/globules	☑
Irregular blotches	☐
Blue-white structures	☑

Fig. 152 Melanoma.

This lesion could be diagnosed as an unusual or atypical solar lentigo because of the moth-like appearance of the border. However, it is very worrisome because there is significant asymmetry of color and structure and the presence of blue-white structures (*circle*), a few irregular streaks (*arrows*), and also irregular dots/globules throughout the lesion. In addition, there are areas with hints of an atypical pigment network. The constellation of findings is virtually diagnostic of a melanoma on moderately sun-damaged skin.

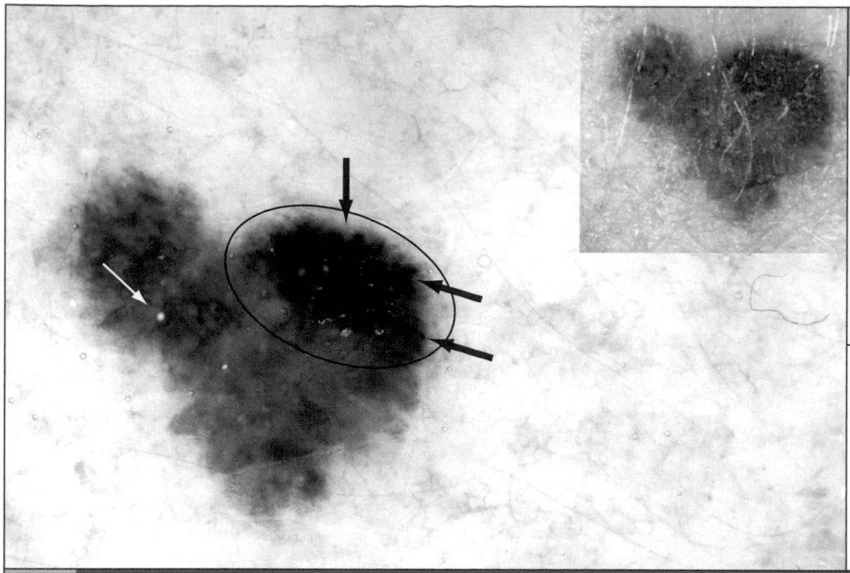

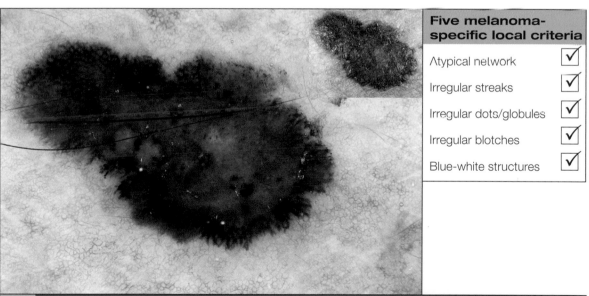

Five melanoma-specific local criteria

Atypical network	☐
Irregular streaks	☑
Irregular dots/globules	☐
Irregular blotches	☑
Blue-white structures	☐

Fig. 153 Melanoma.

The white dots (*white arrow*) are not milia-like cysts but reflection artifacts from the photography of this lesion under oil immersion. This lesion has only two melanoma-specific criteria. One is obvious—the irregular blotch (*circle*), and one is hard to find—irregular streaks within the blotch (*black arrows*). Always focus attention and look for subtle melanoma-specific criteria in a seemingly benign lesion. The very dark and asymmetrically located irregular blotch is worrisome enough by itself to warrant an excision.

Five melanoma-specific local criteria

Atypical network	☑
Irregular streaks	☑
Irregular dots/globules	☑
Irregular blotches	☑
Blue-white structures	☑

Fig. 154 Melanoma.

This melanoma has all of the melanoma-specific criteria from our algorithm and should be easy to diagnose. There are areas with an atypical pigment network, irregular streaks asymmetrically located in the lesion, irregular dots and globules, irregular blotches, and blue-white structures. Clinically this lesion was in the gray zone of suspicion, but this dermoscopic picture leaves no doubt that this is a melanoma.

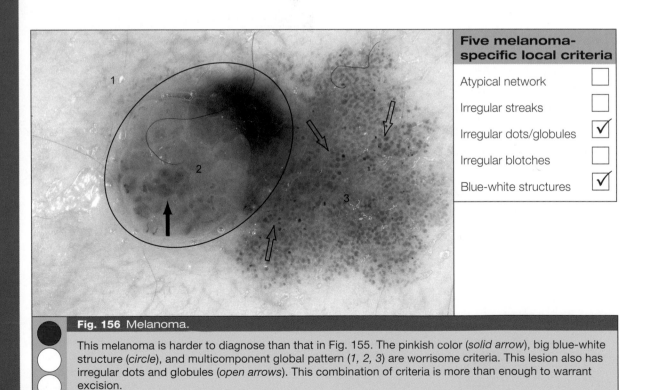

Five melanoma-specific local criteria

Atypical network	☐
Irregular streaks	☑
Irregular dots/globules	☑
Irregular blotches	☑
Blue-white structures	☑

Fig. 155 Melanoma.

The obviously present blue-white structures and irregular dots and globules mean that this is a melanoma. If the irregular streaks and irregular blotches are missed, the significant asymmetry of color and structure plus the presence of two prominent melanoma-specific criteria should be sufficient clues for the novice dermoscopist to remove a lesion that looks like this.

Five melanoma-specific local criteria

Atypical network	☐
Irregular streaks	☐
Irregular dots/globules	☑
Irregular blotches	☐
Blue-white structures	☑

Fig. 156 Melanoma.

This melanoma is harder to diagnose than that in Fig. 155. The pinkish color (*solid arrow*), big blue-white structure (*circle*), and multicomponent global pattern (*1, 2, 3*) are worrisome criteria. This lesion also has irregular dots and globules (*open arrows*). This combination of criteria is more than enough to warrant excision.

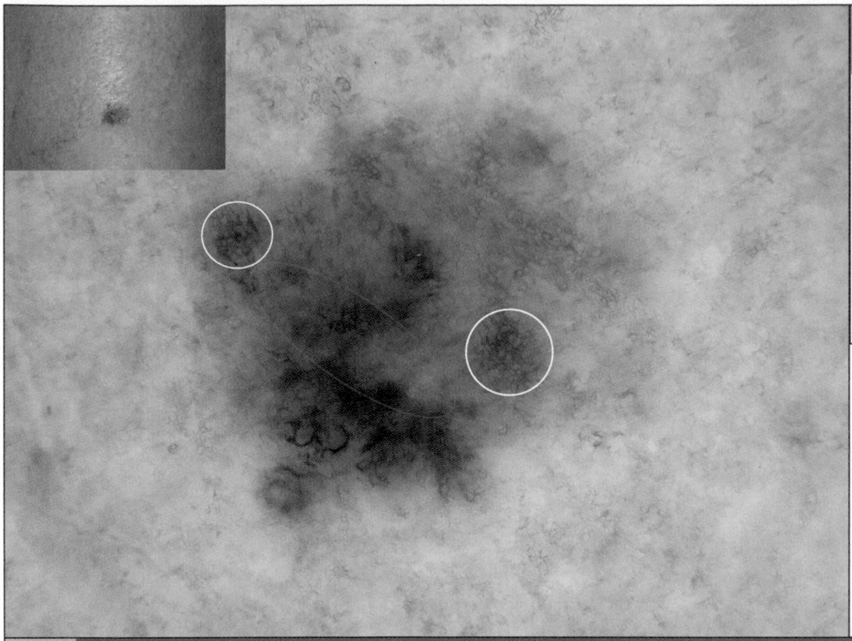

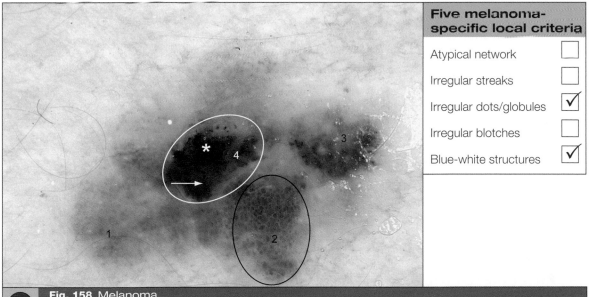

Five melanoma-specific local criteria

Atypical network	☑
Irregular streaks	☐
Irregular dots/globules	☐
Irregular blotches	☐
Blue-white structures	☑

Fig. 157 Melanoma.

This strikingly asymmetric lesion is worrisome already at the first glance, although rarely the histopathology of a lesion like this one will reveal only a dysplastic (Clark) nevus with severe atypia. Our pathologist diagnosed here a melanoma. The melanoma-specific criteria underlining the diagnosis are blue-white structures (*oval*) and few foci of an atypical network (*circles*). Please note that the atypical network could easily be interpreted also as irregular streaks with a tendency to form a network (*arrows*). Some colleagues think that the many morphologic faces observed with dermoscopy could even be used for a Rorschach test!

Five melanoma-specific local criteria

Atypical network	☐
Irregular streaks	☐
Irregular dots/globules	☑
Irregular blotches	☐
Blue-white structures	☑

Fig. 158 Melanoma.

This is a melanoma arising in a nevus. The remnants of the globular pattern of the nevus are still evident (*black circle*). By definition, the dark area would not be considered to be an irregular blotch (*white circle*) because it contains irregular dots and globules (*asterisk*) and a blue-white structure (*arrow*). It should be featureless. Two of five melanoma-specific criteria are present plus a multicomponent global pattern (*1, 2, 3, 4*) and multiple vivid colors. However, no matter how worrisome a dermoscopic picture may look, some of the worst looking lesions turn out to be benign.

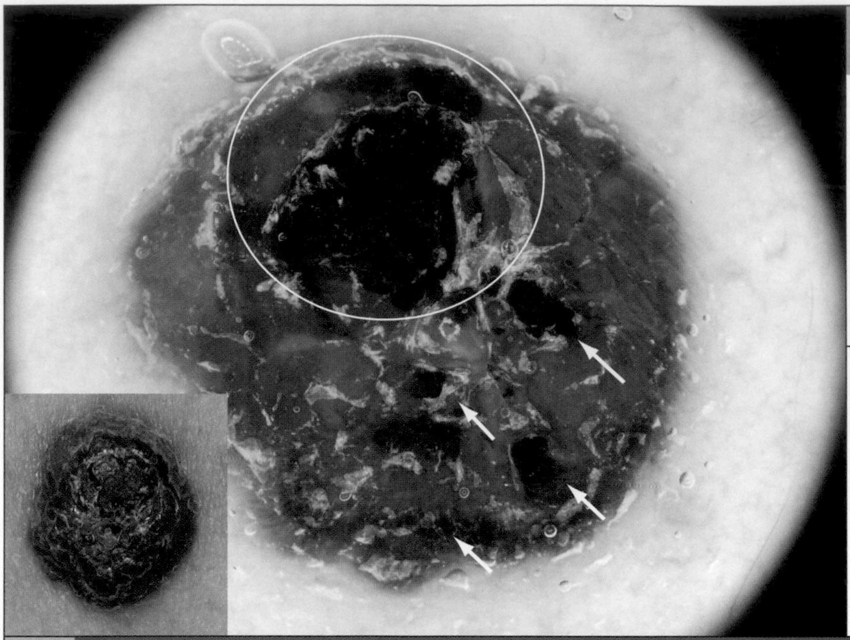

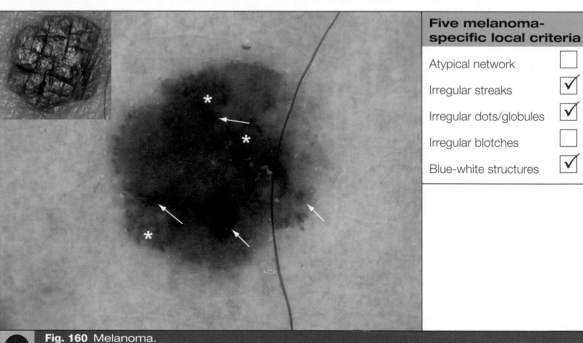

Five melanoma-specific local criteria

Atypical network	☐
Irregular streaks	☐
Irregular dots/globules	☑
Irregular blotches	☑
Blue-white structures	☑

Fig. 159 Melanoma.

This lesion is difficult to diagnose because one can easily interpret it clinically and dermoscopically as irritated seborrheic keratosis. Keep in mind that also a melanoma can be irritated! There is only slight asymmetry in shape and not even a hint of a pigment network. However, there is a large irregular blotch (*circle*) and there are few irregular dots/globules (*arrows*) all probably representing old hemorrhagic crusts of this ulcerated thin nodular melanoma. Please note the blue-whitish structure representing the background of this lesion and note also the thin reddish rim particularly well visible in the left half of the lesion.

Five melanoma-specific local criteria

Atypical network	☐
Irregular streaks	☑
Irregular dots/globules	☑
Irregular blotches	☐
Blue-white structures	☑

Fig. 160 Melanoma.

This is another example of a superficial melanoma which sometimes even histopathologically is very difficult to differentiate from a dysplastic (Clark) nevus with severe atypia. The asymmetry in color and structure due to the presence of irregular streaks (*asterisks*) and irregular dots/globules (*arrows*) leads even the novice to the diagnosis of a melanoma. In addition, there are blue-white structures clearly visible in the central parts of this lesion.

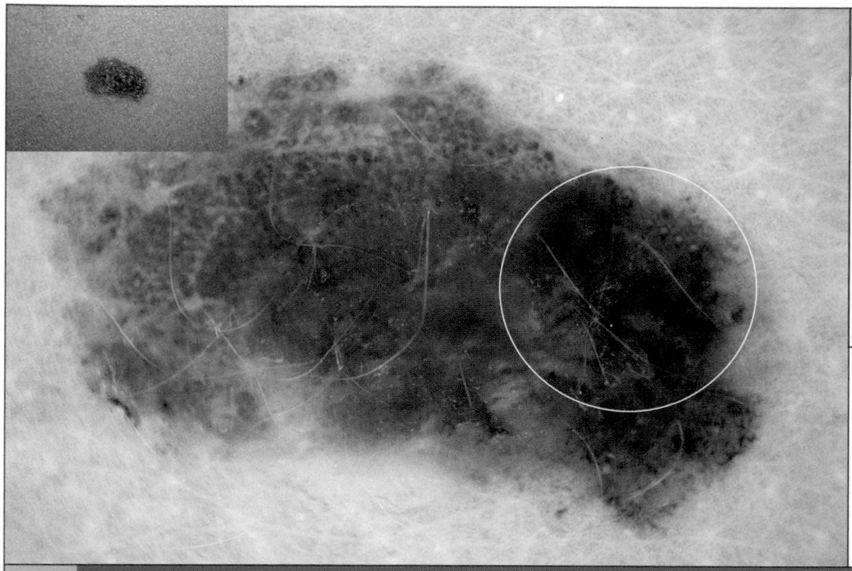

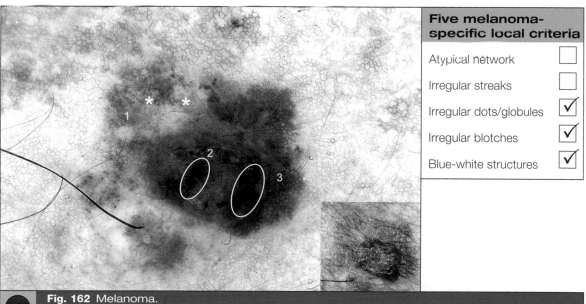

Five melanoma-specific local criteria

Atypical network	☐
Irregular streaks	☐
Irregular dots/globules	☑
Irregular blotches	☑
Blue-white structures	☑

Fig. 161 Melanoma.

It would be very unusual (although not impossible) to see such a vivid blue-white structure and asymmetry of criteria in a benign lesion. There are several black dots and globules at the periphery from 2 to 6 o'clock. There is a large irregular blotch in the right half of the lesion (*circle*). This melanoma has three melanoma-specific criteria; all are easy to see. It is not necessary to identify all five criteria to make here the dermoscopic diagnosis of melanoma with confidence.

Five melanoma-specific local criteria

Atypical network	☐
Irregular streaks	☐
Irregular dots/globules	☑
Irregular blotches	☑
Blue-white structures	☑

Fig. 162 Melanoma.

This is a small lesion but the blue-white structures and irregular blotches (*white circles*) make this worrisome. One could argue whether the pigment network is typical or atypical. There are different areas with irregular dots and globules. Some are black and some are bluish and "pepper-like," representing melanophages (*asterisks*). The multicomponent global pattern (*1, 2, 3*), blue-white structures, and irregular blotches provide more than enough criteria to make the tentative dermoscopic diagnosis of melanoma.

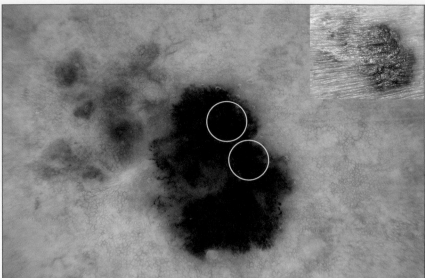

Five melanoma-specific local criteria	
Atypical network	☑
Irregular streaks	☑
Irregular dots/globules	☑
Irregular blotches	☑
Blue-white structures	☑

Fig. 163 Melanoma.

In some instances, the diagnosis of superficial melanomas is very straightforward and should never be missed particularly when dermoscopy is applied. Obviously in the left upper part of this melanoma, regressive changes are observed; otherwise this lesion reveals all stereotypical dermoscopic criteria of a full-blown melanoma. Not uncommonly there is an overlap between irregular streaks and irregular blotches (*circles*). Note that each of the dermoscopic criteria has a wide variation of its morphologic aspects and details. Never forget that melanomas do not read textbooks!

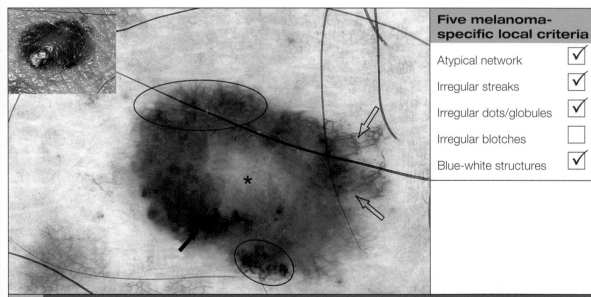

Five melanoma-specific local criteria	
Atypical network	☑
Irregular streaks	☑
Irregular dots/globules	☑
Irregular blotches	☐
Blue-white structures	☑

Fig. 164 Melanoma.

Clinically this is a relatively symmetrical lesion, but there is asymmetry of color and structure when viewed with dermoscopy and there is a multicomponent global pattern. The blue-white structure (*asterisk*) is the most obvious clue that this could be a melanoma. The pigment network is atypical (*circles*), with a hard-to-see focus of streaks (*open arrows*). There are also irregular dots and globules (*solid arrow*). Once again, some criteria are easier to see than others.

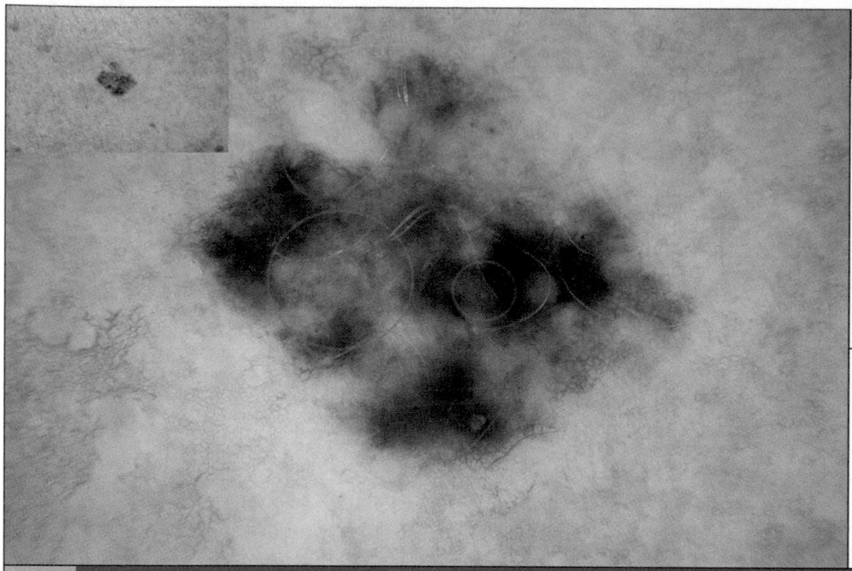

Five melanoma-specific local criteria

Atypical network	☐
Irregular streaks	☐
Irregular dots/globules	☐
Irregular blotches	☑
Blue-white structures	☑

Fig. 165 Melanoma.

This melanoma should not be interpreted as a dysplastic (Clark) nevus, clinically and dermoscopically, and to pick it out in a patient with numerous dysplastic (Clark) nevi might be difficult but not impossible. This lesion is characterized by a patchy reticular pattern along its periphery. The melanoma specific criteria here are irregular blotches and blue-white structures (circle). In addition, the standout features are the many colors and clear-cur asymmetry.

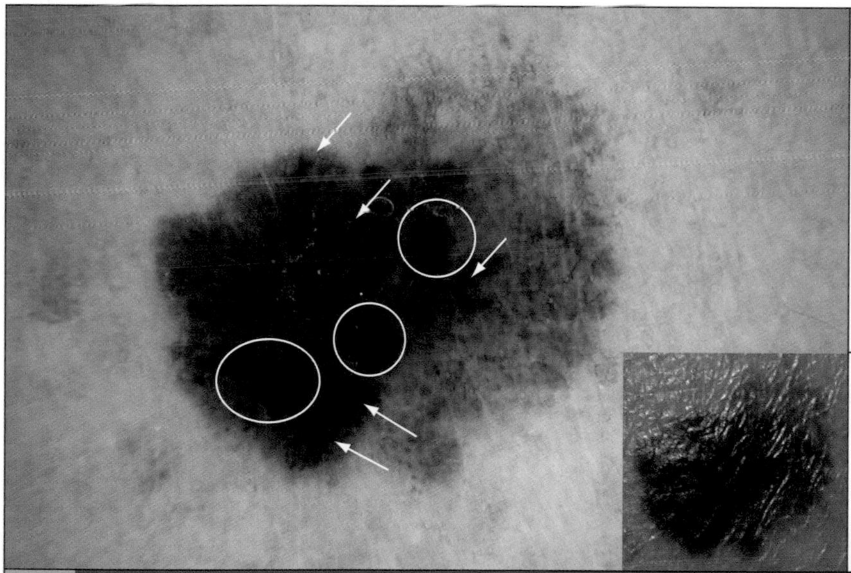

Five melanoma-specific local criteria

Atypical network	☐
Irregular streaks	☑
Irregular dots/globules	☑
Irregular blotches	☑
Blue-white structures	☐

Fig. 166 Melanoma.

This superficial melanoma can be recognized easily even by a beginner because of the striking asymmetry in shape, structure, and color. Closer scrutiny reveals some irregularly outlined black blotches (circles), a few irregular streaks (arrows), and numerous irregular brownish to black dots/globules. Always keep in mind that there are many variations of morphology of the classic dermoscopic criteria as evidenced in this image.

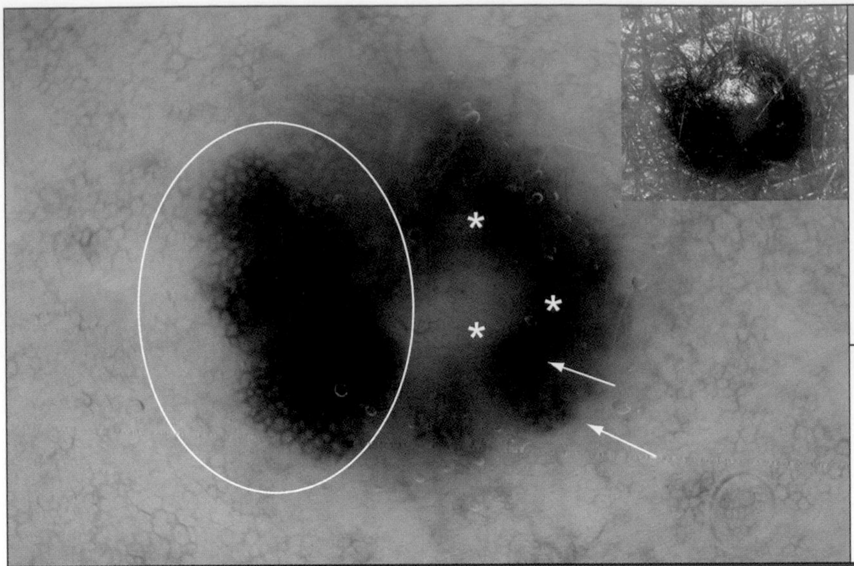

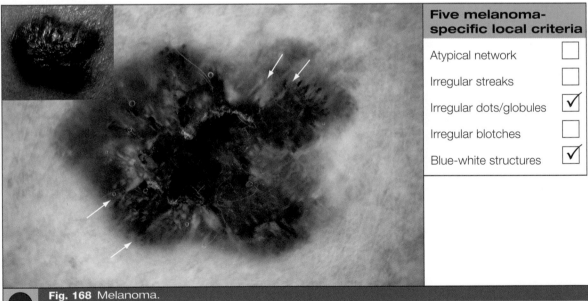

Five melanoma-specific local criteria

Atypical network	☑
Irregular streaks	☐
Irregular dots/globules	☑
Irregular blotches	☐
Blue-white structures	☑

Fig. 167 Melanoma.

This melanoma is rather difficult to diagnose and can be confused with a dysplastic (Clark) nevus despite the fact that there is considerable asymmetry in structure and color. Most probably, the asymmetrically located atypical pigmented network (*circle*) will catch your eye immediately, as will the blue-white structures (*asterisks*) in the right half of the lesion. Completing the list of melanoma-specific criteria, there are irregular dots/globules (*arrows*).

Five melanoma-specific local criteria

Atypical network	☐
Irregular streaks	☐
Irregular dots/globules	☑
Irregular blotches	☐
Blue-white structures	☑

Fig. 168 Melanoma.

This heavily pigmented lesion is easily recognized as a melanoma or a pigmented basal cell carcinoma. A distinction between these two malignant lesions often cannot be ascertained based on dermoscopic criteria alone as evidenced by this observation. Of course, you always err on the side of caution and excise this lesion with utmost priority. Melanoma-specific criteria clearly visible here are blue-white structures and black irregular dots/globules. The many shiny white streaks (*arrows*) strikingly present throughout the lesion indicate that this image has been captured with polarized light. However, the criterion of shiny white streaks (also called chrysalis structures) does not help at all to differentiate between a melanoma and a pigmented basal cell carcinoma.

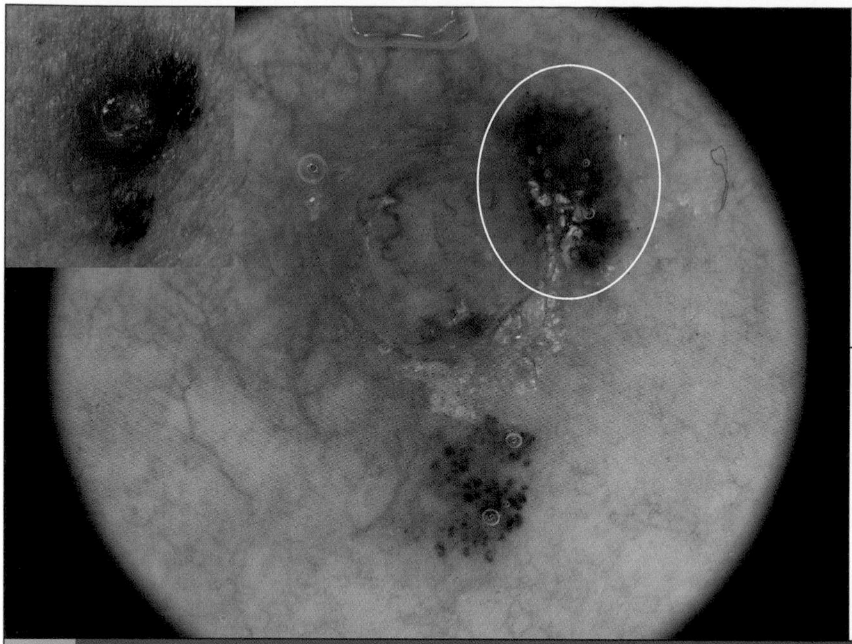

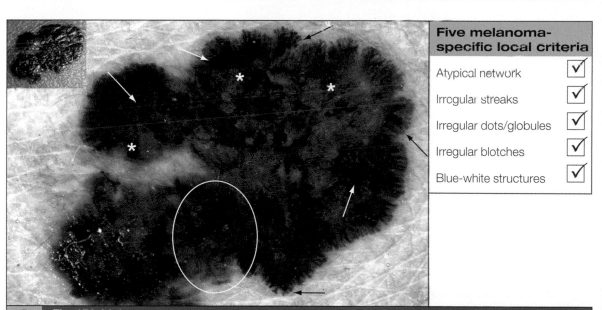

Five melanoma-specific local criteria

Atypical network	☐
Irregular streaks	☑
Irregular dots/globules	☑
Irregular blotches	☐
Blue-white structures	☐

Fig. 169 Melanoma.

This melanoma is characterized by at least three completely different morphologic areas. A dome-shaped skin-colored nodule reminiscent of a dermal nevus, a pigmented area composed of brownish irregular streaks (*circle*), and at 6 o'clock another pigmented patch comprising irregular dots/globules. No doubt that we are dealing with a melanoma. Histopathology revealed that the skin-colored nodule was not a pre-existing dermal nevus, but an amelanotic melanoma with a Breslow index of 2.2 mm. Always be very cautious with nodular lesions within the context of a melanoma.

Five melanoma-specific local criteria

Atypical network	☑
Irregular streaks	☑
Irregular dots/globules	☑
Irregular blotches	☑
Blue-white structures	☑

Fig. 170 Melanoma.

This is a very worrisome dermoscopic picture. Some criteria are very easy to see, while others are camouflaged by intense pigmentation and are harder to find. Areas of atypical pigment network (*circle*) and irregular dots and globules (*asterisks*) are difficult to see but will be found if one searches hard enough. There is no comparison between the irregular streaks (*black arrows*) and irregular blotches (*white arrows*) seen here and those in Fig. 169. There are also well-developed blue-white structures.

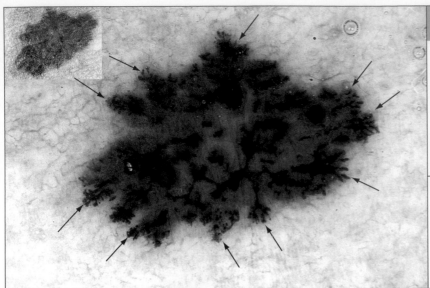

Five melanoma-specific local criteria

Atypical network ☐

Irregular streaks ☑

Irregular dots/globules ☑

Irregular blotches ☑

Blue-white structures ☑

Fig. 171 Melanoma.

Spitzoid, starburst, asymmetry of color and structure—this is therefore melanoma. There are streaks (*arrows*) and areas without streaks. By definition, they are irregular streaks because they are not identified in all areas at the periphery of the lesion. There are also irregular dots and globules and irregular blotches throughout the lesion on a background of blue-white structures.

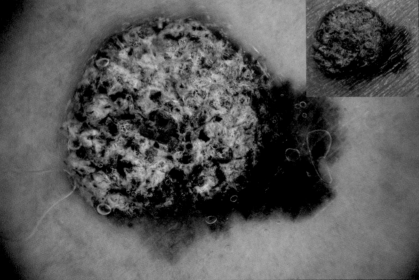

Five melanoma-specific local criteria

Atypical network ☑

Irregular streaks ☐

Irregular dots/globules ☑

Irregular blotches ☐

Blue-white structures ☑

Fig. 172 Melanoma.

This is a verrucous melanoma arising within a pre-existing dysplastic (Clark) nevus. Do not interpret this lesion as a keratotic seborrheic keratosis adjacent to a benign nevus. Follow your intuition and stick with your first impression that this lesion is strikingly asymmetric in shape, structure, and color and needs to be excised with highest priority. When analyzing the morphologic features in detail, you will realize that none of the three criteria mentioned here (see box above) is clearly visible. You do need a bit of imagination to see them. It does not necessarily matter if you do not see them—what is important is that you recognize this verrucous melanoma (Breslow index 3.2 mm) and make the right management decisions.

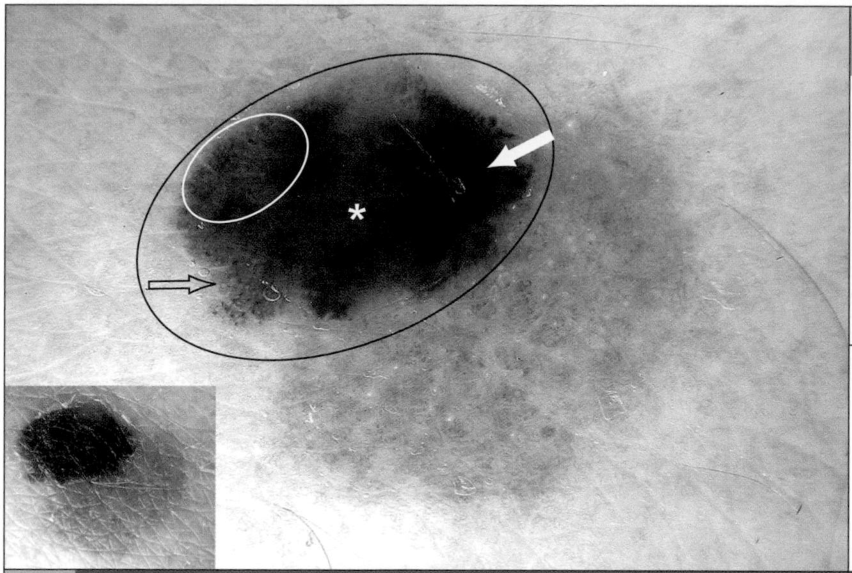

Five melanoma-specific local criteria

Atypical network	☐
Irregular streaks	☐
Irregular dots/globules	☑
Irregular blotches	☑
Blue-white structures	☑

Fig. 173 Melanoma.

Although this is a small lesion, the eccentric area (black circle) indicates the presence of significant activity. The large hypopigmented featureless area is nonspecific. The differential diagnosis includes a Clark (dysplastic) nevus and melanoma. There are small foci of pigment network (*white circle*), irregular dots and globules (*open arrow*), an irregular blotch (*solid arrow*), and a blue-white structure (*asterisk*).

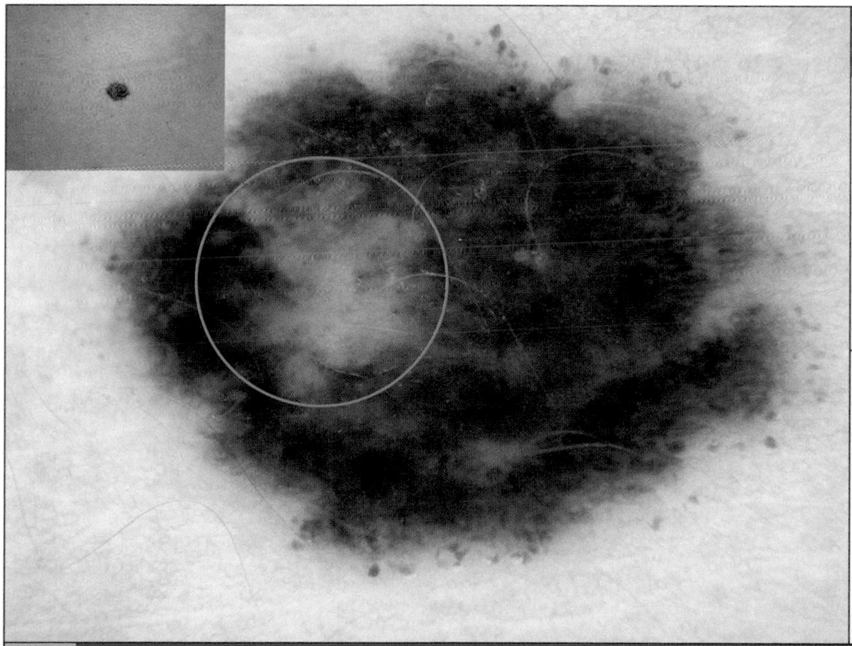

Five melanoma-specific local criteria

Atypical network	☑
Irregular streaks	☑
Irregular dots/globules	☐
Irregular blotches	☐
Blue-white structures	☐

Fig. 174 Melanoma.

This appears to be an easy to diagnose melanoma, with a variation on the theme of atypical pigment network at 9 o'clock and irregular streaks at 2 to 3 o'clock. There are brown and black dots and globules here and there throughout the lesion with one asymmetrically located irregularly outlined white blotch (*circle*). Significant asymmetry of color and structure and multiple vivid colors are striking. The dermoscopic diagnosis of melanoma is not at all difficult if one can recognize the important high-risk criteria.

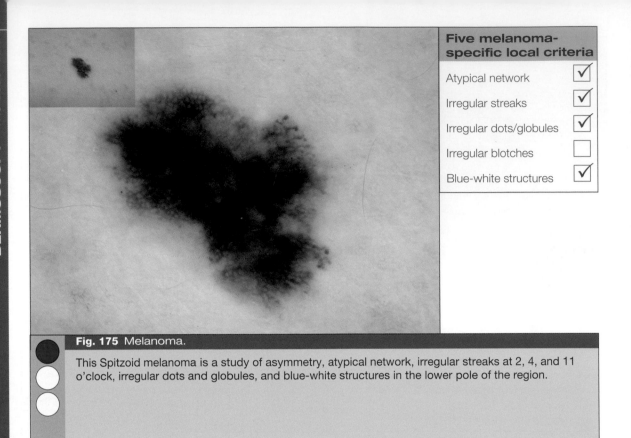

Five melanoma-specific local criteria

Atypical network	☑
Irregular streaks	☑
Irregular dots/globules	☑
Irregular blotches	☐
Blue-white structures	☑

Fig. 175 Melanoma.

This Spitzoid melanoma is a study of asymmetry, atypical network, irregular streaks at 2, 4, and 11 o'clock, irregular dots and globules, and blue-white structures in the lower pole of the region.

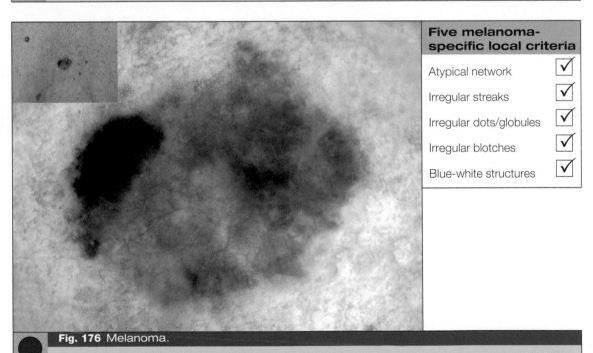

Five melanoma-specific local criteria

Atypical network	☑
Irregular streaks	☑
Irregular dots/globules	☑
Irregular blotches	☑
Blue-white structures	☑

Fig. 176 Melanoma.

This is a superficial melanoma with regression with striking asymmetry in structure and color. We see (with a bit of imagination) all five melanoma-specific local criteria here. At the end of this chapter, we are confident that you also will see most of them and therefore have not placed any annotations on this image. If your pathologist diagnosed this lesion a regressive nevus, we expect you to challenge it—this is a regressive superficial melanoma.

Diagnosis of facial melanoma using four site-specific melanoma-specific criteria

Facial melanomas usually occur in severely sun-damaged skin and is called lentigo maligna when an in situ lesion, and lentigo maligna melanoma when the lesion is invasive. Because of the specific anatomy of facial skin characterized by numerous folliculo-sebaceous units and an effaced epidermis, melanomas on facial skin reveal the following dermoscopic features. These criteria are present in facial melanomas in various combinations and as a rule are not found in non-facial melanomas.

Annular-granular structures

Annular-granular structures are multiple brown or blue-gray dots surrounding the follicular ostia with an annular-granular appearance.

Asymmetrically pigmented follicles

Asymmetrically pigmented follicles are gray circles/rings of pigmentation distributed asymmetrically around follicular ostia. Sometimes, the gray circles may contain an inner gray dot or circle.

Rhomboidal structures

Rhomboid structures are thickened areas of pigmentation surrounding the follicular ostia with a rhomboidal appearance (a rhomboid is a parallelogram with unequal angles and sides).

Gray pseudonetwork

Gray pseudonetwork describes gray pigmentation surrounding the follicular ostia formed by the confluence of annular-granular structures.

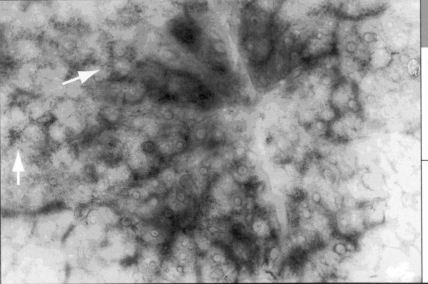

Four site-specific melanoma-specific criteria

Annular-granular structures	☐
Asymmetrically pigmented follicles	☐
Rhomboidal structures	☑
Gray pseudonetwork	☑

Fig. 177 Melanoma.

The default differential diagnosis of lentigo maligna (melanoma in situ on severely sun-damaged skin) clinically, dermoscopically, and sometimes also histopathologically is actinic (solar) lentigo. This diagnostic uncertainty is underlined by the concept of unstable lentigo—an actinic lentigo on the way to a lentigo maligna. Interestingly, this concept has not been widely adopted, maybe because we are used to accepting a benign/malignant dichotomy. The lesion depicted here is a lentigo maligna characterized by a few rhomboidal structures (*circle*) and hints of a gray pseudonetwork (*arrows*).

Four site-specific melanoma-specific criteria

Annular-granular structures	☑
Asymmetrically pigmented follicles	☑
Rhomboidal structures	☐
Gray pseudonetwork	☐

Fig. 178 Melanoma.

Annular-granular structures are present in this lesion (*arrows*). Do not confuse the ostia of the appendages with the milia-like cysts of seborrheic keratosis. Now check the ostia carefully. Some are totally and some are partially ringed by thin layers of pigmentation. The dermoscopic diagnosis of asymmetrically pigmented follicles is made when the rim of pigmentation does not surround the entire ostium. True rhomboidal structures are not formed yet. The vessels should not be confused with those seen in basal cell carcinomas. They correspond to the dermal plexus shining through the thinned epidermis.

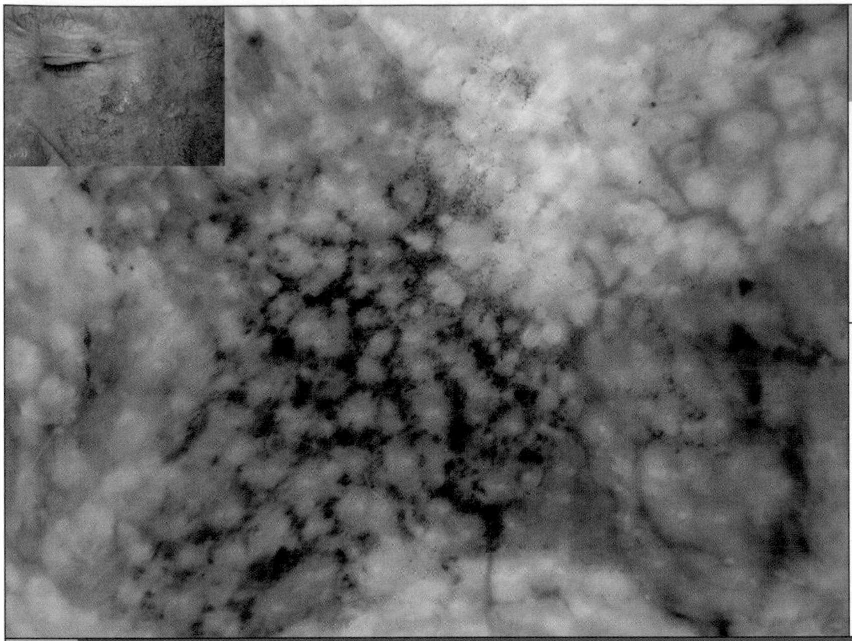

Four site-specific melanoma-specific criteria

Annular-granular structures	☑
Asymmetrically pigmented follicles	☐
Rhomboidal structures	☑
Gray pseudonetwork	☐

Fig. 179 Melanoma.

This lesion shows a variation on the theme of lentigo maligna. Note the asymmetry in structure and color. There are annular-granular structures that are forming rhomboidal structures. The gray granules of the annular-granular structures are hard to see, but are there. In addition, quite a few brown and black globules representing junctional nests of melanocytes can be seen nicely.

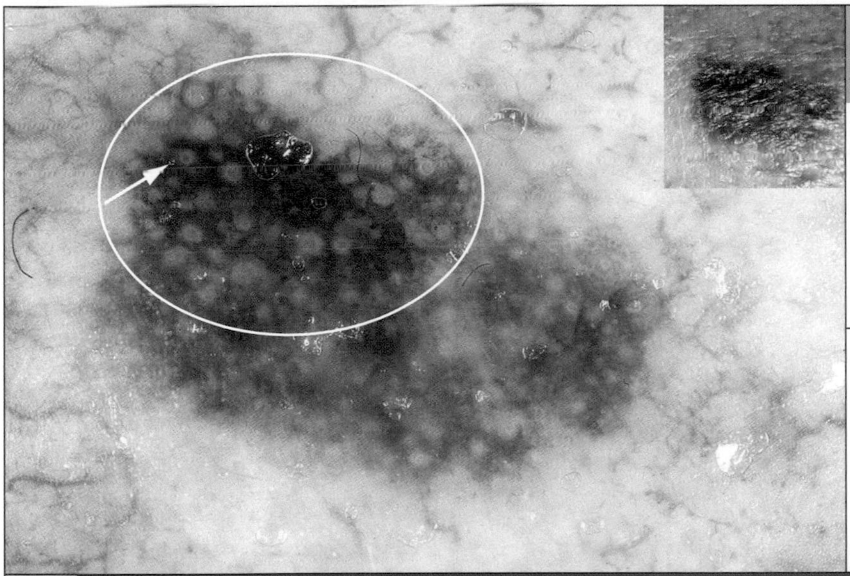

Four site-specific melanoma-specific criteria

Annular-granular structures	☑
Asymmetrically pigmented follicles	☐
Rhomboidal structures	☑
Gray pseudonetwork	☑

Fig. 180 Melanoma.

The asymmetry of color and structure seen here should be more than enough for the novice dermoscopist to increase his or her index of suspicion of a high-risk lesion. The annular-granular structures make up rhomboidal structures (*arrow*). Confluence of rhomboidal structures makes up the gray pseudonetwork (*circle*). Biopsy the darker blotch because it could be an area of invasion. Lentigo maligna melanoma—not lentigo maligna. Do not confuse the follicular ostia with milia-like cysts or comedo-like openings.

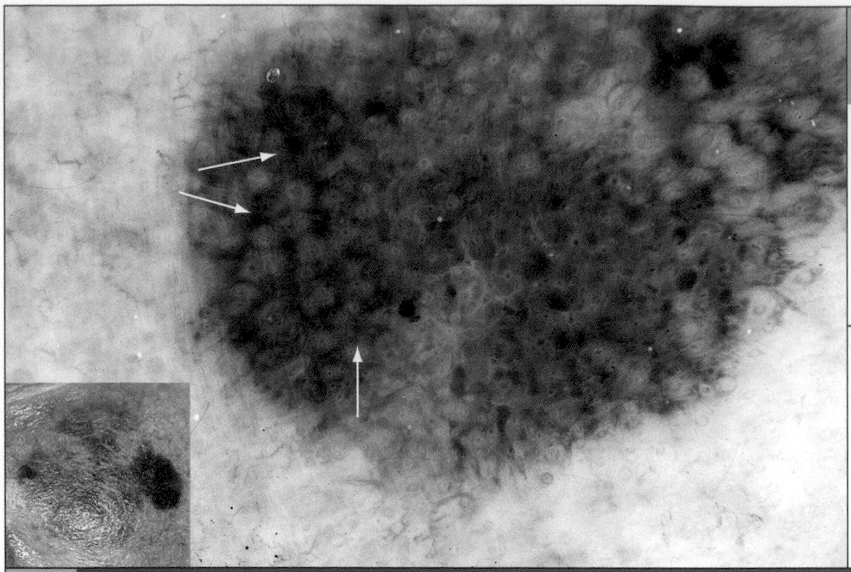

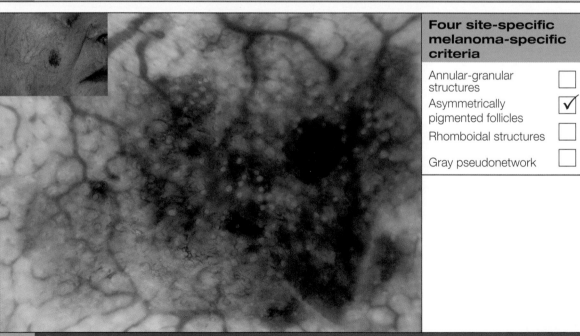

Four site-specific melanoma-specific criteria

Annular-granular structures	☑
Asymmetrically pigmented follicles	☐
Rhomboidal structures	☑
Gray pseudonetwork	☐

Fig. 181 Melanoma.

The asymmetry of color and structure plus vivid colors, including an overall pinkish hue, should raise one's index of suspicion that this is a melanoma. Scan the entire lesion for site-specific, melanoma-specific criteria. There are very small annular-granular structures, but no asymmetrically pigmented follicles. There are also multiple subtle rhomboidal structures (*arrows*) and irregular dots and globules. It is possible to see melanoma-specific criteria for trunk and extremity melanomas on the head and neck.

Four site-specific melanoma-specific criteria

Annular-granular structures	☐
Asymmetrically pigmented follicles	☑
Rhomboidal structures	☐
Gray pseudonetwork	☐

Fig. 182 Melanoma.

This lesion shows a classic appearance of an early lentigo maligna. There is only a slight asymmetry in shape, but there is obvious asymmetry in pigmentation. Dermoscopy shows asymmetrically pigmented hair follicles appearing as gray and brown circles. Today, reflectance confocal microscopy is increasingly used for the noninvasive diagnosis of lentigo maligna.

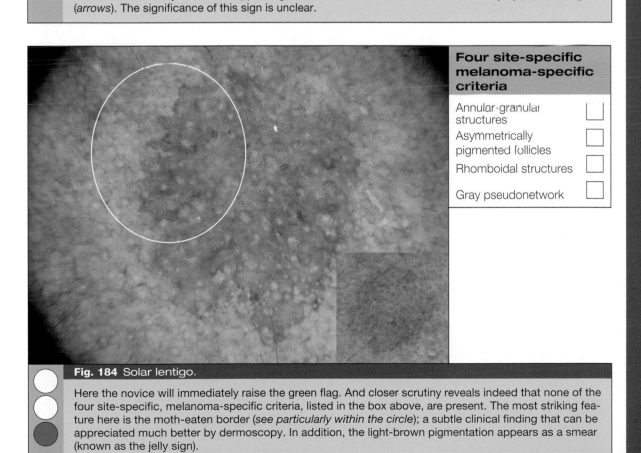

Four site-specific melanoma-specific criteria	
Annular-granular structures	☐
Asymmetrically pigmented follicles	☐
Rhomboidal structures	☐
Gray pseudonetwork	☐

Fig. 183 Pigmented actinic keratosis.

For this strikingly asymmetric lesion (in shape, structure, and color), we are raising immediately the red flag. Closer scrutiny, however, shows that none of the four site-specific, melanoma-specific criteria listed in the box above are present. There are keratin-filled hair follicle openings that appear white encompassed by a superficial brown pseudonetwork suggestive of a pigmented actinic keratosis. There are also rosette-like tiny structures appearing as four white dots, which can be seen only by polarized light (*arrows*). The significance of this sign is unclear.

Four site-specific melanoma-specific criteria	
Annular-granular structures	☐
Asymmetrically pigmented follicles	☐
Rhomboidal structures	☐
Gray pseudonetwork	☐

Fig. 184 Solar lentigo.

Here the novice will immediately raise the green flag. And closer scrutiny reveals indeed that none of the four site-specific, melanoma-specific criteria, listed in the box above, are present. The most striking feature here is the moth-eaten border (*see particularly within the circle*); a subtle clinical finding that can be appreciated much better by dermoscopy. In addition, the light-brown pigmentation appears as a smear (known as the jelly sign).

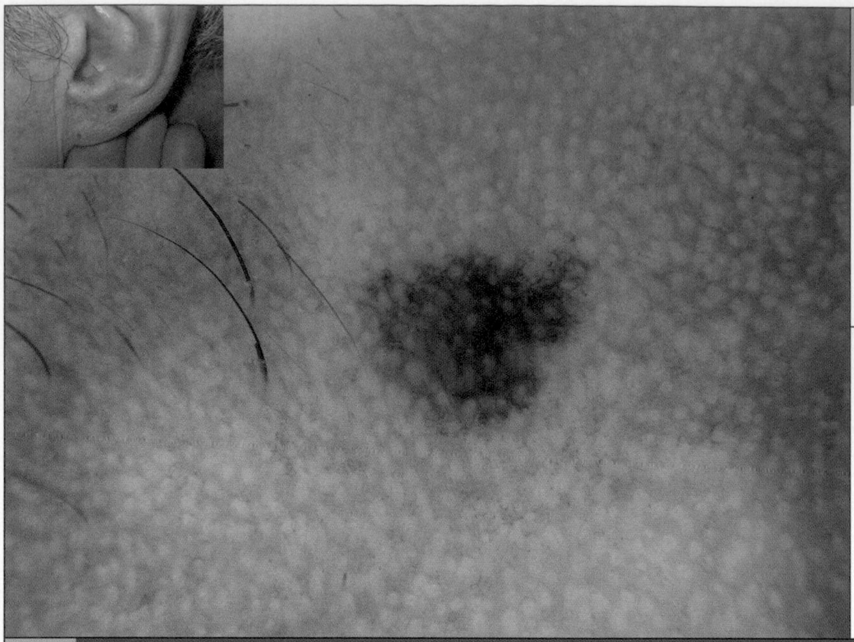

Four site-specific melanoma-specific criteria

Annular-granular structures	☐
Asymmetrically pigmented follicles	☐
Rhomboidal structures	☐
Gray pseudonetwork	☐

Fig. 185 Solar lentigo.

We are raising the orange flag here although none of the four site-specific, melanoma-specific criteria are present. There is only a hint of a moth-eaten border in the upper half of the lesion, and there are a few symmetrically pigmented follicles visible throughout the lesion. Because of the very subtle tinge of gray color, we recommend annual follow-up of this lesion and raise the orange flag. The differential diagnosis here includes a benign nevus.

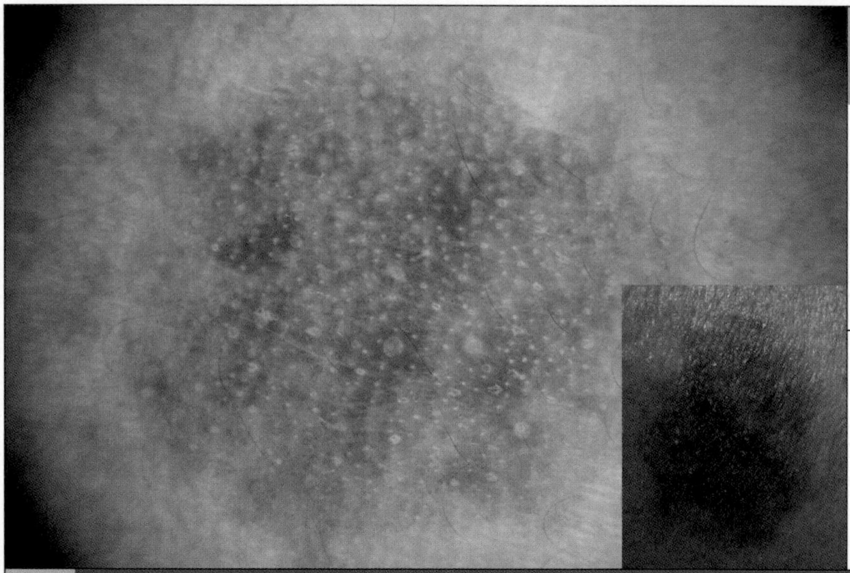

Four site-specific melanoma-specific criteria

Annular-granular structures	☐
Asymmetrically pigmented follicles	☐
Rhomboidal structures	☐
Gray pseudonetwork	☐

Fig. 186 Solar lentigo.

Quickly we are becoming well acquainted with the dermoscopic appearance of a solar lentigo. There are numerous symmetrically pigmented follicles rather evenly distributed throughout the lesion. And there is complete absence of all site-specific, melanoma-specific criteria.

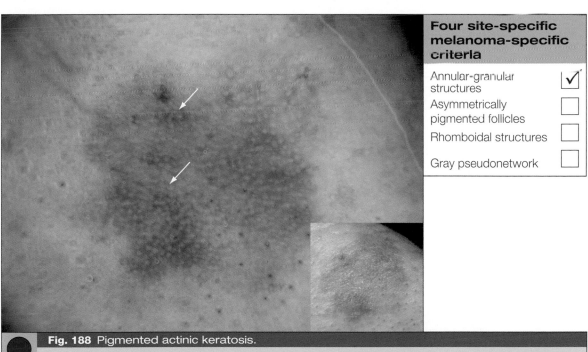

Four site-specific melanoma-specific criteria

Annular-granular structures	☐
Asymmetrically pigmented follicles	☐
Rhomboidal structures	☐
Gray pseudonetwork	☐

Fig. 187 Seborrheic keratosis evolving from an actinic lentigo.

The beginner might raise the orange flag here because of the asymmetry in structure and color. Please note the striking moth-eaten border at the left half of the lesion (*circle*). In the right lower part of the lesion, there are several, medium to dark-brown pigmented, regular broad streaks (also called "fat fingers"). These structures are a rather typical finding for superficial seborrheic keratoses. One needs to see a few examples of this type of seborrheic keratosis arising from an actinic lentigo before making this diagnosis with confidence.

Four site-specific melanoma-specific criteria

Annular-granular structures	☑
Asymmetrically pigmented follicles	☐
Rhomboidal structures	☐
Gray pseudonetwork	☐

Fig. 188 Pigmented actinic keratosis.

The overall architecture of this lesion together with its pinkish coloration is worrisome and we are raising the red flag. Closer scrutiny reveals a mostly brownish pseudonetwork with only delicate shades of gray coloration. There are hints of annular-granular-like structures (*arrows*) and of course we have to take lentigo maligna into our differential diagnostic considerations. However, histopathology confirmed a pigmented actinic keratosis. Sometimes even with dermoscopy, the diagnosis of facial pigmented lesions is rather difficult.

Four patterns for acral melanocytic lesions

The parallel pattern is found exclusively in melanocytic lesions on glabrous skin of palms and soles because of the presence of particular anatomic structures inherent to these locations. The pigmentation may follow the furrows as well as the ridges of glabrous skin but rarely may also be arranged at a right angle to these pre-existing structures:

- the parallel furrow, lattice-like, and fibrillar patterns are commonly found in acral benign nevi;
- the parallel ridge pattern is suggestive of melanomas on acral sites.

General dermoscopic principles for evaluating acral lesions

- First look at the periphery of the lesion to determine where the ridges and furrows are.

- The pigmentation is located in the ridges when the pigmented lines are thicker than the nonpigmented ones and have white dots running along like a string of pearls. It is not always possible to see the string of pearls.
- The appearance of dermoscopic criteria tends to be out of focus on acral areas, owing to the thickness of the skin.
- Other clinical data such as the patient's age and history of the lesion are often essential.

Box 2.1 Four patterns for acral melanocytic lesions
• Parallel furrow
• Parallel ridge
• Lattice-like
• Fibrillar

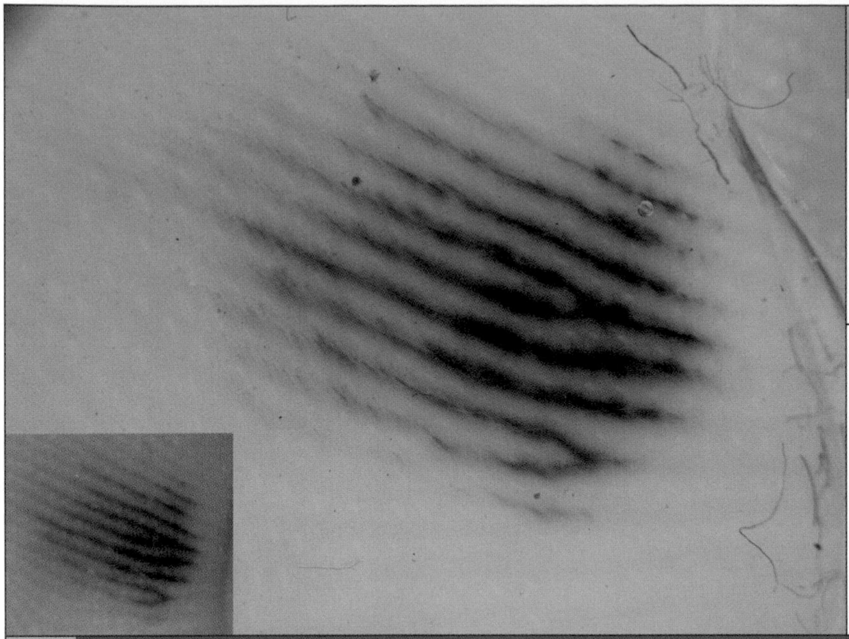

Four patterns for acral melanocytic lesions

Parallel furrow	☑
Parallel ridge	☐
Lattice-like	☐
Fibrillar	☐

Fig. 189 Nevus.

This is the parallel furrow pattern of an acral nevus. The dermoscopic hallmark of this lesion is the presence of several parallel pigmented lines in the sulci (or furrows) of glabrous skin. Please note that the lines in the right half of the lesion are more pigmented than the ones in the left half. It is not always easy to determine whether the linear band of pigmentation is in the ridges or the furrows. A helpful clue is that the pigmentation in the furrows is smaller than the pigmentation following the ridges. See also Fig. 199 and 200.

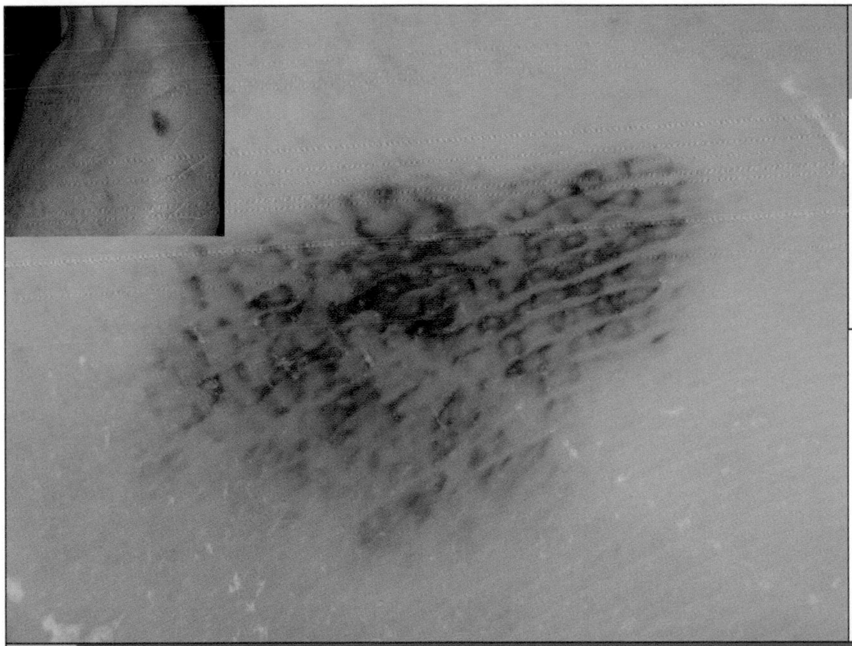

Four patterns for acral melanocytic lesions

Parallel furrow	☐
Parallel ridge	☐
Lattice-like	☑
Fibrillar	☐

Fig. 190 Nevus.

This is a variation on the theme of the lattice-like pattern of an acral nevus. It is characterized by a lattice-like structure formed by a rectangular network of brownish lines punctuated by several whitish dots, which look like a string of pearls. The whitish dots represent the openings of the eccrine ducts situated in the ridges of the skin. Without specific knowledge of the various dermoscopic patterns of acral nevi, this benign lesion could easily be called as early acral melanoma, and we have therefore raised the orange flag.

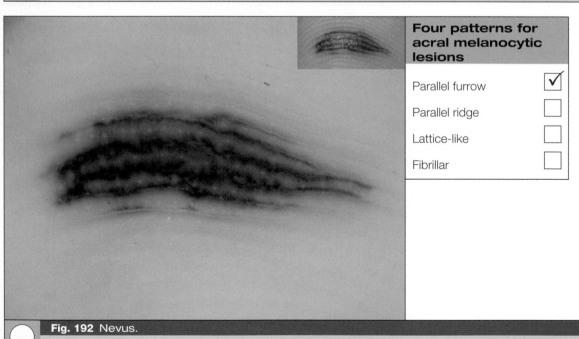

Four patterns for acral melanocytic lesions

Parallel furrow	✓
Parallel ridge	☐
Lattice-like	☐
Fibrillar	☐

Fig. 191 Nevus.

This lesion shows a variation of the morphology seen with the parallel furrow pattern, and there are many. There are only a few linear bands of pigmentation following the furrows of the acral skin. Note the double contour of the linear pigmentation (*arrows*) following the furrows in the lower half of this nevus. The management of acral lesions is strongly influenced by the ability to differentiate the benign parallel furrow pattern from the malignant parallel ridge pattern.

Four patterns for acral melanocytic lesions

Parallel furrow	✓
Parallel ridge	☐
Lattice-like	☐
Fibrillar	☐

Fig. 192 Nevus.

Here is another parallel furrow type of acral nevus with a subtle superimposed globular component. This lesion has four prominent parallel pigmented lines in the furrows. The bands of pigmentation are superimposed by few dark-brown to black dots. Between the pigmented bands, there are several tiny whitish dots arranged like a string of pearls corresponding to the eccrine ducts reaching the surface on the ridges. Whatever form the pigment takes in an acral nevus, if it is determined to be in the furrows, the lesion is benign. There can be single lines, single rows of dots and globules, and even double rows of lines or double rows of dots and globules. Just ensure the pigmentation is not in the ridges. Here we scored this lesion to be of moderate risk (orange traffic light) because the furrow pattern is difficult to recognize.

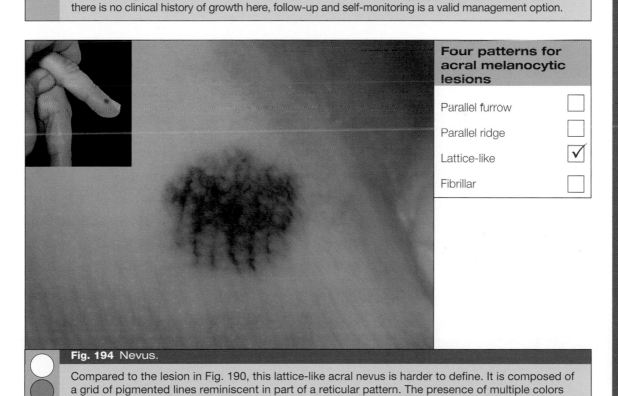

Four patterns for acral melanocytic lesions

Parallel furrow	☐
Parallel ridge	☐
Lattice-like	☑
Fibrillar	☐

Fig. 193 Nevus.

This lesion provides another variation on the theme of the lattice-like pattern. Here the pigmented grid is distorted due to a swirl shape in the underlying ridges and furrows. Numerous whitish dots represent the openings of eccrine ducts. The pigmented lines follow the furrows of the acral skin. Thinner pigmented lines are arranged perpendicularly to the thicker lines to form the lattice-like pattern. The presence of multiple colors (brown, black, and blue-gray), with irregularly distributed black dots, make this lesion difficult to classify. However, the advice "if in doubt, cut it out" is not always appropriate on acral surfaces. If there is no clinical history of growth here, follow-up and self-monitoring is a valid management option.

Four patterns for acral melanocytic lesions

Parallel furrow	☐
Parallel ridge	☐
Lattice-like	☑
Fibrillar	☐

Fig. 194 Nevus.

Compared to the lesion in Fig. 190, this lattice-like acral nevus is harder to define. It is composed of a grid of pigmented lines reminiscent in part of a reticular pattern. The presence of multiple colors (light brown, dark brown, and blue-gray), a poorly defined grid, and few brownish dots and globules makes this a difficult lesion to classify. Again, the advice "if in doubt, cut it out" is not always so easy to follow on acral sites. If there is no clinical history of growth here, follow-up and self-monitoring is a valid management option.

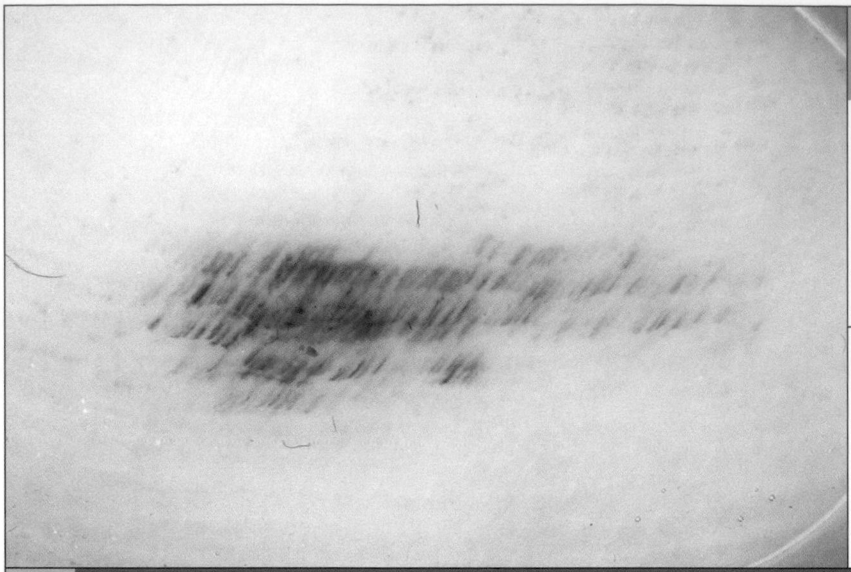

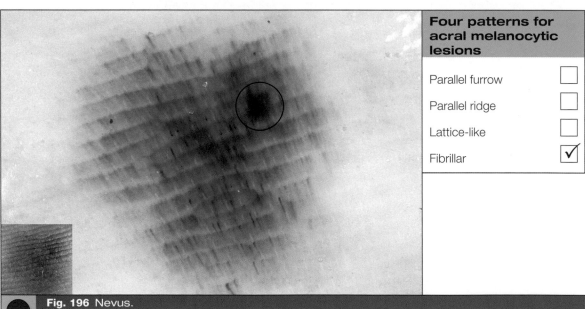

Four patterns for acral melanocytic lesions

Parallel furrow	☐
Parallel ridge	☐
Lattice-like	☐
Fibrillar	☑

Fig. 195 Nevus.

This lesion is out of focus and is a stereotypical example of the fibrillar pattern seen in acral nevi. It is characterized by numerous short and thin brown lines that not only have a parallel arrangement, but also run oblique to the ridges and furrows of the acral skin. The parallel furrow, lattice-like and fibrillar patterns are those seen in benign acral melanocytic lesions. Furrow, lattice or fibrillar = benign nevus.

Four patterns for acral melanocytic lesions

Parallel furrow	☐
Parallel ridge	☐
Lattice-like	☐
Fibrillar	☑

Fig. 196 Nevus.

This shows a variation of the fibrillar pattern of acral nevus, and it is hard to differentiate this from the parallel ridge pattern. It is composed of numerous, obliquely arranged, smudged, pigmented, thin, short lines. There is also a blotch (*circle*). Numerous light-brown parallel lines are also found in the furrows of the skin. This lesion is difficult to evaluate; therefore it should be excised. It could easily be mistaken for the parallel ridge pattern, even by an experienced dermoscopist.

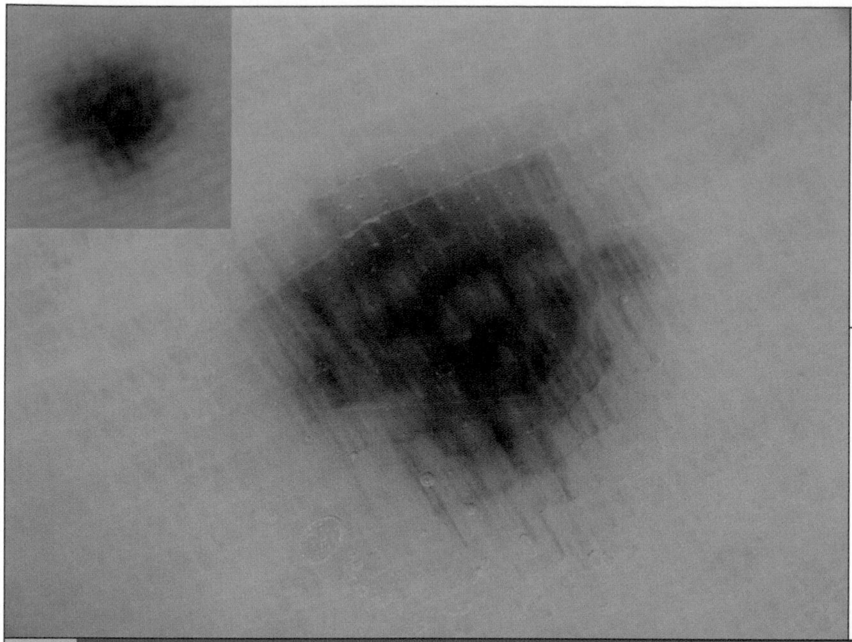

Four patterns for acral melanocytic lesions

Parallel furrow	☐
Parallel ridge	☐
Lattice-like	☐
Fibrillar	☑

Fig. 197 Nevus.

This lesion provides a rather typical example of a fibrillar pattern. This pattern is observed particularly in the pressure areas of the plantar surfaces. Because there is some degree of variation in pigmentation, the orange flag might be raised here. Still, we felt comfortable not to excise this lesion and recommended annual follow-up.

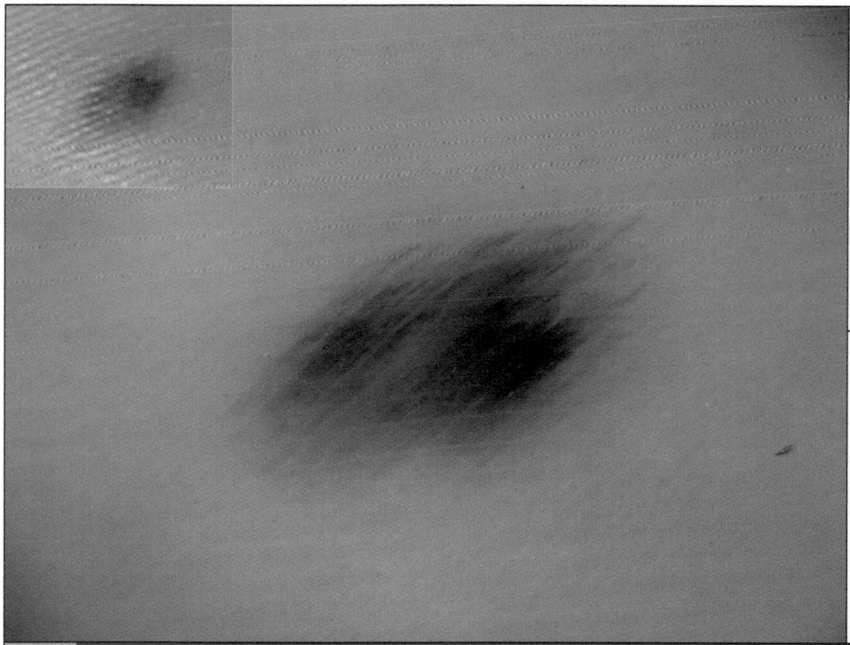

Four patterns for acral melanocytic lesions

Parallel furrow	☐
Parallel ridge	☐
Lattice-like	☐
Fibrillar	☑

Fig. 198 Nevus.

This is another example of an acral nevus with fibrillar pattern. As in the case above, there is some degree of uneven pigmentation that also leads to asymmetry in color. Because of this asymmetric pigmentation, the lesion was interpreted as suspicious, the orange flag was raised, and the lesion was excised. The histopathologic examination confirmed the diagnosis of benign acral nevus. In hindsight, we could have well decided to just follow up this lesion with striking fibrillar pattern.

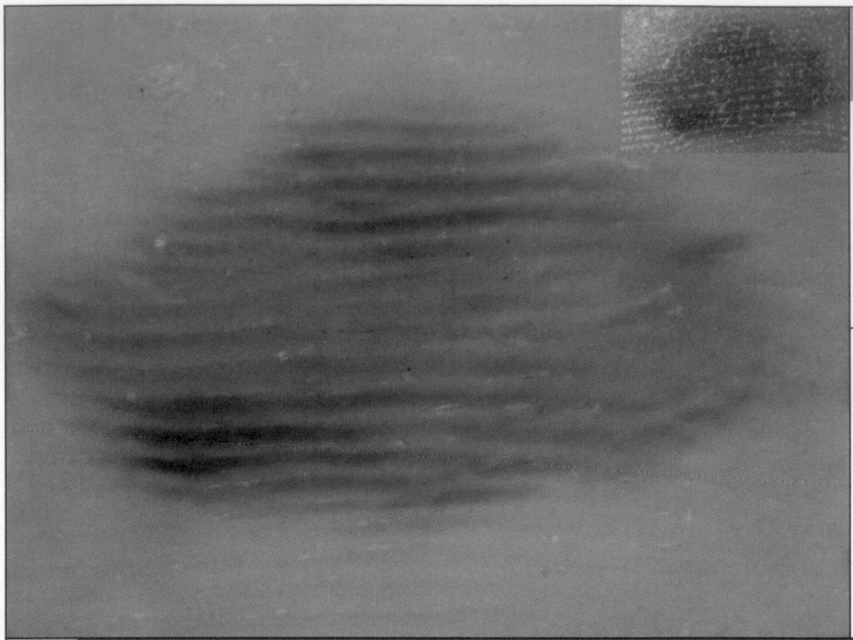

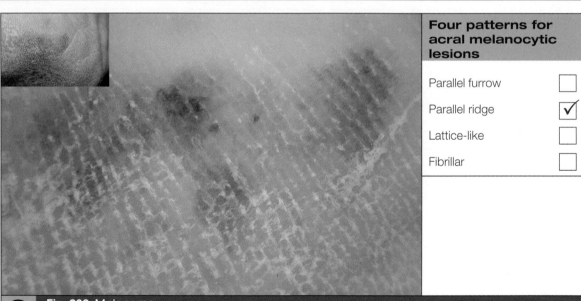

Four patterns for acral melanocytic lesions

Parallel furrow	☐
Parallel ridge	☑
Lattice-like	☐
Fibrillar	☐

Fig. 199 Melanoma.

This is an acral melanocytic proliferation with a pronounced parallel pattern. Please note that the pigmented bands are broader than the whitish lines in between. This is suggestive of a parallel-ridge pattern, and therefore this lesion was excised without any delay. The histopathologic examination confirmed the diagnosis of an acral-lentiginous melanoma in situ.

Four patterns for acral melanocytic lesions

Parallel furrow	☐
Parallel ridge	☑
Lattice-like	☐
Fibrillar	☐

Fig. 200 Melanoma.

This image shows an acral melanoma with a very subtle parallel ridge pattern. This asymmetrical lesion is composed of several brown, thickened lines in the ridges of the skin and very few isolated large globules. Because of the pronounced keratosis, even the dermoscopic assessment of the lesion is very difficult, and this type of lesion can easily be missed. Remember that the parallel ridge pattern is pathognomonic for acral melanoma. The major pitfall is that the parallel ridge pattern might be interpreted as a parallel furrow pattern and the melanoma might not be diagnosed.

Six criteria for diagnosing non-melanocytic lesions

To diagnose non-melanocytic pigmented skin lesions, there should be an absence of criteria for melanocytic lesions (pigment network, globules, streaks, homogeneous and parallel patterns) and the presence of criteria considered specific for basal cell carcinoma, seborrheic keratosis, hemangioma, or dermatofibroma.

Blue-gray blotches

Blue-gray blotches are structureless areas that are round to oval and often irregular in shape. The color ranges from brownish-gray to blue-gray. Histopathologically they represent heavily pigmented, solid aggregations of basaloid cells in the papillary dermis of superficial or nodular basal cell carcinoma. Blue-gray blotches are a pathognomonic finding in pigmented basal cell carcinoma, especially when associated with arborizing vessels and an absence of criteria seen in melanocytic lesions.

Arborizing vessels

Arborizing vessels are discrete, thickened, and branched red blood vessels that are similar in appearance to the branches of a tree. Histopathologically they represent dilated arterial circulation that feeds the tumor. Arborizing vessels are 99% diagnostic of basal cell carcinoma. Rarely they can be found in intradermal nevi or featureless melanomas.

Milia-like cysts

Milia-like cysts are variously sized, white or yellowish, round structures. Histopathologically, they represent intraepidermal horn globules, also called horn pseudocysts, a common histopathologic finding in acanthotic seborrheic keratosis. Multiple milia-like cysts are predominantly found in seborrheic keratoses, but they can also be seen in papillomatous dermal nevi, and rarely a few milia-like cysts are seen in melanomas.

Comedo-like openings

Comedo-like openings refer to brownish-yellow or brown-black, irregularly shaped, sharply circumscribed structures. Histopathologically, they represent keratin plugs within dilated follicular openings. Due to oxidation of the keratinous material, they often have a yellowish-brown or dark-brown to black color. Comedo-like openings are found predominantly in seborrheic keratoses, but they can also be seen in papillomatous dermal nevi. At times it is difficult to differentiate dark comedo-like openings from the globules seen in melanocytic lesions.

Red-blue lacunae

Red lacunae appear as sharply demarcated, round to oval structures. The color can vary from red, red-blue, dark-red to black. A whitish color is also often seen in vascular lesions. Histopathologically, red lacunae represent dilated vascular spaces located in the upper dermis. Lacunae with dark-red to black color represent vascular spaces that are partially or completely thrombosed. Red lacunae are the stereotypical criterion of hemangiomas and angiokeratomas. Structures similar in appearance can also be seen in subungual and subcorneal hematomas.

Central white patch

The central white patch diagnostic of dermatofibromas is a well-circumscribed, round-to-oval, sometimes irregularly outlined, bony-milky-white area usually in the center of a firm lesion. There are many variations of the morphology of this criterion.

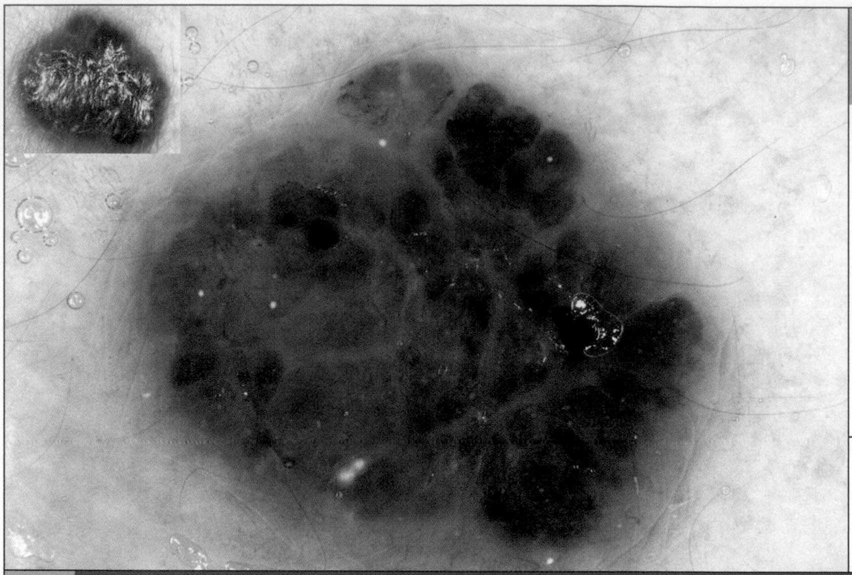

Six criteria for non-melanocytic lesions

Blue-gray blotches	☑
Arborizing vessels	☐
Milia-like cysts	☐
Comedo-like openings	☐
Red-blue lacunae	☐
Central white patch	☐

Fig. 201 Basal cell carcinoma.

Arborizing vessels characteristic of a basal cell carcinoma are hard to see; therefore this could easily be mistaken for a melanoma. The blue-white structures and blue-gray blotches also favor a diagnosis of melanoma, but in this case, it turned out to be a basal cell carcinoma. Blue-white structures are found not only in melanomas but also in basal cell carcinomas. It is not always possible to differentiate melanoma from basal cell carcinoma with dermoscopy.

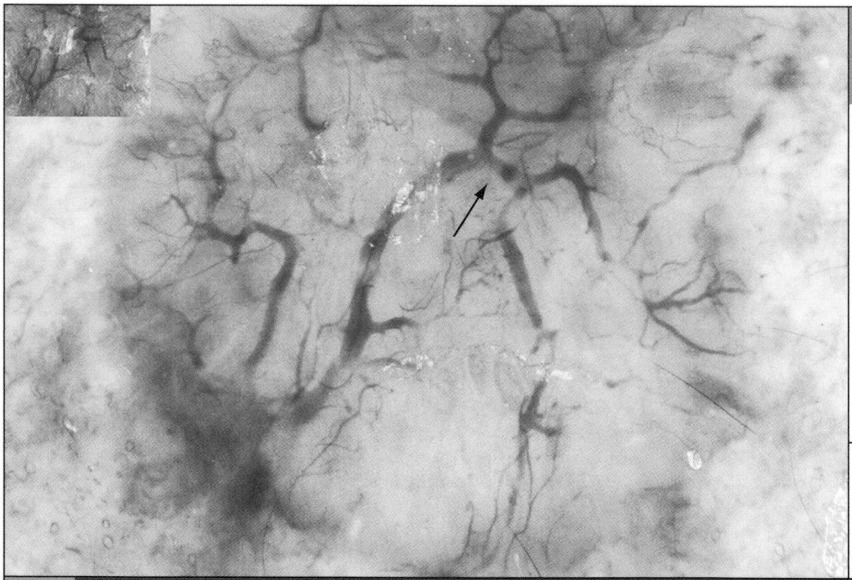

Six criteria for non-melanocytic lesions

Blue-gray blotches	☐
Arborizing vessels	☑
Milia-like cysts	☐
Comedo-like openings	☐
Red-blue lacunae	☐
Central white patch	☐

Fig. 202 Basal cell carcinoma.

Do not press down hard on a lesion with vessels like this because they may blanch out. This is a classic dermoscopic picture of a basal cell carcinoma with arborizing vessels (*arrow*) — like the branches of a big tree. Rarely amelanotic melanoma looks like this. Other criteria are not needed to make the dermoscopic diagnosis of basal cell carcinoma.

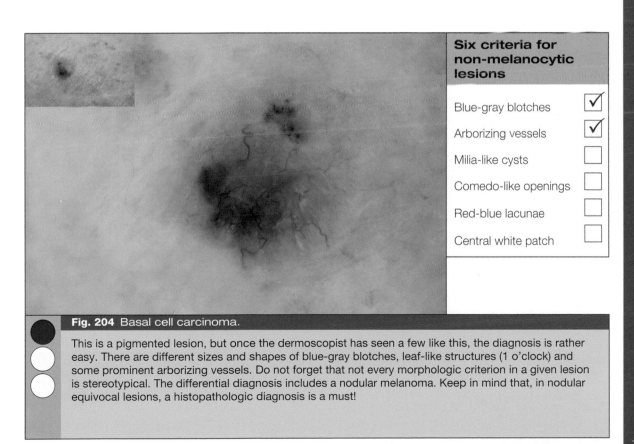

Six criteria for non-melanocytic lesions

Blue-gray blotches	☑
Arborizing vessels	☑
Milia-like cysts	☐
Comedo-like openings	☐
Red-blue lacunae	☐
Central white patch	☐

Fig. 203 Basal cell carcinoma.

There is an absence of criteria in this lesion to diagnose a melanocytic lesion; therefore, look for criteria to diagnose a non-melanocytic lesion. Arborizing vessels (*arrows*) and a blue-gray blotch (*circle*) lead to the diagnosis of basal cell carcinoma.

Six criteria for non-melanocytic lesions

Blue-gray blotches	☑
Arborizing vessels	☑
Milia-like cysts	☐
Comedo-like openings	☐
Red-blue lacunae	☐
Central white patch	☐

Fig. 204 Basal cell carcinoma.

This is a pigmented lesion, but once the dermoscopist has seen a few like this, the diagnosis is rather easy. There are different sizes and shapes of blue-gray blotches, leaf-like structures (1 o'clock) and some prominent arborizing vessels. Do not forget that not every morphologic criterion in a given lesion is stereotypical. The differential diagnosis includes a nodular melanoma. Keep in mind that, in nodular equivocal lesions, a histopathologic diagnosis is a must!

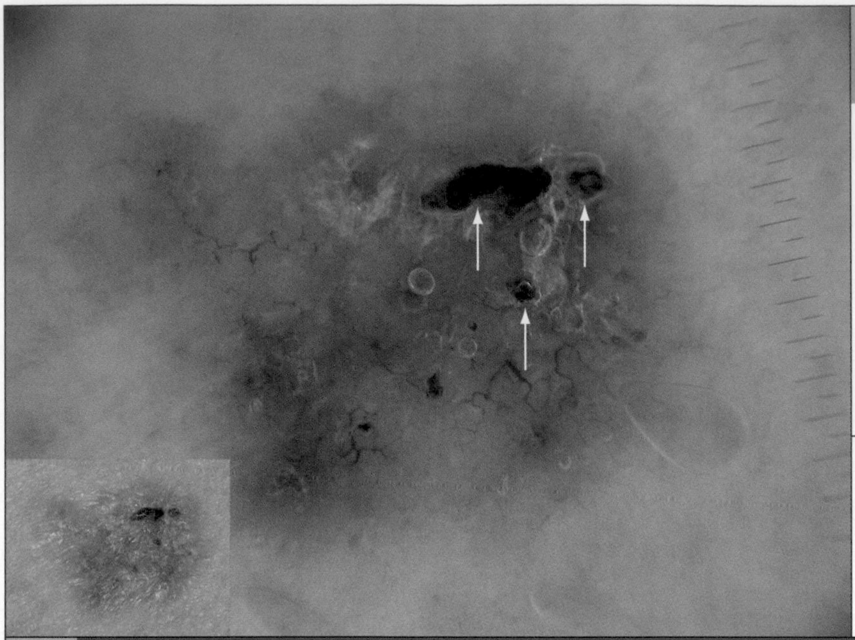

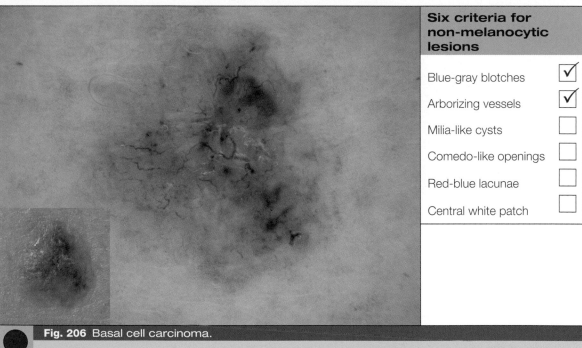

Six criteria for non-melanocytic lesions

Blue-gray blotches	☐
Arborizing vessels	☐
Milia-like cysts	☐
Comedo-like openings	☐
Red-blue lacunae	☐
Central white patch	☐

Fig. 205 Basal cell carcinoma.

Pink color—beware. Develop a dermoscopic differential diagnosis because not all cases are clear-cut. There is an absence of criteria to diagnose a melanocytic lesion; therefore, the next step is to consider which non-melanocytic lesion this is. It does not look like seborrheic keratosis, dermatofibroma, or hemangioma; therefore, it could be a basal cell carcinoma. There are some foci with ulceration covered with crusts (*arrows*), which favor a diagnosis of basal cell carcinoma. The lesion lacks prominent arborizing vessels, but fine microarborizing vessels are scattered throughout the lesion supporting the diagnosis of a basal cell carcinoma. Rarely a melanoma could also look like this.

Six criteria for non-melanocytic lesions

Blue-gray blotches	☑
Arborizing vessels	☑
Milia-like cysts	☐
Comedo-like openings	☐
Red-blue lacunae	☐
Central white patch	☐

Fig. 206 Basal cell carcinoma.

Sometimes the diagnosis is straightforward, as is the case in this basal cell carcinoma. There are delicate but typical arborizing and microarborizing vessels, and there are many variations of the morphology seen with blue-gray blotches. Basically there is no differential diagnosis here.

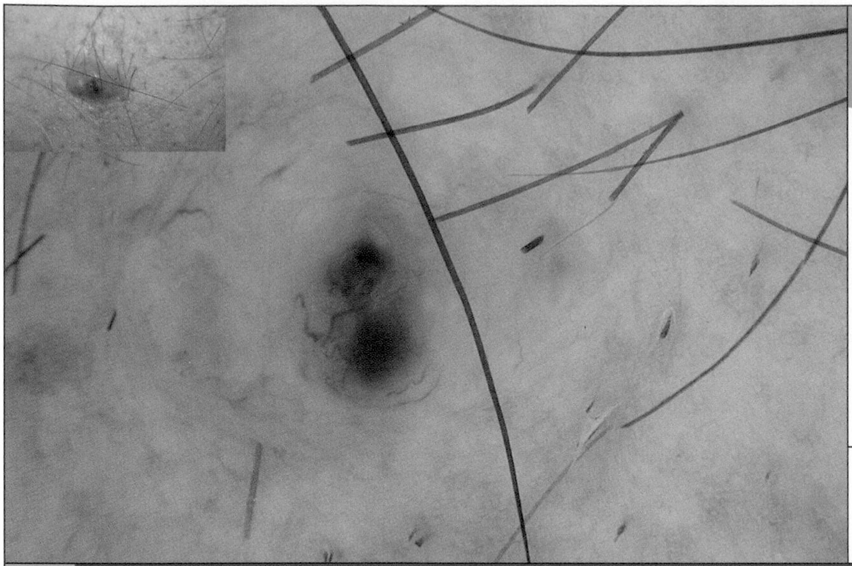

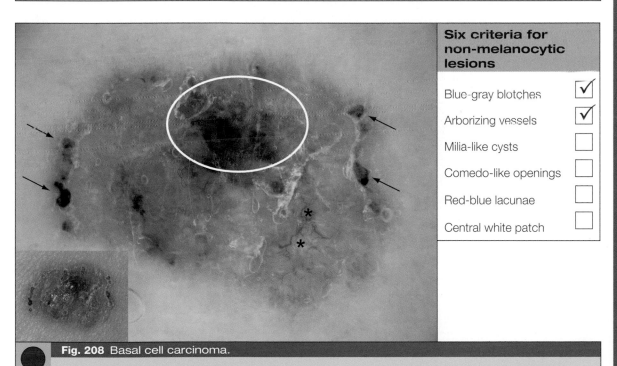

Fig. 207 Basal cell carcinoma.

This is a stereotypical basal cell carcinoma with arborizing vessels and blue-gray blotches. The differential diagnosis includes a nodular melanoma, but this is less likely.

Fig. 208 Basal cell carcinoma.

Once again, this is a stereotypical example of a basal cell carcinoma with large blotch of blue-gray pigmentation (*circle*) and some foci of arborizing vessels (*asterisks*). In addition, there are, particularly in the periphery, foci of ulcerations covered with crusts (*arrows*). Even the dermoscopy beginner will diagnose this basal cell carcinoma with confidence!

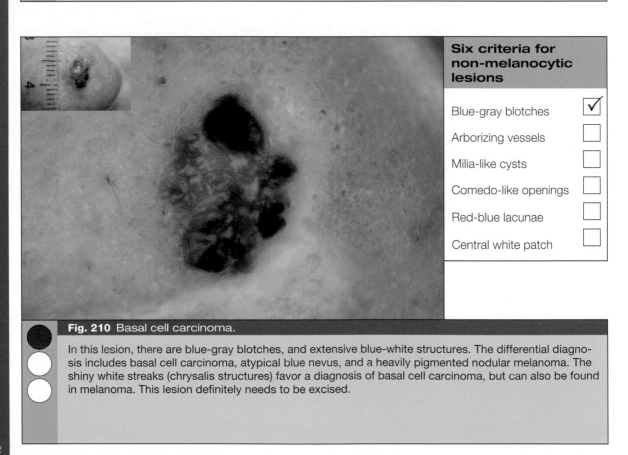

Six criteria for non-melanocytic lesions

Blue-gray blotches	☑
Arborizing vessels	☐
Milia-like cysts	☐
Comedo-like openings	☐
Red-blue lacunae	☐
Central white patch	☐

Fig. 209 Basal cell carcinoma.

This heavily pigmented lesion has two criteria diagnostic of a basal cell carcinoma—leaf-like structures, and blue-gray blotches. In this particular case, there is morphological overlap between these two features, which makes the diagnosis less straightforward. The differential diagnosis here is a superficial melanoma.

Six criteria for non-melanocytic lesions

Blue-gray blotches	☑
Arborizing vessels	☐
Milia-like cysts	☐
Comedo-like openings	☐
Red-blue lacunae	☐
Central white patch	☐

Fig. 210 Basal cell carcinoma.

In this lesion, there are blue-gray blotches, and extensive blue-white structures. The differential diagnosis includes basal cell carcinoma, atypical blue nevus, and a heavily pigmented nodular melanoma. The shiny white streaks (chrysalis structures) favor a diagnosis of basal cell carcinoma, but can also be found in melanoma. This lesion definitely needs to be excised.

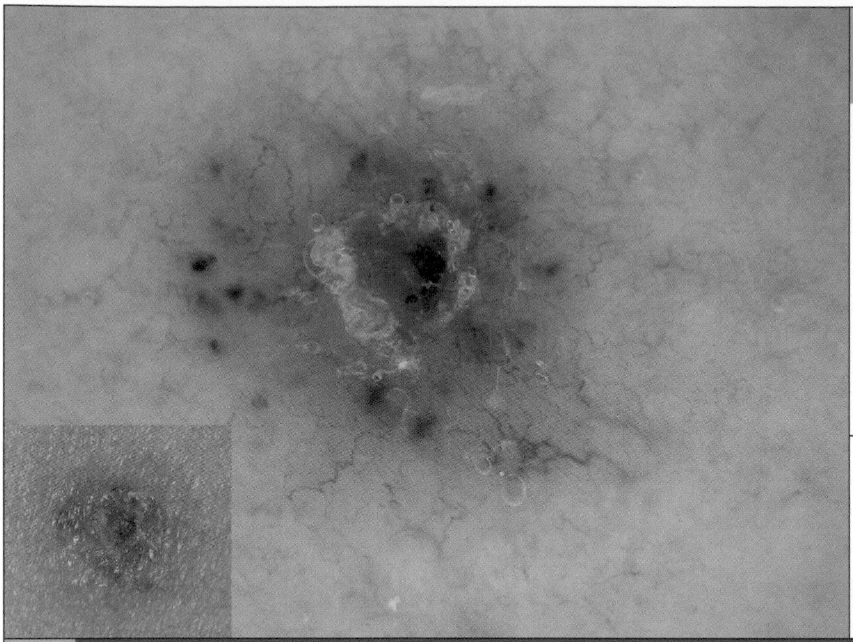

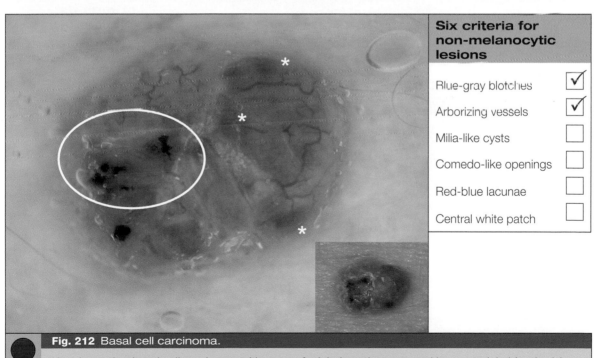

Six criteria for non-melanocytic lesions

Blue-gray blotches	☑
Arborizing vessels	☑
Milia-like cysts	☐
Comedo-like openings	☐
Red-blue lacunae	☐
Central white patch	☐

Fig. 211 Basal cell carcinoma.

This is another small nodular basal cell carcinoma characterized by numerous clearly visible blue-gray blotches. There are also hints of arborizing vessels; however, this criterion does not work very well in this instance, as some of the arborizing vessels are present even outside the lesion. Criteria to diagnose a melanocytic lesion are lacking. Still, the clinical appearance should be sufficient to warrant a histopathologic diagnosis. Please never forget that hypomelanotic melanomas may deceive sometimes even the expert dermoscopist.

Six criteria for non-melanocytic lesions

Blue-gray blotches	☑
Arborizing vessels	☑
Milia-like cysts	☐
Comedo-like openings	☐
Red-blue lacunae	☐
Central white patch	☐

Fig. 212 Basal cell carcinoma.

Here is another basal cell carcinoma with areas of mini-ulcerations covered by crusts (*circle*), arborizing blood vessels, and blue-gray blotches (*asterisks*). This is a rather clear-cut example of basal cell carcinoma, but do not forget to develop a dermoscopic differential diagnosis because there will be surprises from time to time.

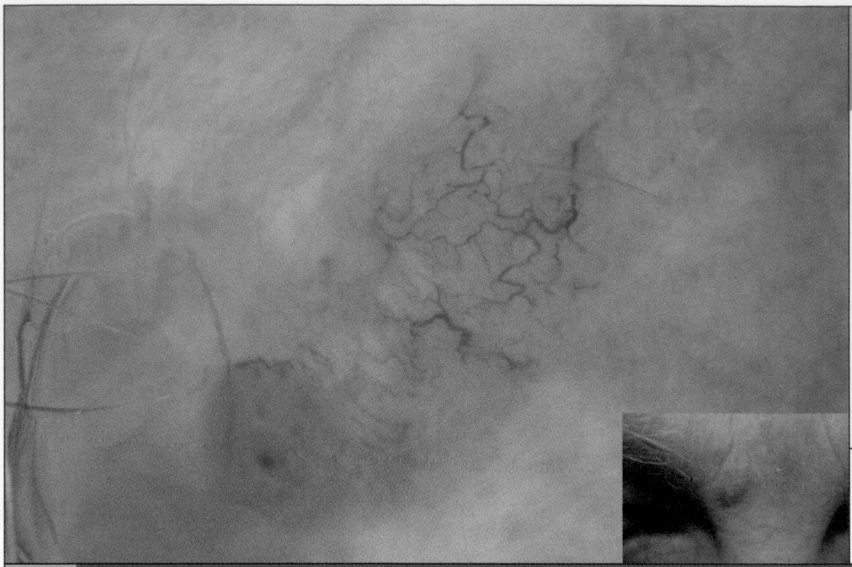

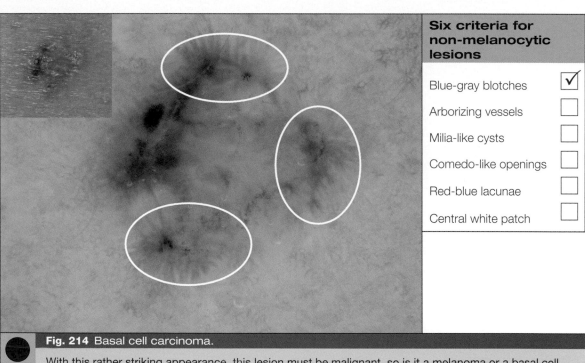

Six criteria for non-melanocytic lesions

Blue-gray blotches	☐
Arborizing vessels	☑
Milia-like cysts	☐
Comedo-like openings	☐
Red-blue lacunae	☐
Central white patch	☐

Fig. 213 Basal cell carcinoma.

This shows another variation of the morphology seen with a nodular basal cell carcinoma, characterized by numerous arborizing vessels. Please note, the vessels should be in sharp focus for a basal cell carcinoma, as in this example. This dermoscopic picture is virtually diagnostic for a basal cell carcinoma.

Six criteria for non-melanocytic lesions

Blue-gray blotches	☑
Arborizing vessels	☐
Milia-like cysts	☐
Comedo-like openings	☐
Red-blue lacunae	☐
Central white patch	☐

Fig. 214 Basal cell carcinoma.

With this rather striking appearance, this lesion must be malignant, so is it a melanoma or a basal cell carcinoma? There are gray-blue blotches throughout most of the periphery of the lesion in a ring-like alignment but no hint of arborizing vessels. The more experienced dermoscopist will recognize the so-called leaf-like structures (*circles*), a classic criterion for pigmented basal cell carcinoma, whereas the beginner might interpret these structures as irregular streaks of a melanoma. Never mind, this lesion needs to be excised!

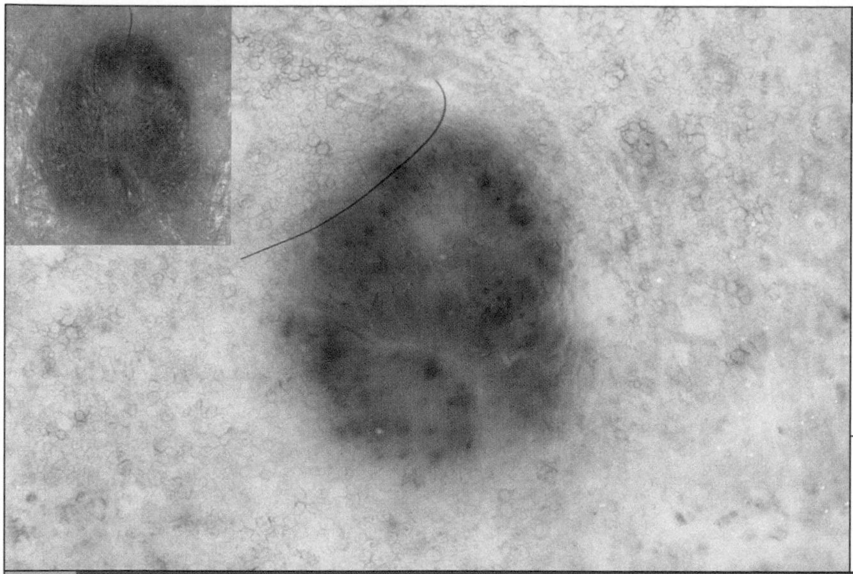

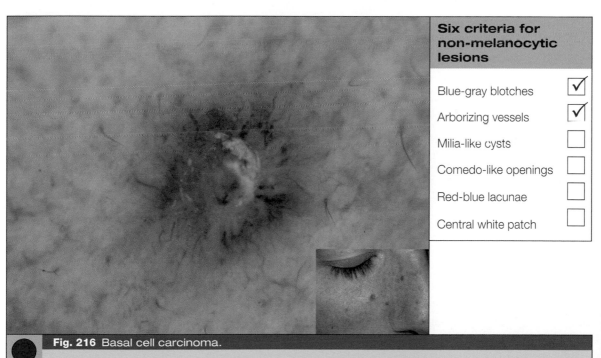

Six criteria for non-melanocytic lesions	
Blue-gray blotches	☑
Arborizing vessels	☐
Milia-like cysts	☐
Comedo-like openings	☐
Red-blue lacunae	☐
Central white patch	☐

Fig. 215 Basal cell carcinoma.

This small pink lesion has subtle blue-gray blotches, small linear, non-arborizing vessels, and blue-white structures. Once again the absence of criteria needed to diagnose a melanocytic lesion point toward the dermoscopic diagnosis of a basal cell carcinoma. As long as it is realized that this lesion is not benign, dermoscopy has served its purpose. This is a gray-zone lesion and a hypomelanotic melanoma needs to be excluded.

Six criteria for non-melanocytic lesions	
Blue-gray blotches	☑
Arborizing vessels	☑
Milia-like cysts	☐
Comedo-like openings	☐
Red-blue lacunae	☐
Central white patch	☐

Fig. 216 Basal cell carcinoma.

Some of this lesion is covered by a scale-crust due to ulceration. There are also small arborizing vessels and multiple blue-gray blotches and peppering. The pigmentation seen in basal cell carcinomas can be brown, gray, or blue. It can form well-defined ovoid structures or be indistinct. The more lesions a dermoscopist diagnoses, the better he or she will understand this basic dermoscopic principle. There are numerous variations of all dermoscopic criteria.

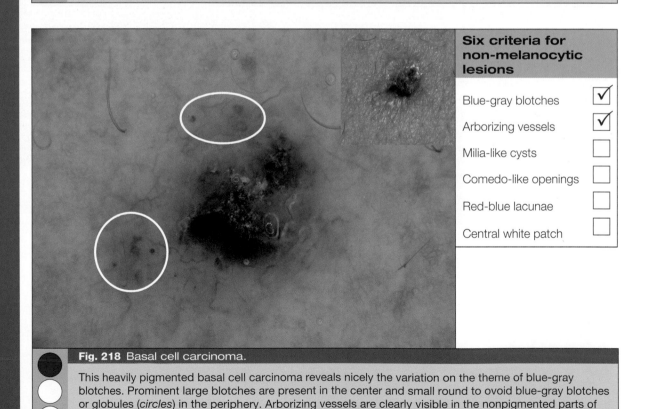

Six criteria for non-melanocytic lesions

Blue-gray blotches	☑
Arborizing vessels	☑
Milia-like cysts	☐
Comedo-like openings	☐
Red-blue lacunae	☐
Central white patch	☐

Fig. 217 Basal cell carcinoma.

This is a very nonspecific pinkish lesion. This lesion is as difficult to diagnose for the dermoscopy beginner as for the dermoscopy expert. The subtle blue-gray blotches at 3 o'clock and the barely-visible microarborizing vessels at 12 o'clock are the only subtle hint for a basal cell carcinoma. There are however shiny white lines (chrysalis structures) in the center of the lesion. This lesion cannot be differentiated with certainty from a hypomelanotic melanoma, therefore you have to manage this lesion as a melanoma.

Six criteria for non-melanocytic lesions

Blue-gray blotches	☑
Arborizing vessels	☑
Milia-like cysts	☐
Comedo-like openings	☐
Red-blue lacunae	☐
Central white patch	☐

Fig. 218 Basal cell carcinoma.

This heavily pigmented basal cell carcinoma reveals nicely the variation on the theme of blue-gray blotches. Prominent large blotches are present in the center and small round to ovoid blue-gray blotches or globules (*circles*) in the periphery. Arborizing vessels are clearly visible in the nonpigmented parts of this basal cell carcinoma.

DERMOSCOPY – The Essentials

116

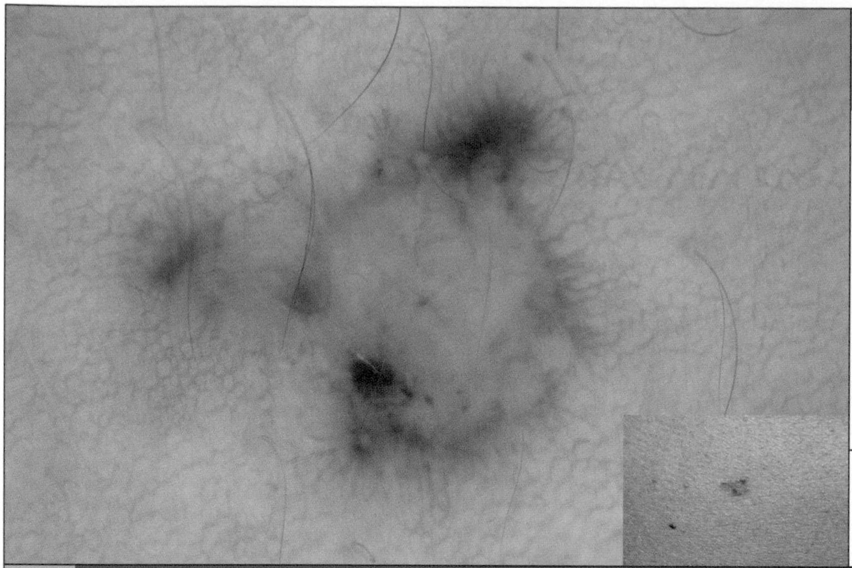

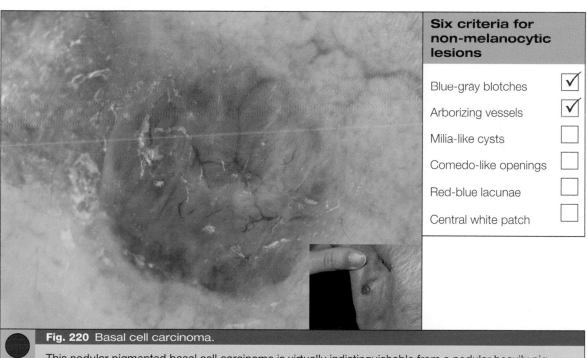

Six criteria for non-melanocytic lesions

Blue-gray blotches	☑
Arborizing vessels	☐
Milia-like cysts	☐
Comedo-like openings	☐
Red-blue lacunae	☐
Central white patch	☐

Fig. 219 Basal cell carcinoma.

This is another pink basal cell carcinoma reminiscent of a hypomelanotic melanoma. Some foci with leaf-like structures at 1 o'clock are noted and allow the diagnosis of basal cell carcinoma to be made, along with prominent blue-gray blotches. The classic criterion for basal cell carcinoma on which we focus in this dermoscopy primer, namely arborizing vessels, are not visible in this basal cell carcinoma.

Six criteria for non-melanocytic lesions

Blue-gray blotches	☑
Arborizing vessels	☑
Milia-like cysts	☐
Comedo-like openings	☐
Red-blue lacunae	☐
Central white patch	☐

Fig. 220 Basal cell carcinoma.

This nodular pigmented basal cell carcinoma is virtually indistinguishable from a nodular heavily pigmented melanoma. There are numerous confluent blue-gray blotches present throughout the lesion—a finding also observed in a nodular melanoma. However, there are also several arborizing vessels that point to the diagnosis of basal cell carcinoma. Please do not forget that in this clinical setting the correct management decision is more relevant than the diagnosis.

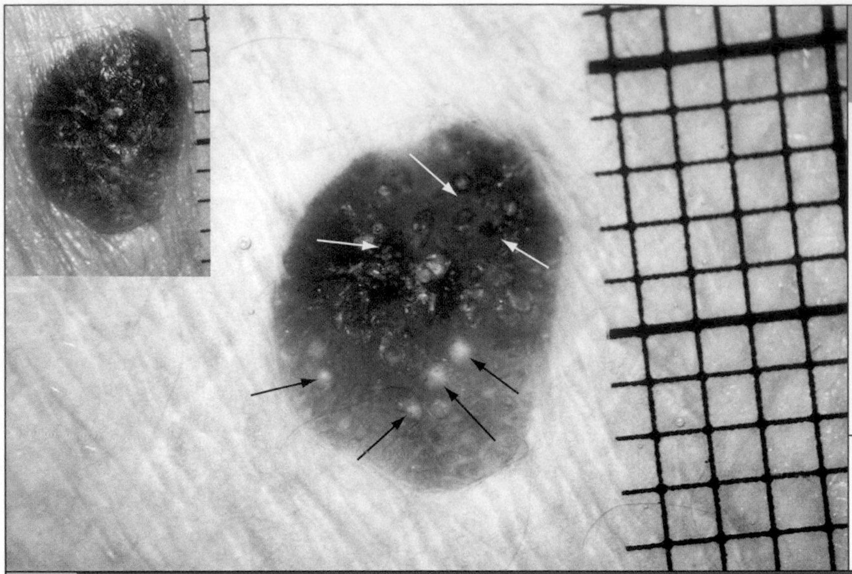

Six criteria for non-melanocytic lesions

Blue-gray blotches ☐
Arborizing vessels ☐
Milia-like cysts ☑
Comedo-like openings ☑
Red-blue lacunae ☐
Central white patch ☐

Fig. 221 Seborrheic keratosis.

The main dermoscopic criteria in this flat plaque are milia-like cysts (*black arrows*) and comedo-like openings (*white arrows*), which are diagnostic of a seborrheic keratosis. Using these criteria, this is an easy case to diagnose.

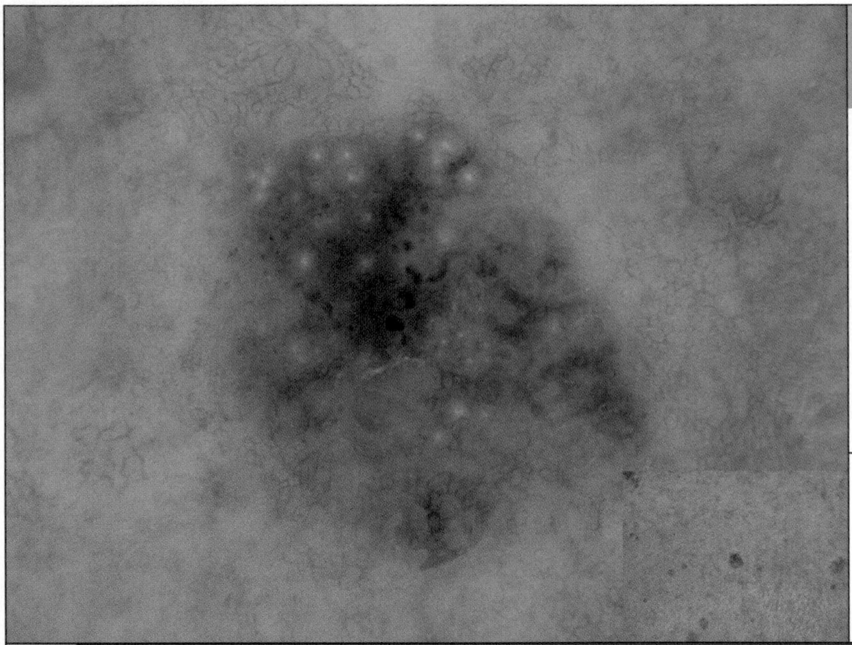

Six criteria for non-melanocytic lesions

Blue-gray blotches ☐
Arborizing vessels ☐
Milia-like cysts ☑
Comedo-like openings ☑
Red-blue lacunae ☐
Central white patch ☐

Fig. 222 Seborrheic keratosis.

In this seborrheic keratosis, a few comedo-like openings, milia-like cysts, and yellow keratin plugs are clearly seen. The dull gray zone in the upper half of the lesion and the absence of criteria specific for melanocytic lesions argue against the differential diagnosis of a papillomatous melanocytic nevus.

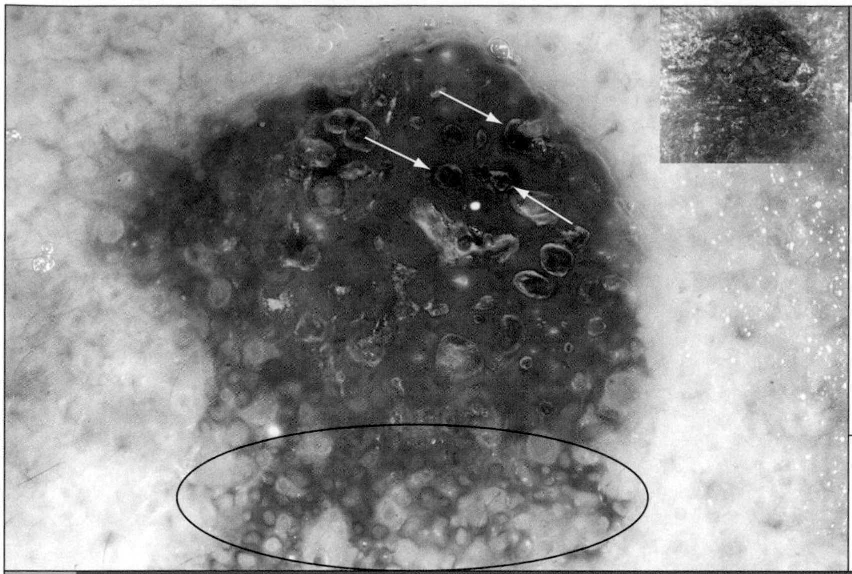

Fig. 223 Seborrheic keratosis.

This lesion shows good examples of well-developed comedo-like openings (*arrows*) and a few milia-like cysts. Is there a pigment network in the lower part of the lesion (*circle*)? No—it is a pseudonetwork formed by the openings of follicles on the face (site-specific criterion). They are not forming the rhomboidal structures of a lentigo maligna.

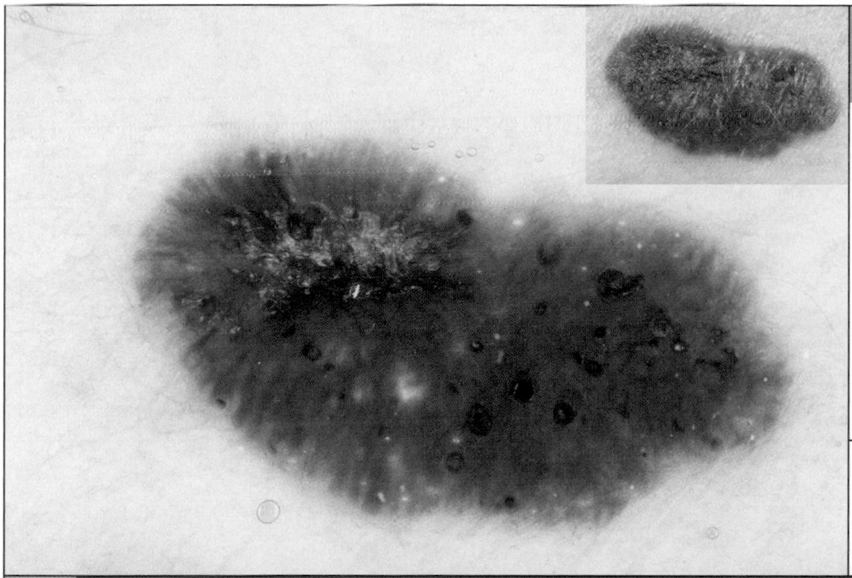

Fig. 224 Seborrheic keratosis.

This flat plaque is characterized by multiple comedo-like openings and some milia-like cysts. Looking carefully at the borders of the lesion, one might think that there is a starburst pattern of a Spitz nevus. Comedo-like openings and milia-like cysts are as a rule not seen in a Spitz nevus. Perhaps it could be described as a pseudostarburst pattern.

Six criteria for non-melanocytic lesions

Blue-gray blotches ☐
Arborizing vessels ☐
Milia-like cysts ☑
Comedo-like openings ☑
Red-blue lacunae ☐
Central white patch ☐

Six criteria for non-melanocytic lesions

Blue-gray blotches ☐
Arborizing vessels ☐
Milia-like cysts ☑
Comedo-like openings ☑
Red-blue lacunae ☐
Central white patch ☐

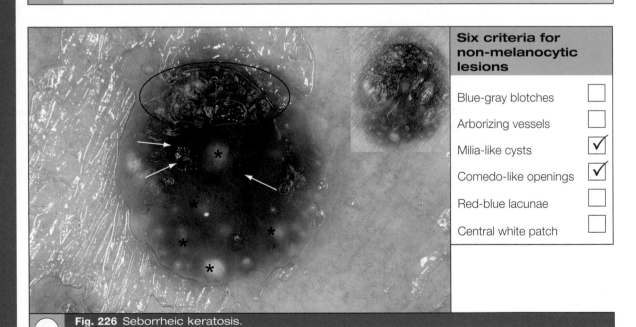

Six criteria for non-melanocytic lesions

Blue-gray blotches	☐
Arborizing vessels	☐
Milia-like cysts	☑
Comedo-like openings	☑
Red-blue lacunae	☐
Central white patch	☐

Fig. 225 Seborrheic keratosis.

Sometimes seborrheic keratoses are strikingly asymmetric in shape, structure, and color, and the clinical image strongly supports this observation. Dermoscopy clearly reveals several comedo-like openings (*circles*) and, in addition, few tiny milia-like cysts (*arrows*). Very rarely comedo-like openings and milia-like cysts are found also in superficial melanomas, and therefore we raise the orange flag. It is better to shave one seborrheic keratosis than miss one melanoma!

Six criteria for non-melanocytic lesions

Blue-gray blotches	☐
Arborizing vessels	☐
Milia-like cysts	☑
Comedo-like openings	☑
Red-blue lacunae	☐
Central white patch	☐

Fig. 226 Seborrheic keratosis.

Opaque color, milia-like cysts (*asterisks*), and comedo-like openings (*arrows*) are seen in this lesion with a verrucous surface (*circle*). This lesion should prove easy to diagnose dermoscopically as a seborrheic keratosis by now.

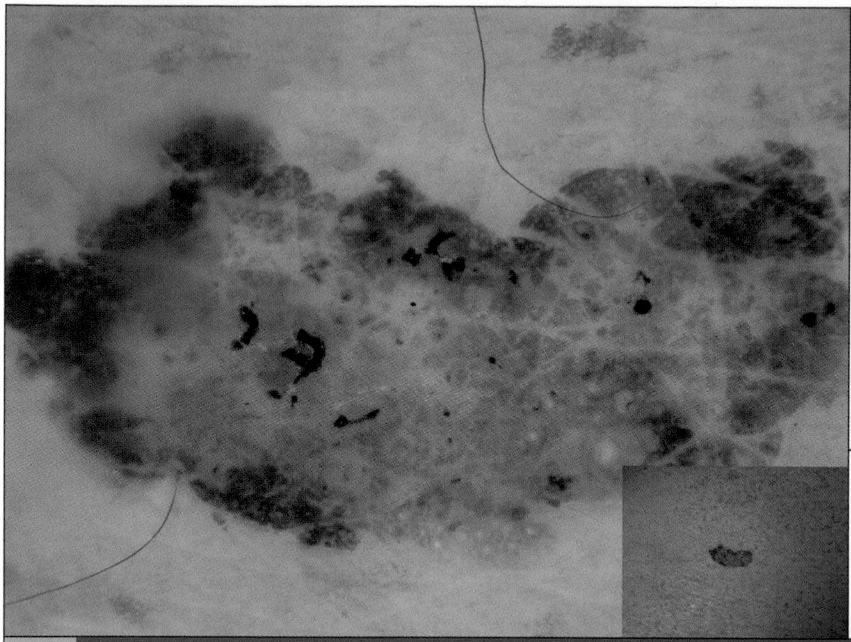

Six criteria for non-melanocytic lesions

Blue-gray blotches	☐
Arborizing vessels	☐
Milia-like cysts	☑
Comedo-like openings	☑
Red-blue lacunae	☐
Central white patch	☐

Fig. 227 Seborrheic keratosis.

Compared to the case shown in Fig. 226, this is not so easy to diagnose. This lesion is separated by a few furrows, and there are few comedo-like openings. Do not confuse them with the globules of a melanocytic lesion. Subtle milia-like cysts at 6'oclock are difficult to find. There is also a large central hypopigmented area, which may be seen in seborrheic keratosis. Because of the asymmetry of this lesion, a diagnostic excision to rule out a melanoma is recommended.

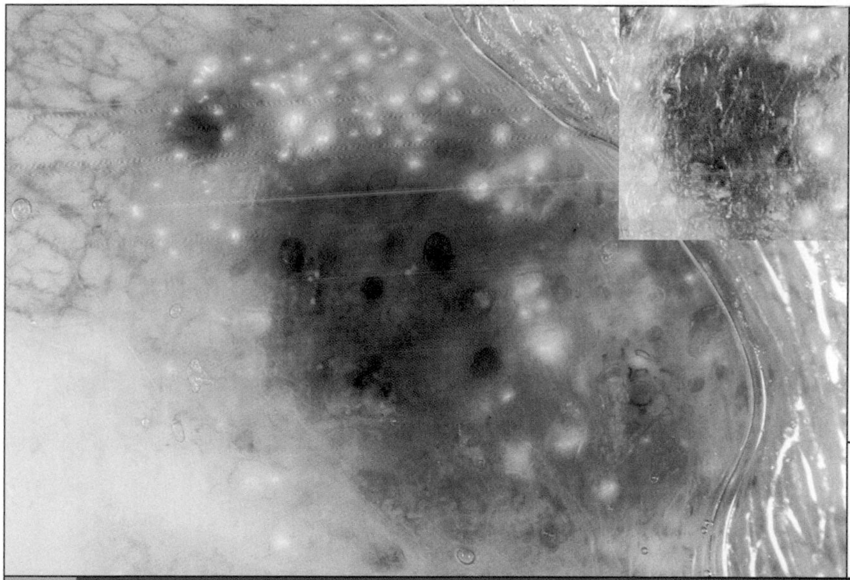

Six criteria for non-melanocytic lesions

Blue-gray blotches	☑
Arborizing vessels	☐
Milia-like cysts	☑
Comedo-like openings	☑
Red-blue lacunae	☐
Central white patch	☐

Fig. 228 Seborrheic keratosis.

A clear-cut case of seborrheic keratosis with numerous milia-like cysts and a few comedo-like openings. Because of these straightforward criteria we are raising the green flag despite the evident asymmetry of this lesion.

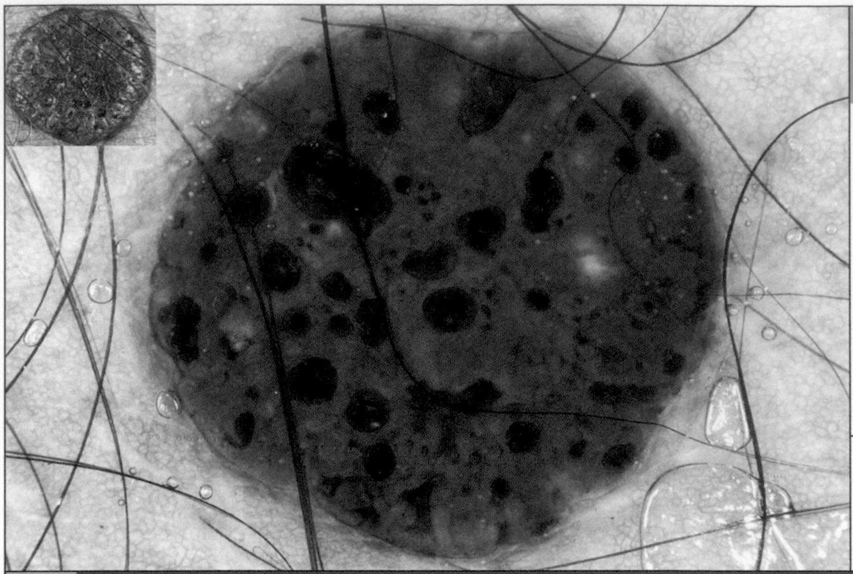

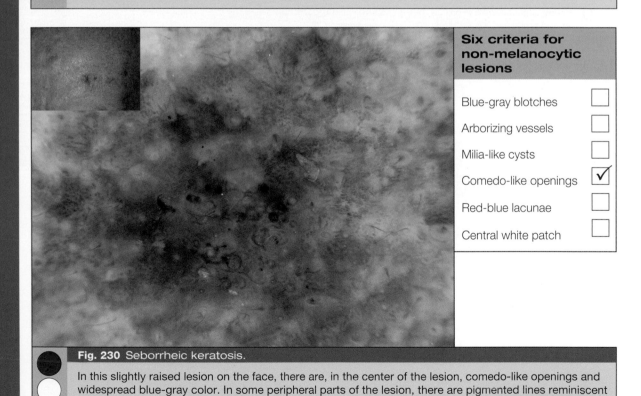

Six criteria for non-melanocytic lesions

Blue-gray blotches	☐
Arborizing vessels	☐
Milia-like cysts	☑
Comedo-like openings	☑
Red-blue lacunae	☐
Central white patch	☐

Fig. 229 Seborrheic keratosis.

This is another stereotypical seborrheic keratosis characterized by numerous comedo-like openings and only a few milia-like cysts. Criteria for a melanocytic lesion are absent.

Six criteria for non-melanocytic lesions

Blue-gray blotches	☐
Arborizing vessels	☐
Milia-like cysts	☐
Comedo-like openings	☑
Red-blue lacunae	☐
Central white patch	☐

Fig. 230 Seborrheic keratosis.

In this slightly raised lesion on the face, there are, in the center of the lesion, comedo-like openings and widespread blue-gray color. In some peripheral parts of the lesion, there are pigmented lines reminiscent of fingerprint-like structures. The differential diagnosis here includes lentigo maligna, so we recommend a diagnostic shave biopsy.

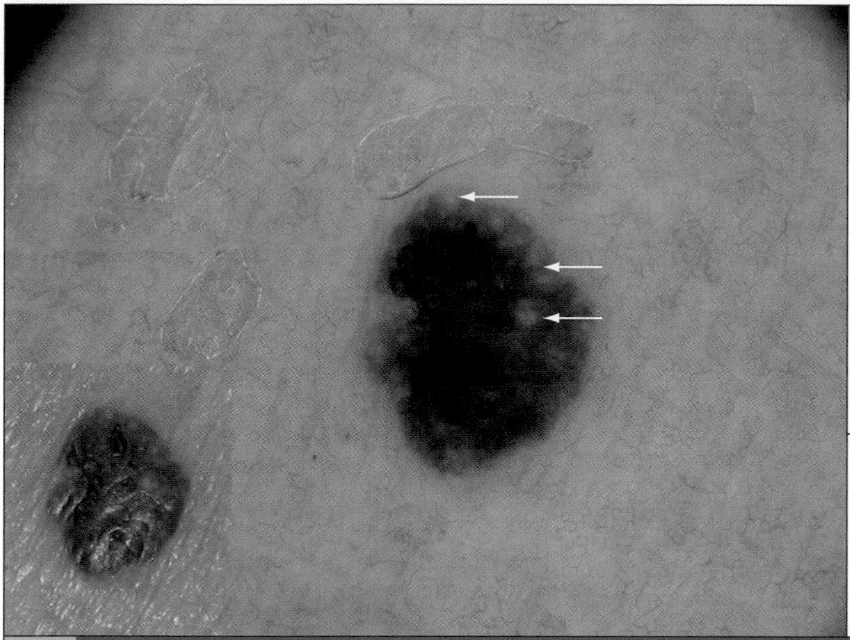

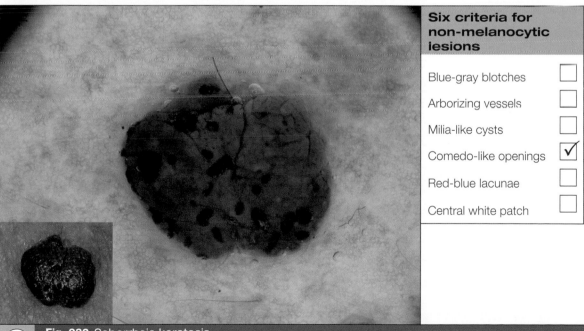

Six criteria for non-melanocytic lesions

Blue-gray blotches	☐
Arborizing vessels	☐
Milia-like cysts	☑
Comedo-like openings	☑
Red-blue lacunae	☐
Central white patch	☐

Fig. 231 Seborrheic keratosis.

This is a rather straightforward example of an acanthotic type of seborrheic keratosis characterized by several comedo-like openings (no annotations because clearly evident) and few milia-like cysts (*arrows*). There is also a hint of a blue-white veil and therefore we are raising the orange flag. As evidenced by this example, there are many variations of seborrheic keratosis. Remember, when in doubt, "shave" it out. In more elegant words, perform an excisional shave biopsy with subsequent histopathologic examination.

Six criteria for non-melanocytic lesions

Blue-gray blotches	☐
Arborizing vessels	☐
Milia-like cysts	☐
Comedo-like openings	☑
Red-blue lacunae	☐
Central white patch	☐

Fig. 232 Seborrheic keratosis.

This rather stereotypical example of a seborrheic keratosis is slightly asymmetric in structure because the several well-developed comedo-like openings are distributed unevenly throughout the lesion. In addition, the clinical image displays well the stuck-on appearance of a classic seborrheic keratosis. The only relevant differential diagnosis here is a benign papillomatous dermal nevus and therefore we are raising the green flag.

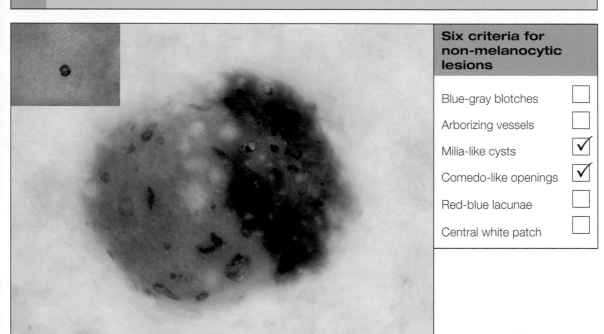

Six criteria for non-melanocytic lesions

Blue-gray blotches	☐
Arborizing vessels	☐
Milia-like cysts	☐
Comedo-like openings	☐
Red-blue lacunae	☐
Central white patch	☐

Fig. 233 Seborrheic keratosis.

This seborrheic keratosis is composed of a more or less diffuse pigmented area with a grayish color and numerous reddish dots reminiscent of dotted vessels. Classic comedo-like openings and milia-like cysts are not visible even to the expert dermoscopist. Based on clinico-dermoscopic correlation, we are confident that this is superficial seborrheic keratosis and raise the green flag. Please remember if you are not so confident and want to rule out a lentigo maligna or a pigmented basal cell carcinoma, perform a diagnostic biopsy.

Six criteria for non-melanocytic lesions

Blue-gray blotches	☐
Arborizing vessels	☐
Milia-like cysts	☑
Comedo-like openings	☑
Red-blue lacunae	☐
Central white patch	☐

Fig. 234 Seborrheic keratosis.

Despite the clear-cut asymmetrical, off-center dark zone, the presence of multiple milia-like cysts and comedo-like openings in this lesion are virtually diagnostic of a seborrheic keratosis. However, because of the large black blotch and subtle polymorphous vessels we raised the orange flag and performed a shave biopsy to rule out an unusual verrucous melanoma.

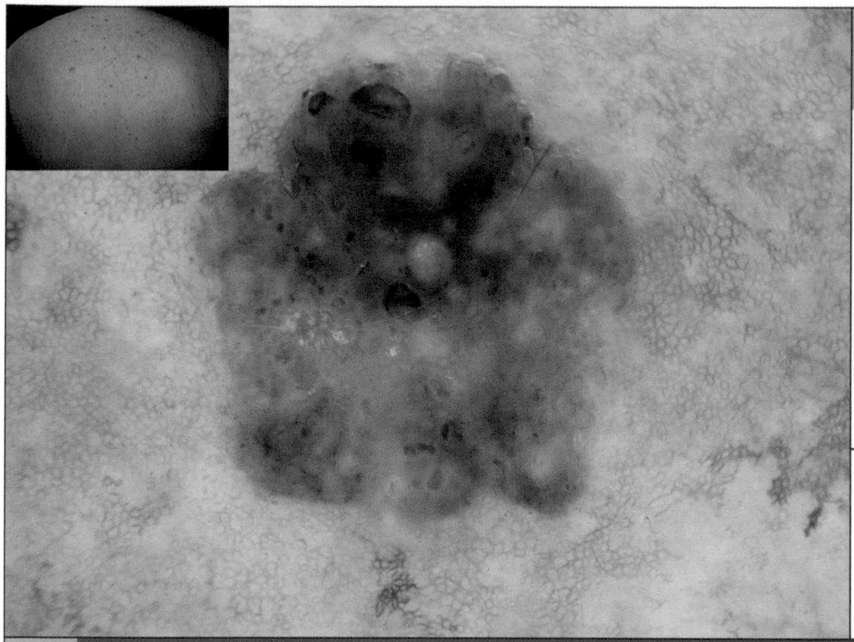

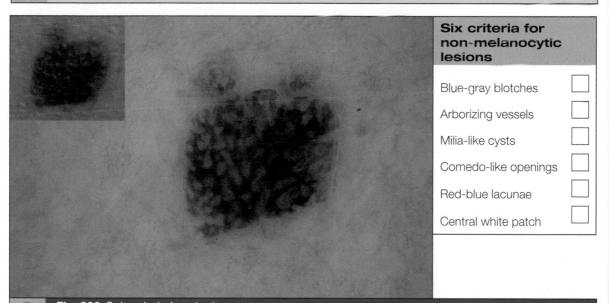

Six criteria for non-melanocytic lesions

Blue-gray blotches	☐
Arborizing vessels	☐
Milia-like cysts	☑
Comedo-like openings	☑
Red-blue lacunae	☐
Central white patch	☐

Fig. 235 Seborrheic keratosis.

This is a typical dermoscopic feature of seborrheic keratosis. Please note the many solar lentigines on moderately to severely sun-damaged skin surrounding this seborrheic keratosis. There are few comedo-like openings and several milia-like cysts, one of which is very large and in the center of the lesion. The asymmetry in pigmentation could lead one astray to the diagnosis of a superficial melanoma. Nevertheless, we raised the green flag as we were confident about the diagnosis of seborrheic keratosis. However, you are in charge of your patients and if you are not sure, then shave it out! We cannot over-emphasize this basic principle.

Six criteria for non-melanocytic lesions

Blue-gray blotches	☐
Arborizing vessels	☐
Milia-like cysts	☐
Comedo-like openings	☐
Red-blue lacunae	☐
Central white patch	☐

Fig. 236 Seborrheic keratosis.

This is a rather straightforward seborrheic keratosis despite the lack of the classic criteria like milia-like cysts and comedo-like openings. This lesion is characterized by a variation on the theme of a brown pseudonetwork and several fat fingers are sticking out at the periphery. We are raising the green flag here and with a bit of experience you will also confidently do the same in a morphologically similar lesion.

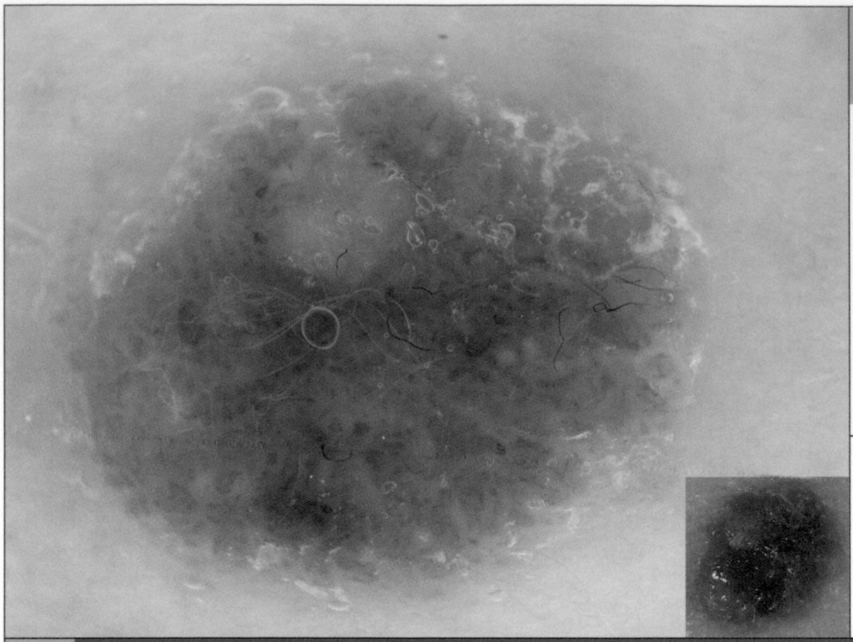

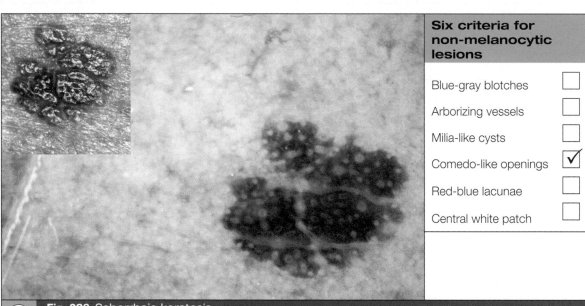

Six criteria for non-melanocytic lesions

Blue-gray blotches	☐
Arborizing vessels	☐
Milia-like cysts	☐
Comedo-like openings	☐
Red-blue lacunae	☐
Central white patch	☐

Fig. 237 Seborrheic keratosis.

This is a very unusual irritated seborrheic keratosis with bluish and pink coloration lacking any classic criteria for seborrheic keratosis. In a lesion like this, you have to be very objective and conclude that there is asymmetry in structure and color as even dermoscopically there is no hint of any diagnostic category. And remember, although the diagnosis is very difficult here, the management is pretty straightforward. A deep shave biopsy or an excisional biopsy with a small margin—both will do the job! Always err on the side of caution and excise equivocal lesions with a confusing dermoscopic picture.

Six criteria for non-melanocytic lesions

Blue-gray blotches	☐
Arborizing vessels	☐
Milia-like cysts	☐
Comedo-like openings	☑
Red-blue lacunae	☐
Central white patch	☐

Fig. 238 Seborrheic keratosis.

This shows yet another variation of the morphology seen in seborrheic keratosis located on the face. Are the multiple light yellow circles comedo-like openings or follicular openings? It is hard to make the differentiation, but we favor comedo-like openings. Clinically, it looks like a seborrheic keratosis, and with dermoscopy, there are no high-risk criteria suggestive of lentigo maligna.

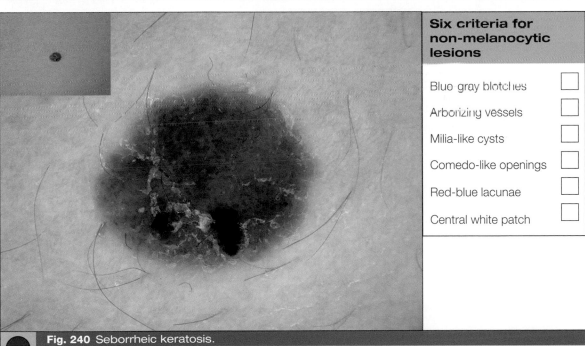

Six criteria for non-melanocytic lesions

Blue-gray blotches	☐
Arborizing vessels	☐
Milia-like cysts	☐
Comedo-like openings	☐
Red-blue lacunae	☐
Central white patch	☐

Fig. 239 Seborrheic keratosis.

This is another example of a seborrheic keratosis lacking the classic dermoscopic criteria, namely, milia-like cysts and comedo-like openings. The differential diagnosis of this superficial reticular type of seborrheic keratosis represents a benign reticular nevus. The sharp demarcation of the reticulation at the periphery here favors a seborrheic keratosis; in melanocytic nevi, the network fades out toward the periphery. Obviously this distinction is merely an academic exercise. We can easily raise the green flag here.

Six criteria for non-melanocytic lesions

Blue-gray blotches	☐
Arborizing vessels	☐
Milia-like cysts	☐
Comedo-like openings	☐
Red-blue lacunae	☐
Central white patch	☐

Fig. 240 Seborrheic keratosis.

This is the last case in a series of seborrheic keratoses and obviously we like to share an equivocal example with you. Similar to Fig. 233, this seborrheic keratosis is composed of a diffuse pigmented area with blue-gray areas and numerous reddish dots reminiscent of dotted vessels around the periphery of the lesion. Typical comedo-like openings and milia-like cysts are lacking, but there are two asymmetric black blotches and some hairpin and irregular linear vessels. There are also whitish scales visible throughout the lesion. Again based on clinico-dermoscopic correlation, we are confident that this is seborrheic keratosis. However, because of the prominent blue-gray areas, black blotches and the pinkish peripheral coloration, we raise the red flag. We would not like to miss a melanoma or a pigmented basal cell carcinoma!

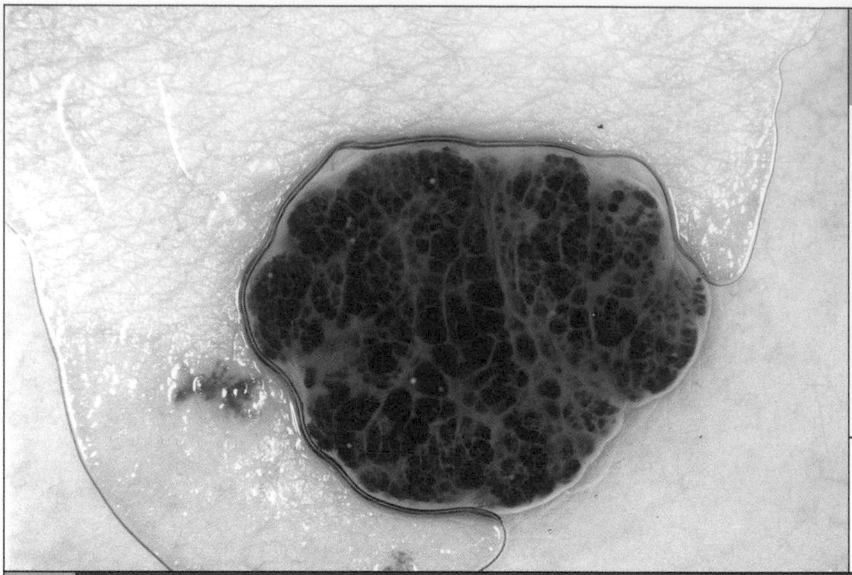

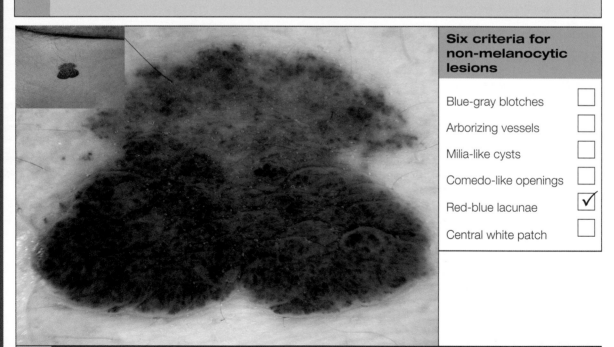

Six criteria for non-melanocytic lesions	
Blue-gray blotches	☐
Arborizing vessels	☐
Milia-like cysts	☐
Comedo-like openings	☐
Red-blue lacunae	☑
Central white patch	☐

Fig. 241 Hemangioma.

This is a classic hemangioma with multiple red lacunae. They are well-demarcated, reddish, round-to-polygonal structures that correspond to the dilated vessels in the upper dermis. White color is commonly found in hemangiomas; in this case, it has a reticular pattern. There is no doubt of the dermoscopic diagnosis in this case.

Six criteria for non-melanocytic lesions	
Blue-gray blotches	☐
Arborizing vessels	☐
Milia-like cysts	☐
Comedo-like openings	☐
Red-blue lacunae	☑
Central white patch	☐

Fig. 242 Hemangioma.

This vascular lesion is characterized by multiple red and purplish lacunae. It is possible to confuse the blue to purplish color with a blue-white structure. It is unusual to find two colors in a hemangioma, however, despite raising the orange flag, we are still confident this is a hemangioma and decided not to excise it. Remember, the patient is your responsibility, so if you have any doubts, then act appropriately.

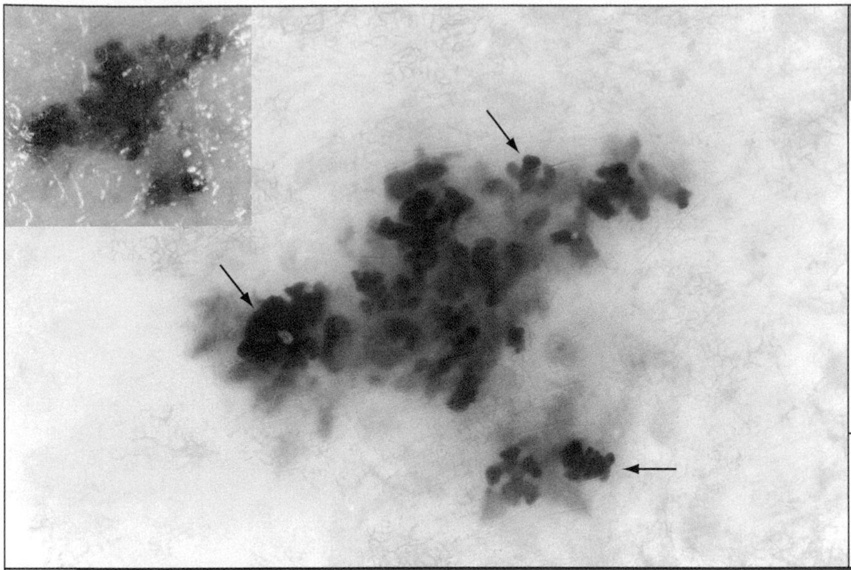

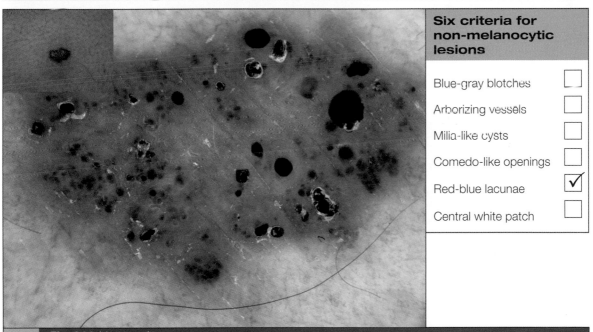

Six criteria for non-melanocytic lesions	
Blue-gray blotches	☐
Arborizing vessels	☐
Milia-like cysts	☐
Comedo-like openings	☐
Red-blue lacunae	☑
Central white patch	☐

Fig. 243 Hemangioma.

This is another stereotypical example of cherry (senile) hemangioma and has numerous well-circumscribed red-blue lacunae (*arrows*). Remember that, to diagnose the lacunae, they should have sharp borders. They should be clear and not out of focus or blurred.

Six criteria for non-melanocytic lesions	
Blue-gray blotches	☐
Arborizing vessels	☐
Milia-like cysts	☐
Comedo-like openings	☐
Red-blue lacunae	☑
Central white patch	☐

Fig. 244 Hemangioma.

This hemangioma displays a diffuse blue-white color that mimics blue-white structures. Closer scrutiny reveals a few clear-cut red-blue lacunae, and in hindsight of the histopathologic diagnosis of a hemangioma with prominent fibrosis, also clear-cut red-blue lacunae are present. The black round to oval areas represent thrombosed vascular spaces. Because of the equivocal dermoscopic appearance, we raised the orange flag and excised this lesion.

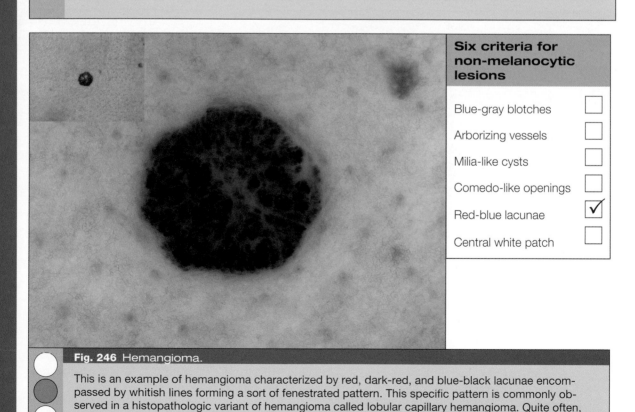

Six criteria for non-melanocytic lesions

Blue-gray blotches	☐
Arborizing vessels	☐
Milia-like cysts	☐
Comedo-like openings	☐
Red-blue lacunae	☑
Central white patch	☐

Fig. 245 Fibroangioma.

This is a fibroangioma characterized by a diffuse reddish-whitish color, which is the hallmark of the lesion. There are several red lacunae throughout the lesion. The fenestrated whitish lines represent fibrosis encompassing the angioma lobules. Pyogenic granuloma, Kaposi's sarcoma, and amelanotic melanoma could have a similar dermoscopic appearance; therefore, the red flag was raised and the lesion was excised.

Six criteria for non-melanocytic lesions

Blue-gray blotches	☐
Arborizing vessels	☐
Milia-like cysts	☐
Comedo-like openings	☐
Red-blue lacunae	☑
Central white patch	☐

Fig. 246 Hemangioma.

This is an example of hemangioma characterized by red, dark-red, and blue-black lacunae encompassed by whitish lines forming a sort of fenestrated pattern. This specific pattern is commonly observed in a histopathologic variant of hemangioma called lobular capillary hemangioma. Quite often, dark-colored hemangiomas mimic melanoma or melanoma metastasis clinically. Dermoscopy usually is very helpful, as in this example, in making the correct diagnosis. Still we raised the orange flag here and excised the lesion.

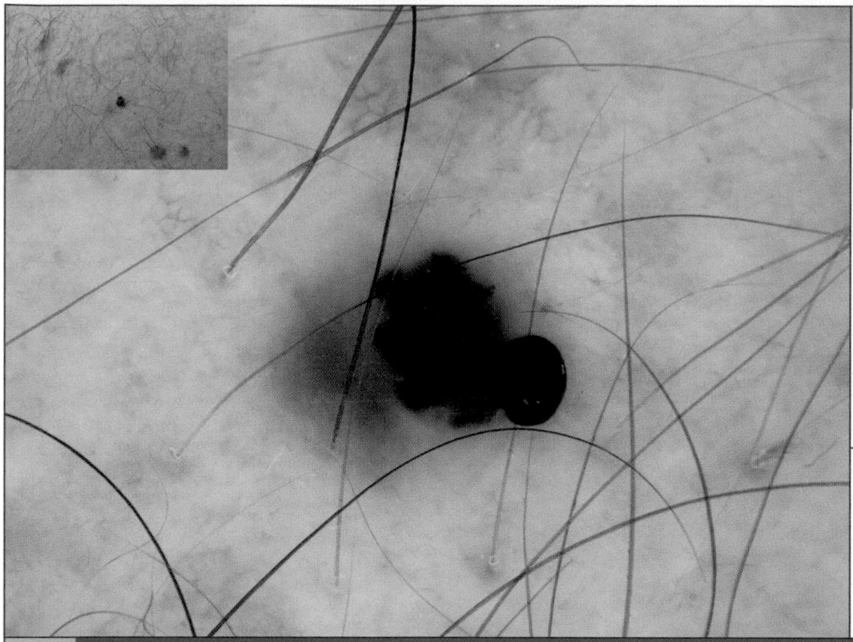

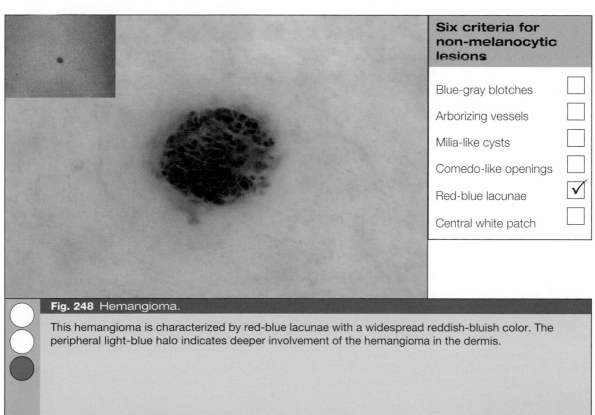

Six criteria for non-melanocytic lesions

Blue-gray blotches	☐
Arborizing vessels	☐
Milia-like cysts	☐
Comedo-like openings	☐
Red-blue lacunae	☑
Central white patch	☐

Fig. 247 Hemangioma.

This hemangioma is partially thrombosed. The reddish-black areas in the right half of the lesion represent thrombosed vascular spaces and not the blotches of a melanoma. The dark red and blue-black lacunae also point to a benign hemangioma. However, because of the several different colors, we raise here the orange flag.

Six criteria for non-melanocytic lesions

Blue-gray blotches	☐
Arborizing vessels	☐
Milia-like cysts	☐
Comedo-like openings	☐
Red-blue lacunae	☑
Central white patch	☐

Fig. 248 Hemangioma.

This hemangioma is characterized by red-blue lacunae with a widespread reddish-bluish color. The peripheral light-blue halo indicates deeper involvement of the hemangioma in the dermis.

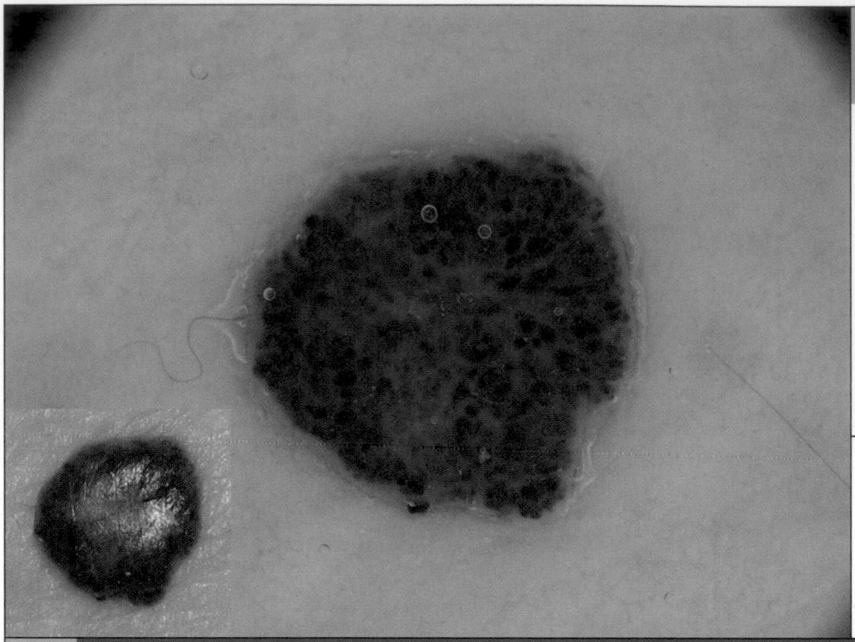

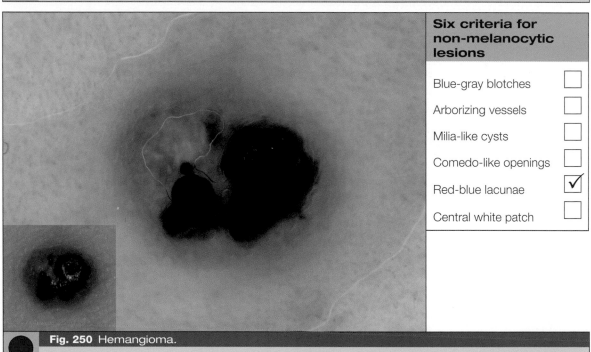

Six criteria for non-melanocytic lesions

Blue-gray blotches	☐
Arborizing vessels	☐
Milia-like cysts	☐
Comedo-like openings	☐
Red-blue lacunae	☑
Central white patch	☐

Fig. 249 Hemangioma.

This is another classic example of cherry hemangioma. In contrast to Fig. 241, the coloration is darker. The fenestrated whitish pattern reflects the fibrosis encompassing the hemangioma lobules. In a case like this, even the beginner can make the diagnosis of a hemangioma. There is no need to perform a biopsy in a clear-cut example like this one.

Six criteria for non-melanocytic lesions

Blue-gray blotches	☐
Arborizing vessels	☐
Milia-like cysts	☐
Comedo-like openings	☐
Red-blue lacunae	☑
Central white patch	☐

Fig. 250 Hemangioma.

Although the expert dermoscopist favors here a thrombosed hemangioma, there is no doubt that this lesion is worrisome. There are dark-red to black lacunae corresponding to the thrombosed areas and bluish-white areas most probably corresponding to dermal fibrosis. The differential diagnosis here includes an ulcerated melanoma and an ulcerated basal cell carcinoma. A diagnostic excision is definitely warranted.

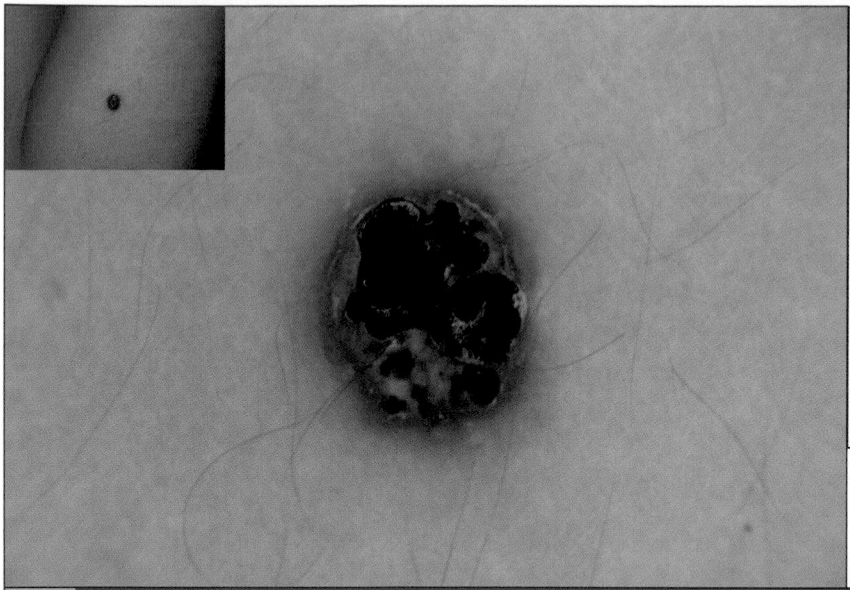

Six criteria for non-melanocytic lesions

Blue-gray blotches	☐
Arborizing vessels	☐
Milia-like cysts	☐
Comedo-like openings	☐
Red-blue lacunae	☑
Central white patch	☐

Fig. 251 Hemangioma.

The clinical and dermoscopic images of this lesion are quite alarming and therefore we raised the orange flag. However, this lesion shows a variation of the morphology that can be seen with a partially fibrosed hemangioma with a large thrombosed area. It is characterized by several tiny red-blue to blue-black lacunae throughout the lesion, and additionally, a diffuse blue-whitish hue is present. There are many faces of vascular lesions, and the red to purplish color around the lower pole of the lesion is key to making the diagnosis here. But remember, if in doubt, cut or shave it out.

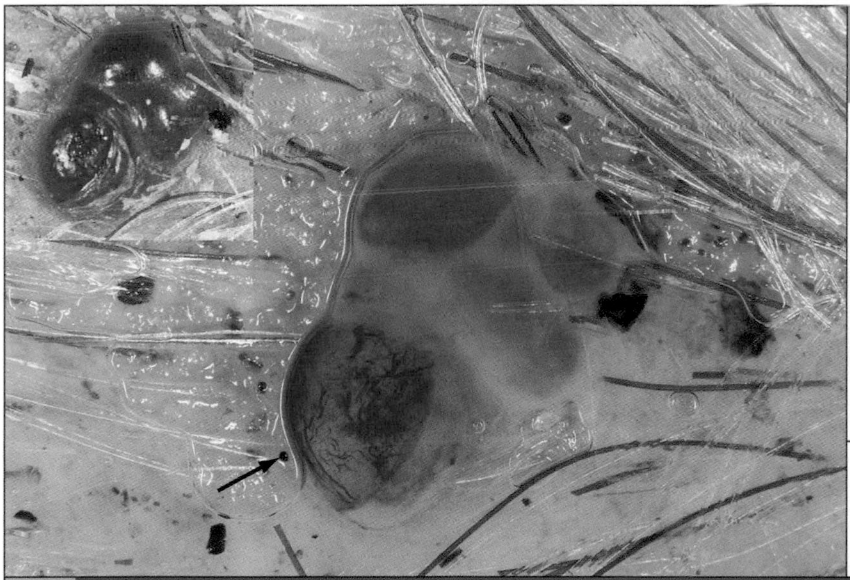

Six criteria for non-melanocytic lesions

Blue-gray blotches	☐
Arborizing vessels	☐
Milia-like cysts	☐
Comedo-like openings	☐
Red-blue lacunae	☑
Central white patch	☐

Fig. 252 Pyogenic granuloma.

This is a vascular lesion because it has large red lacunae. Numerous telangiectasias are also present (*arrow*). The diagnosis of a pyogenic granuloma can be made only on clinical or histopathologic grounds because precise differentiation from a hemangioma is difficult with dermoscopy. Remember that amelanotic melanoma, the great masquerader, is always in the differential diagnosis of a pyogenic granuloma.

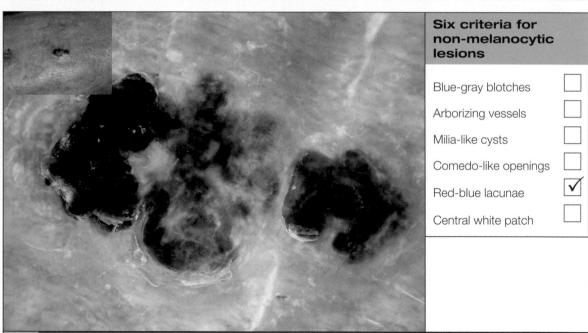

Six criteria for non-melanocytic lesions	
Blue-gray blotches	☐
Arborizing vessels	☐
Milia-like cysts	☐
Comedo-like openings	☐
Red-blue lacunae	☑
Central white patch	☐

Fig. 253 Kaposi's sarcoma.

The dermoscopic appearance of this vascular nodule is nonspecific and similar to the pyogenic granuloma shown in Fig. 252 and the fibroangioma shown in Fig. 245. There are red lacunae and whitish areas of fibrosis (*asterisks*). Important historical and clinical data might be needed to help diagnose certain vascular-appearing lesions.

Six criteria for non-melanocytic lesions	
Blue-gray blotches	☐
Arborizing vessels	☐
Milia-like cysts	☐
Comedo-like openings	☐
Red-blue lacunae	☑
Central white patch	☐

Fig. 254 Hemangioma.

This is another example where the clinical and dermoscopic images are very suspicious, so we have raised the red flag here. As in the previous figures, this vascular lesion exhibits red-blue lacunae with pronounced whitish areas of fibrosis and large, black thrombosed areas at both left and right poles of the lesion. The dermoscopic differential diagnosis includes amelanotic melanoma, Kaposi sarcoma, and an unusual fibrosing pyogenic granuloma. As a rule, the dermoscopic aspect of a lesion should be part of the overall clinical assessment of the patient. This is another basic dermoscopic principle that cannot be overemphasized. The histopathologic diagnosis was a heavily ulcerated and irritated hemangioma. Sometimes it is wise to raise the red flag unnecessarily and act accordingly, as happened here.

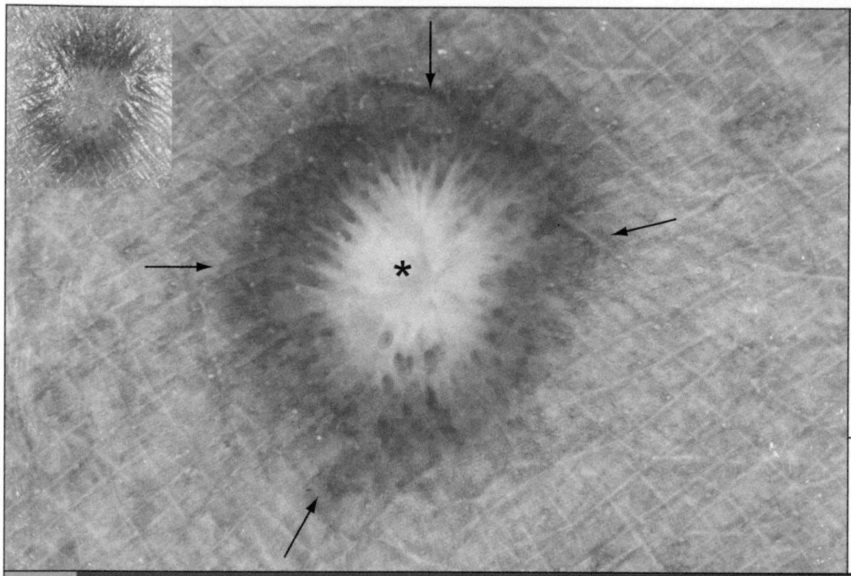

Six criteria for non-melanocytic lesions

Blue-gray blotches	☐
Arborizing vessels	☐
Milia-like cysts	☐
Comedo-like openings	☐
Red-blue lacunae	☐
Central white patch	☑

Fig. 255 Dermatofibroma.

This stereotypical dermatofibroma, with a central white patch (*asterisk*), is surrounded by a very subtle pigment network (*arrows*). Dermatofibromas are one of the few non-melanocytic lesions that can have a pigment network.

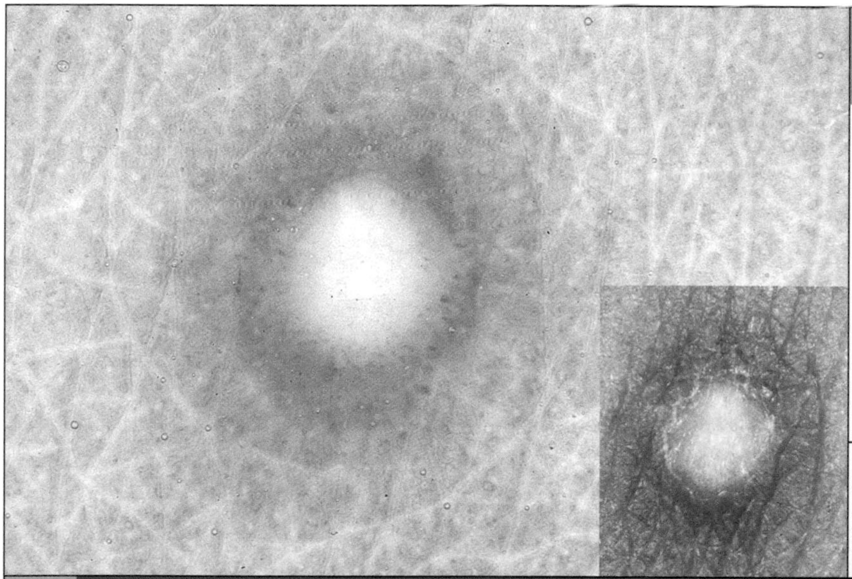

Six criteria for non-melanocytic lesions

Blue-gray blotches	☐
Arborizing vessels	☐
Milia-like cysts	☐
Comedo-like openings	☐
Red-blue lacunae	☐
Central white patch	☑

Fig. 256 Dermatofibroma.

In this dermatofibroma, the central white patch predominates. Light pigmentation, but not a network, can be seen at the periphery. Palpating this firm papule will help in making the diagnosis. There are numerous variations of the white patch seen in dermatofibromas.

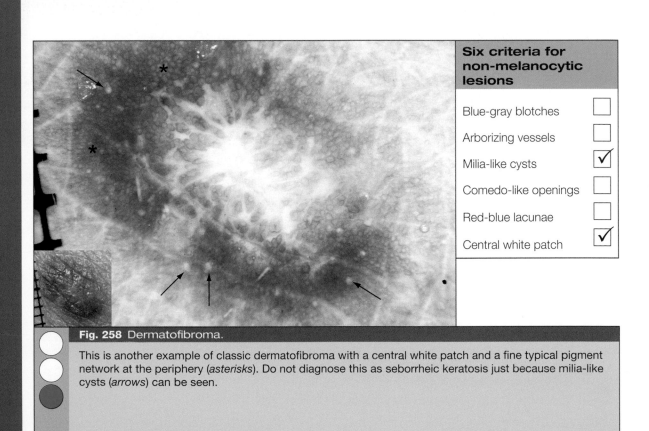

Six criteria for non-melanocytic lesions	
Blue-gray blotches	☐
Arborizing vessels	☐
Milia-like cysts	☐
Comedo-like openings	☐
Red-blue lacunae	☐
Central white patch	☑

Fig. 257 Dermatofibroma.

This dermatofibroma has a reticular depigmentation (*circle*), which is a variation of the central white patch. A very subtle pigment network can also be seen at the periphery (*arrows*). A reticular white color is commonly seen in dermatofibromas.

Six criteria for non-melanocytic lesions	
Blue-gray blotches	☐
Arborizing vessels	☐
Milia-like cysts	☑
Comedo-like openings	☐
Red-blue lacunae	☐
Central white patch	☑

Fig. 258 Dermatofibroma.

This is another example of classic dermatofibroma with a central white patch and a fine typical pigment network at the periphery (*asterisks*). Do not diagnose this as seborrheic keratosis just because milia-like cysts (*arrows*) can be seen.

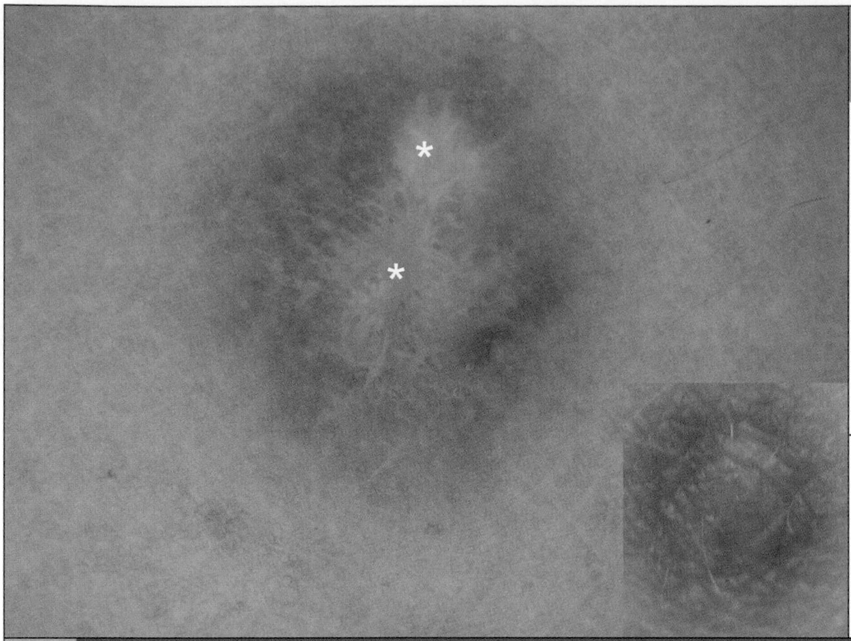

Six criteria for non-melanocytic lesions

Blue-gray blotches	☐
Arborizing vessels	☐
Milia-like cysts	☐
Comedo-like openings	☐
Red-blue lacunae	☐
Central white patch	☑

Fig. 259 Dermatofibroma.

This is a stereotypical example of dermatofibroma with a central white patch (*asterisks*) and a well-detectable but subtle pigment network at the periphery. In a case like this, the beginner will have no problems to raise the green flag and also to diagnose this lesion as dermatofibroma. Of course, palpating this lesion will help in the diagnostic process.

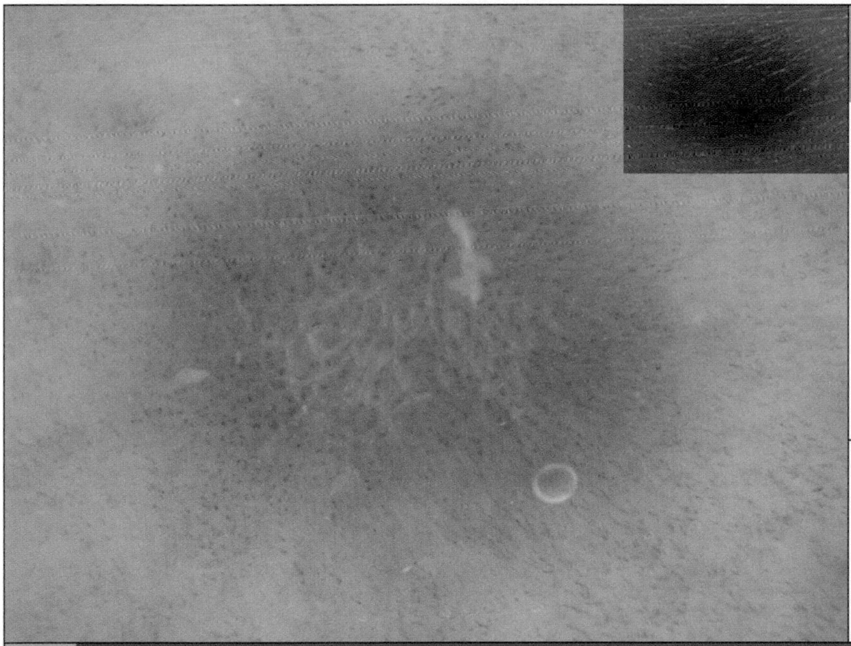

Six criteria for non-melanocytic lesions

Blue-gray blotches	☐
Arborizing vessels	☐
Milia-like cysts	☐
Comedo-like openings	☐
Red-blue lacunae	☐
Central white patch	☐

Fig. 260 Dermatofibroma.

Sometimes dermoscopy does not support the diagnosis of dermatofibroma as is the case in this pink lesion here. There are numerous dotted vessels rather evenly distributed throughout the lesion. The differential diagnosis includes a Spitz nevus and an amelanotic melanoma. Even palpation does not help here as a desmoplastic melanoma may give the same result upon palpation. Beware pink lesions, raise the red flag and perform a diagnostic excision.

Common clinical scenarios

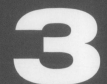

Side-by-side comparisons of similar-appearing lesions that are benign or malignant

Introduction

When you examine a skin lesion with dermoscopy, it might be obviously benign or malignant. There is also a gray zone of equivocal lesions. Gray-zone lesions will commonly be encountered by the novice dermoscopist. To help deal with this common situation, we offer a few suggestions. Learn the basics, practice the technique as often as possible, and develop a dermoscopic differential diagnosis.

You have to be able to think things through logically, weighing the pros and cons for each criterion or pattern that you see. Coming up with a tentative dermoscopic diagnosis, or in many cases, a dermoscopic differential diagnosis, is the end of the process.

For example, are the round to oval yellow dots and globules you see the milia-like cysts of a seborrheic keratosis or the follicular ostia of a melanocytic lesion? What a difference that distinction could make. You could be dealing with a seborrheic keratosis or a lentigo maligna. Are those the brown dots and globules of a melanocytic lesion, or the pigmented follicular openings of a seborrheic keratosis? You notice that the lesion has some blood vessels. Are they the thickened branched vessels of a basal cell carcinoma or the irregular linear vessels that can be found in melanomas?

We regret to inform you that you will encounter difficult lesions—lesions that even the most experienced dermoscopist will not feel confident about. That is the state of the art as it exists today. There are infinite variations of criteria, patterns, and lesions. The scenarios in this final chapter demonstrate the dermoscopic thought process we employ. Focus your attention, use what you have learned in the first two chapters of the book, and you will find that you will learn and grow with each case. Do not be intimidated by what you see. We guarantee that you can master this technique. You will develop your own style of dermoscopic analysis and find that dermoscopy will become an essential part of your practice. You will not be able to practice without it!

Pediatric scenario

General principles

- Melanoma in childhood is exceedingly rare, and the great majority of melanocytic skin lesions in prepubertal children are benign and do not require any special attention. The dermoscopic criteria of childhood nevi are the same as in other age groups, but in most cases, childhood nevi reveal a globular pattern.
- The most problematic skin tumors in the pediatric patient are large to giant congenital melanocytic nevi and atypical Spitz tumors.
- Large to giant congenital nevi represent the most important risk factors for melanoma in prepubertal children, although the risk is still low (<1%). Because melanoma associated with large to giant congenital melanocytic nevi often develops deep in the dermis or in the central nervous system, dermoscopy is of limited benefit in the early diagnosis of melanoma.
- The risk for melanoma in small to medium congenital melanocytic nevi is not established, but they should be kept under regular surveillance. Biopsy is indicated in the case of significant atypical structural changes.
- There are no definitive guidelines about the management of Spitz nevi, and there are controversies about whether to follow up or excise these nevi. However, flat pigmented Spitz nevi (commonly also called Reed nevi) with a stereotypical dermoscopic starburst pattern, appearing below the age of puberty, can be managed conservatively and can be regularly followed up as there is a well-documented tendency of involution.
- Atypical Spitz tumors and rare childhood melanomas commonly present as rapidly growing, pigmented or nonpigmented nodules. Immediate excision of any lesion showing these clinical characteristics is indicated.

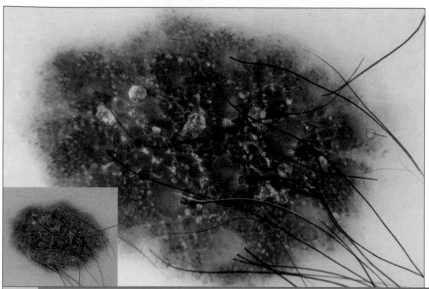

Fig. 261 Congenital nevus.

This congenital nevus revealing some irregularity of color and structure is located on the forearm of a 3-year-old child. Closer scrutiny of the central area displays large and somewhat angulated brown-gray globules (also called cobblestone pattern), which are surrounded by smaller brown globules; characteristic is also the presence of numerous terminal hairs showing either a perifollicular hyperpigmentation or hypopigmentation. Despite the worrisome aspect of this lesion, we raise with confidence the green flag and recommend annual follow-up.

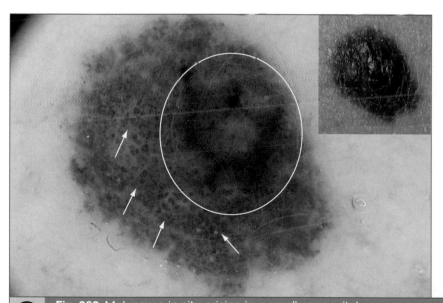

Fig. 262 Melanoma in situ arising in a small congenital nevus.

While melanoma before puberty is very uncommon, the risk increases after puberty. This lesion is located on the shoulder of a 15-year-old girl, who noticed a recent change of color in the preexisting nevus characterized by numerous brown-gray globules resembling cobblestones (*arrows*). Dermoscopically, the melanoma appears as an irregular blue-gray blotch (*circle*) in paracentral location of an otherwise regularly pigmented globular (cobblestone) nevus.

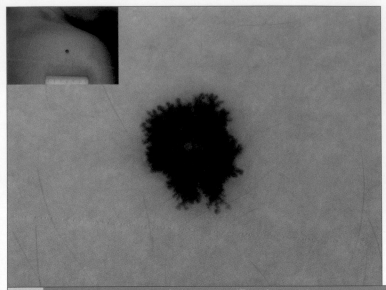

Fig. 263 Pigmented Spitz nevus (Reed nevus).

This is a stereotypical example of a flat pigmented Spitz nevus located on the shoulder of a 5-year-old girl. The dermoscopic hallmarks of a pigmented Spitz nevus (commonly also called Reed nevus) are regularly distributed peripheral streaks and pseudopods that arise from a heavily pigmented area, along with a depigmentation in the center of the lesion. During follow-up, these nevi enlarge symmetrically until the disappearance of peripheral streaks indicates stabilization of growth. At this stage, the nevus reveals a homogeneous black-bluish dark brown to black pigmentation. The management decision here, excision versus monitoring, is influenced by the parent's level of concern and is best decided jointly. We are raising here the orange flag appreciating that the management of these lesions is complex.

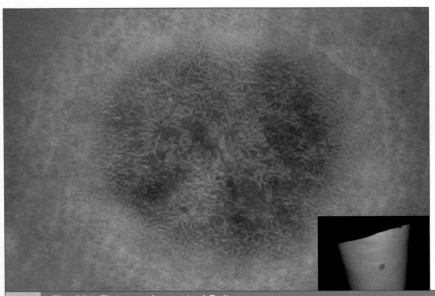

Fig. 264 Flat nonpigmented Spitz nevus.

This flat or plaque-like reddish nevus is located on the thigh of a 10-year-old boy. Dermoscopically, nonpigmented Spitz nevi display regularly distributed dotted vessels over a milky-red background as evidenced by this image. Typically a reticular depigmentation can be seen appearing as white net-like lines between the dotted vessels. Because of the lack of both general guidelines and well-documented cases of involution, nonpigmented Spitz nevi should be excised even in children. Remember our slogan, "pink lesion beware," and raise the red flag.

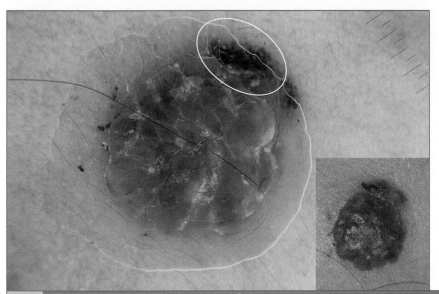

Fig. 265 Atypical nonpigmented Spitz tumor.

This reddish nodule was located on the cheek of an 11-year-old girl and revealed a history of rapid growth within a few months. Despite a brown residual pseudonetwork (*circle*), the nonpigmented nodule lacks any specific pattern and exhibits only pink to red homogeneous areas. No doubt we have to raise the red flag here. The lesion was excised and revealed also histopathologically highly conflicting features. The final histopathologic diagnosis was atypical Spitz tumor, and follow-up after 3 years revealed no recurrence.

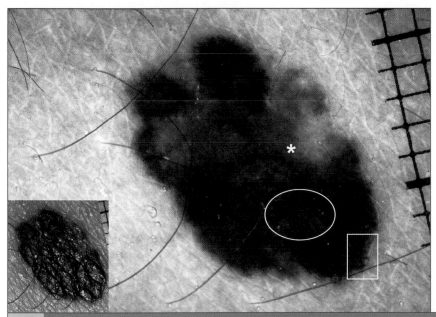

Fig. 266 Melanoma.

This is a melanoma on a 14-year-old child. It has melanoma-specific criteria—a blue-white structure (*asterisk*), which is easy to see; subtle streaks (*square*); and irregular dots and globules (*circle*). Young patients do get melanoma and die from their disease, so it is necessary to increase one's index of suspicion for pediatric patients.

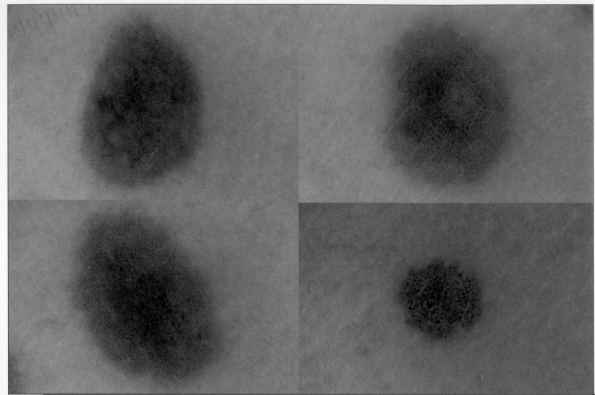

Fig. 267 Common nevi.

This 7-year-old boy reveals some nevi on his back. All nevi are characterized by a uniform pigmentation and by a globular pattern. These nevi do not require any special further attention, and we are raising the green flag with confidence here.

Black lesions

General principles

- Clinically, black color is not always ominous.
- Black color with dermoscopy is also not always ominous.

- The differential diagnosis of a single black macule or papule could be melanocytic or nonmelanocytic, benign or malignant.
- What should be done on finding a black lesion? Check it out with dermoscopy before making another move.

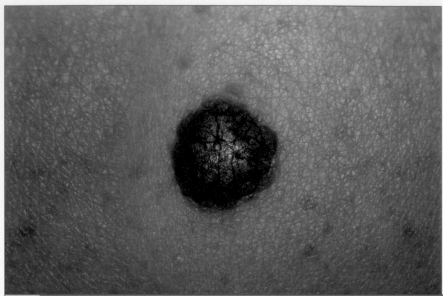

Fig. 268 What is your clinical diagnosis?

This clinically nonspecific nodular dark brown to black lesion looks similar to that in Fig. 269. There is no way to know for sure which of the two lesions is benign and which is malignant. What should be done? Cut it out or check it out? (See Fig. 270.)

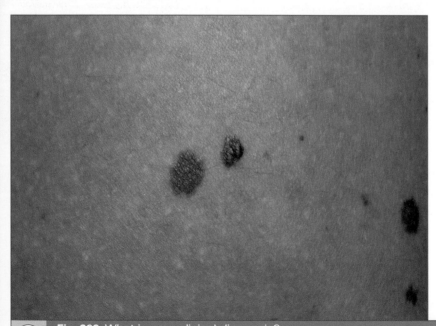

Fig. 269 What is your clinical diagnosis?

This clinically nonspecific dark brown to black lesion (*right*) looks somewhat lighter than the example in Fig. 268 but clearly darker than another lesion (*left*) close by. There is no way to know for sure which is benign and which is malignant. What should be done? Cut it out or check it out? (See Fig. 271.)

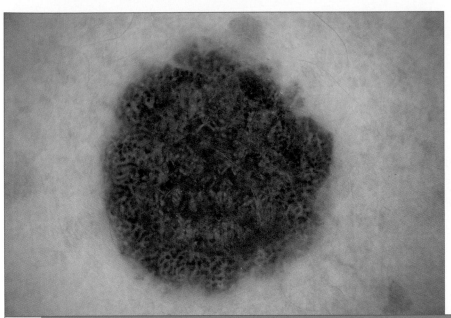

Fig. 270 Melanoma.

This is the dermoscopic image of the lesion in Fig. 268. Step 1—is it melanocytic or nonmelanocytic? It is a melanocytic lesion because there are brown to black globules in the peripheral zone. Step 2—is it benign or malignant? Can melanoma-specific criteria be identified? The large central blue-white structure, shiny white streaks, and some irregular black globules are enough to warrant excision as soon as possible.

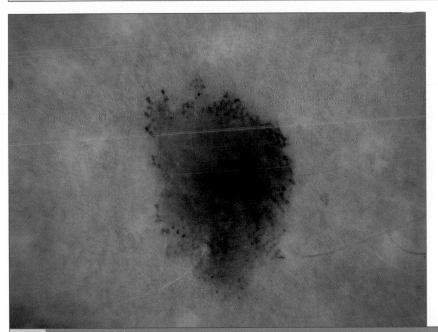

Fig. 271 Melanoma.

This is the dermoscopic image of the lesion in Fig. 269. Surprise! It's also a melanoma. It has three melanoma-specific criteria: an atypical pigment network with thickened and smudged lines at 12–2 o'clock, irregular globules at the periphery from 8–12 o'clock, and a subtle blue-white structure in the upper pole of the lesion.

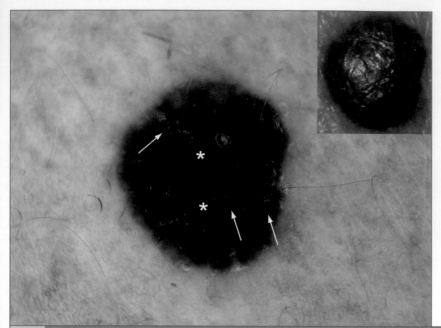

Fig. 272 Seborrheic keratosis.

Is there a blue-white structure (*asterisks*) here? Maybe there are some subtle streaks at the periphery of the lesion. And there might be a few comedo-like openings (*arrows*). So, this lesion has melanoma-specific criteria and criteria seen in a seborrheic keratosis. Sometimes an acanthotic seborrheic keratosis may be heavily pigmented and nearly devoid of any typical criteria. In a case like this, the expert raises the green flag and the beginner might be more cautious and raise the orange flag and excise the lesion. Remember, if in doubt, cut or shave it out.

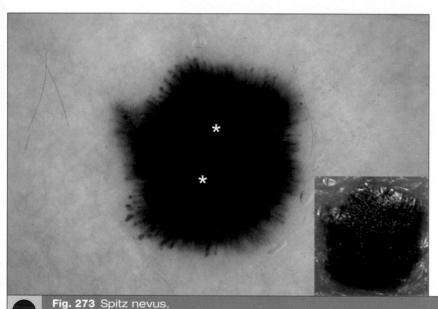

Fig. 273 Spitz nevus.

The differential diagnosis for this Spitzoid appearance should include pigmented Spitz nevus (also called Reed nevus) and melanoma. There is a central rather subtle blue-white structure (*asterisks*) and symmetrically oriented streaks around the lesion. These features favor the diagnosis of a Spitz (Reed) nevus. If a lesion like this one is found in a patient after puberty, a diagnostic excision needs to be performed. Because this lesion was located on the dorsal hand of an adult woman and, in addition, there was also a history of rapid growth, this lesion was excised.

Inkspot lentigo

General principles

- Clinically and dermoscopically inkspot (or reticular) lentigines have a very characteristic appearance.
- Typically, an inkspot lentigo is black and sharply demarcated with a bizarre-looking pigment network filling the lesion. There is an absence of other criteria.
- Individuals with inkspot lentigines commonly have fair skin, light hair, and light eyes and are at risk of developing melanoma. Do not forget to do a comprehensive skin examination to look for high-risk pigmented skin lesions.
- Inkspot lentigines are usually located on the upper trunk and extremities and are surrounded by regular or large sunburn freckles.
- On seeing an "inkspot lentigo," try not to miss seeing the presence of any melanoma-specific criteria.
- If in doubt, cut or shave it out.

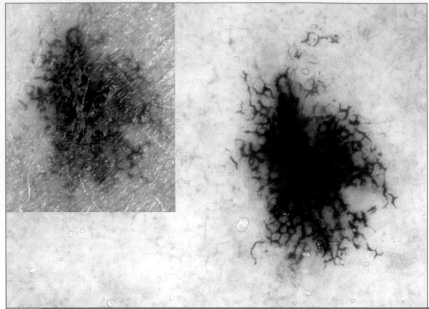

Fig. 274 Inkspot lentigo.

This is a variation of the morphology seen in an inkspot lentigo characterized by a bizarre pigment network. There is also a large homogeneous area with a gray color representing melanophages in the papillary dermis.

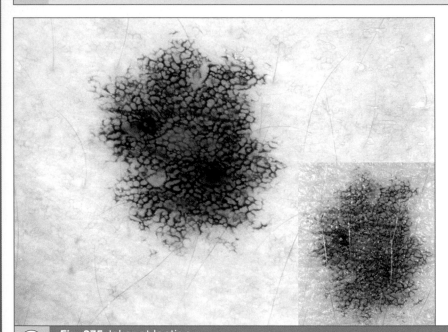

Fig. 275 Inkspot lentigo.

This is a stereotypical inkspot lentigo. The network is commonly black.

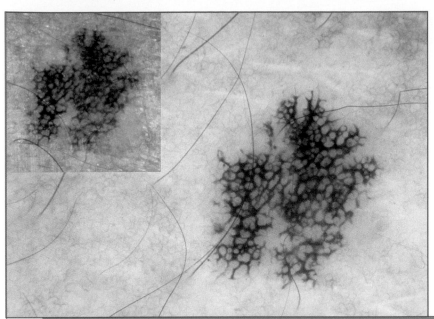

Fig. 276 Inkspot lentigo.

A third variation of the appearance of inkspot lentigo. The clinical appearance, dark color, bizarre shape of the pigment network, and absence of other criteria suggest the correct diagnosis.

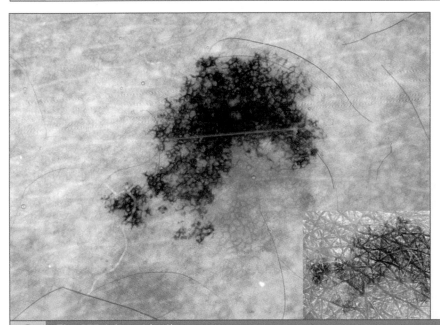

Fig. 277 Inkspot lentigo.

This picture is worrisome because of the asymmetry of color and structure, the irregular dots and globules, and the irregular blotch. It is not wrong to biopsy a lesion that looks like this.

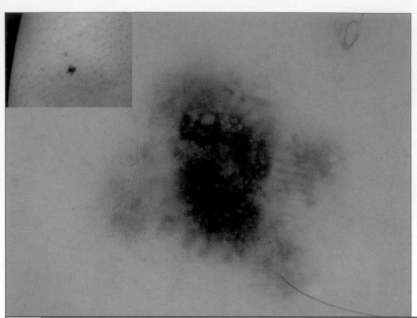

Fig. 278 Clark (dysplastic) nevus.

The quality of the pigment network is suggestive of a reticular type of Clark (dysplastic) nevus. The pigment network is atypical, with variation in line thickness, and the color is blotchy. Therefore, excision or short-term digital follow-up (in the literature commonly referred to as sequential digital dermoscopy imaging or SDDI) is recommended. When the lesion is excised, the final histopathologic diagnosis depends on the judgment of the pathologist, and may range from slight to moderate to severe atypia.

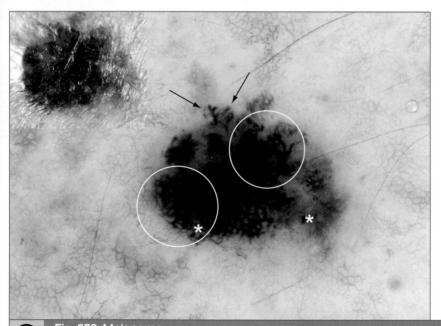

Fig. 279 Melanoma.

This lesion is black with a pigment network, but these are the only features this melanoma has in common with an inkspot lentigo. This lesion has prominent melanoma-specific criteria—an atypical pigment network (*circles*), irregular dots and globules (*asterisks*), and rather typical streaks (*arrows*).

Blue lesions

General principles

- Blue color can be seen in benign and malignant lesions. They are not all blue nevi.
- Blue color indicates that melanin is deep in the dermis.

- It is imperative to develop a complete differential diagnosis for blue lesions.
- If you see a lesion with blue color but it also has other criteria, it should be evaluated like any other lesion.
- Blue lesions can be tricky. If in doubt, do not hesitate—cut it out.

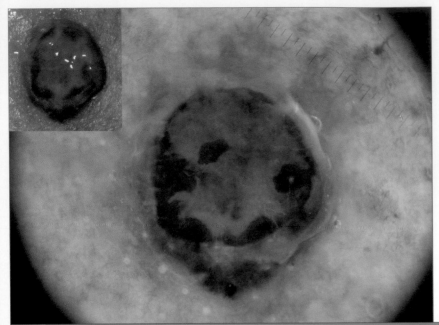

Fig. 280 Nodular melanoma on the face.

This rather expophytic, ulcerated, and hemorrhagic tumor shows structureless blue-white color in the absence of any specific criteria of a melanocytic or nonmelanocytic tumor. Although structureless blue color may be seen also in blue nevi, the irregular distribution of colors together with the ulceration and bleeding represents a high-risk dermoscopic image and must be removed. In fact, it turned out to be a nodular melanoma.

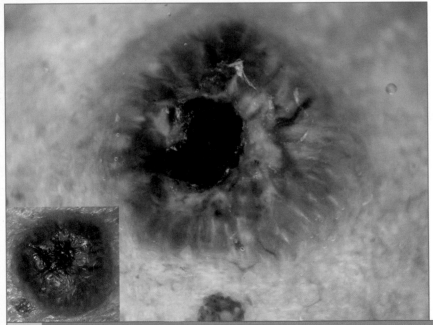

Fig. 281 Basal cell carcinoma.

Another example of a blue-whitish ulcerated nodule prompting us to immediately raise the red flag. There are evident focused vessels and some isolated gray globules as well as a large central ulceration. The experienced dermoscopist might favor a basal cell carcinoma but will insist on a diagnostic excision with high priority because a nodular melanoma cannot be ruled out with certainty.

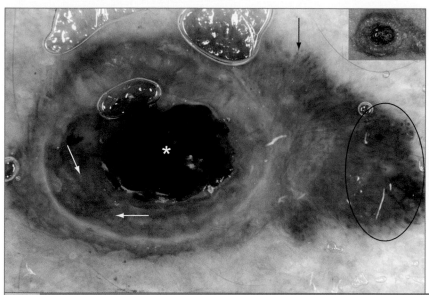

Fig. 282 Melanoma.

One's first opinion might be that this is a basal cell carcinoma because of the ulceration (*asterisk*) and vessels (*white arrows*). Scan the lesion for all criteria. It actually has dots and globules (*circle*), so it is melanocytic. Now it is looking like a melanoma because of the blue-white structure, asymmetrically located irregular dots and globules, and irregular streaks (*black arrow*). This lesion therefore needs a diagnostic excision with a high-level of priority. The dermoscopic picture will help in planning the surgical approach. It is important not to shave through this invasive melanoma.

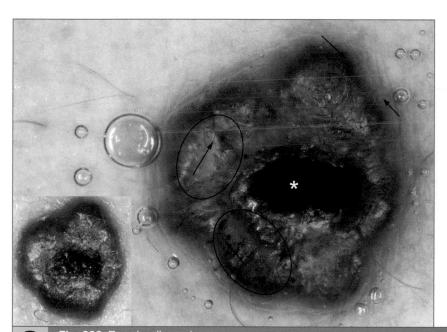

Fig. 283 Basal cell carcinoma.

This lesion is remarkably similar to that shown in Fig. 282. Features include ulceration (*asterisk*), blue-white structures (*circles*), and a few irregular dots and globules (*arrows*). This lesion is melanocytic by definition if the rules are strictly followed, although it turned out to be a basal cell carcinoma. The important point is that this dermoscopic picture needs a diagnostic excision with a high-level of priority.

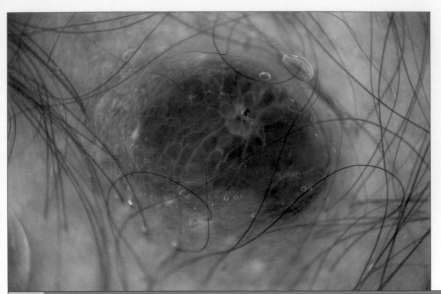

Fig. 284 Melanoma metastasis.

The differential diagnosis of this bluish nodule in the axilla is a blue nevus on one hand and a nodular melanoma or a melanoma metastasis on the other. No doubt the history of the given tumor is of high importance; blue nevi usually have a very stable history in contrast to melanoma or melanoma metastasis, which grow rapidly. In this case, the nodule developed rapidly in a patient with a previous primary melanoma. This along with the dermoscopic aspect should always lead to biopsy—here it was a melanoma metastasis.

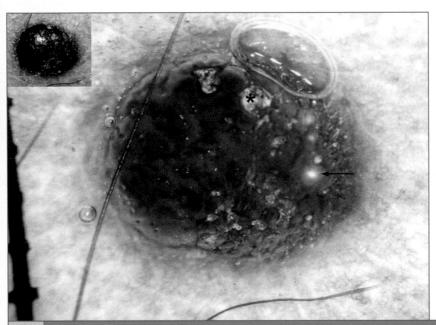

Fig. 285 Blue nevus.

This is a good example of a blue nevus with relatively homogeneous blue color. It is dry and scaly (*asterisk*) with milia-like cysts (*arrow*). Do not forget that the differential diagnosis includes nodular and cutaneous metastatic melanoma. The entire clinical picture will help one decide on the management of this lesion.

Reticular lesions

General principles

- Take a bird's-eye (global) view of the entire lesion to get a first impression.

- Reticular pattern = significant areas with pigment network.
- Is the pigment network typical or atypical?
- What other criteria are there to make the dermoscopic diagnosis?

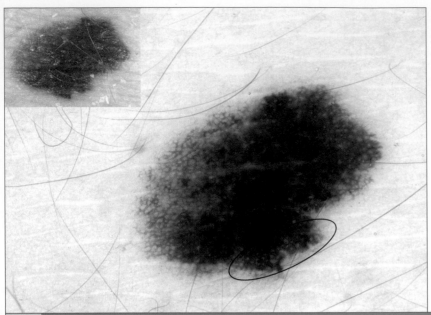

Fig. 286 Melanoma in situ.

Surprisingly this turned out to be an in situ melanoma. It does not look that worrisome. There is enough pigment network to say it has a reticular pattern, and the pigment network is slightly atypical. The subtle irregular streaks (*circle*) push this lesion over the edge to be malignant. Statistically, a lesion with this dermoscopic picture would not be a melanoma but a Clark (dysplastic) nevus. It is suspicious enough to warrant a histopathologic diagnosis.

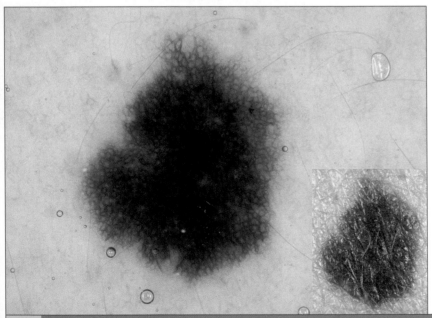

Fig. 287 Clark (dysplastic) nevus.

The pigment network fills most of this lesion. It has more of a reticular pattern than that shown in Fig. 286. The pigment network and dots and globules are questionably atypical but not strikingly worrisome. Differentiate this benign nevus from the in situ melanoma in Fig. 286. Here the network lines are thin and fade out at the periphery, in contrast to the previous case.

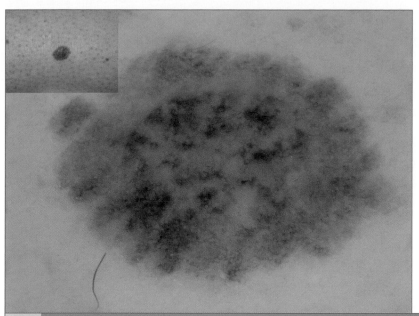

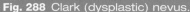

Fig. 288 Clark (dysplastic) nevus.

The pigment network is slightly atypical in this lesion because the line segments are thicker, branched, broken up, and vary in color. The central area of hypopigmentation is reminiscent of blue-white structures, and in combination with the slightly atypical pigment network we cannot rule out a superficial melanoma. We excised this lesion, and our pathologist reported it as a Clark (dysplastic) nevus with severe atypia; however, we are well aware that other pathologists would report this lesion as a melanoma.

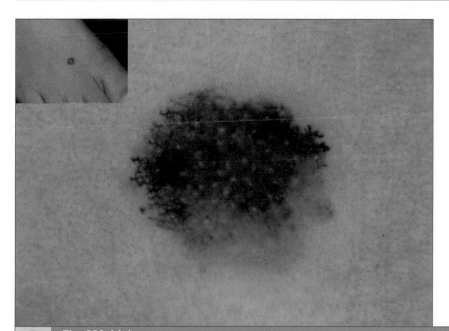

Fig. 289 Melanoma.

This lesion looks more ominous with a reticular pattern forming a simulant of a starburst pattern. There are branched streaks along the periphery from 8–2 o'clock. This favors the diagnosis of a melanoma. This diagnosis is supported by the blue-white structures in the center and lower right of the lesion. A further melanoma-specific criterion is the presence of subtle irregular dots and globules at the center of the lesion. Excise this lesion.

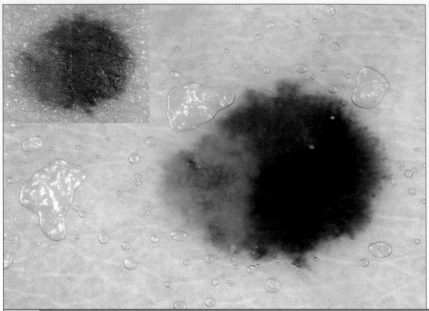

Fig. 290 Melanoma.

Imagination is needed to recognize the streaks and atypical pigment network that classify this as a reticular pattern. The dermoscopist should realize that this is a high-risk lesion because of the clear-cut asymmetry of color and structure. As is the case here, an early in situ melanoma may be hard to diagnose.

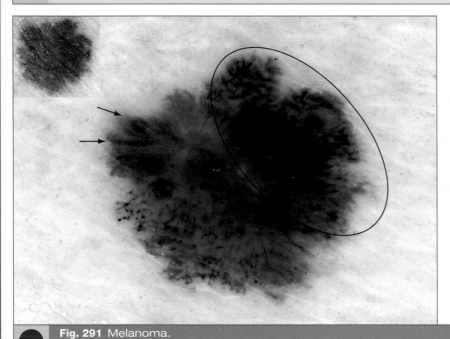

Fig. 291 Melanoma.

This bizarre dermoscopic picture shows areas with very atypical pigment network (*circle*), irregular streaks (*arrows*), and irregular dots and globules in the left lower part of this lesion. Never tell a patient that they definitely have a melanoma based on the dermoscopic picture, no matter how ominous it looks. The result of the histopathologic examination sometimes may surprise you.

Spitzoid lesions

General principles

- Spitzoid means similar in appearance to a starburst pattern.
- Spitzoid differential diagnosis includes Clark (dysplastic) nevus, Spitz nevus, and melanoma.
- Spitzoid morphology comprises a light-dark or blue central area and dots and globules or streaks at the periphery.
- Symmetrical Spitzoid pattern = benign lesion.

- Asymmetrical Spitzoid pattern = rule out melanoma.
- The stereotypical starburst pattern is seen more frequently than the globular pattern, which is more common than the nonspecific Spitzoid pattern.

Caution

Deaths have occurred secondary to metastatic "Spitz" nevi that were in reality melanomas. Excise the vast majority of Spitzoid lesions. It is better to be safe than sorry.

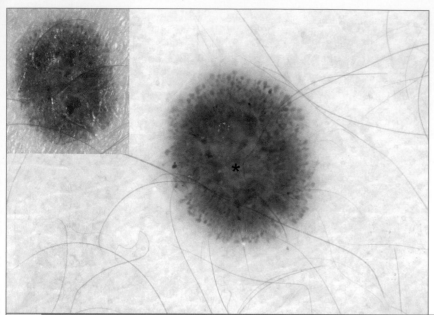

Fig. 292 Spitz nevus.

This is a classic symmetrical Spitzoid pattern. In the center of the lesion there is a subtle blue-white structure (*asterisk*). The rim of dots and globules at all points along the periphery of the lesion allows this dermoscopic diagnosis. On looking carefully, there are also some streaks at the periphery.

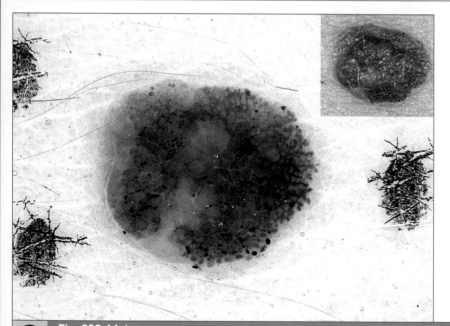

Fig. 293 Melanoma.

Compared to the lesion shown in Fig. 292, this lesion demonstrates significant asymmetry of color and structure with several melanoma-specific criteria. Why then is this Spitzoid? There is subtle central blue-white structure with irregular dots and globules and streaks at the periphery. They are trying to form a starburst pattern, but the criteria are not at all evenly distributed at the periphery of the lesion. This constellation of findings raises the red flag, and the lesion was diagnosed histopathologically as melanoma.

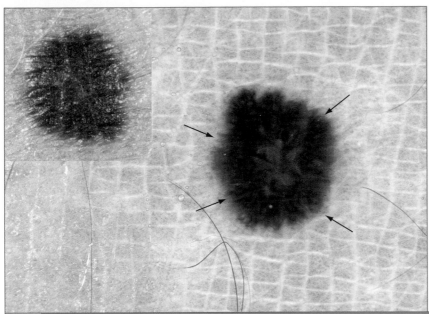

Fig. 294 Spitz nevus.

It is important to recognize symmetry and asymmetry in Spitzoid lesions. This lesion is very symmetrical, with subtle radially oriented streaks (*arrows*) at all points along the periphery of the lesion. Remember, the criteria are not always easy to see, so practice dermoscopy as much as possible to be able to see subtle patterns. The central blue-white structure is commonly found in Spitz nevi.

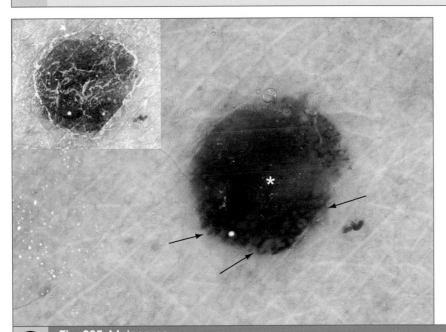

Fig. 295 Melanoma.

It is necessary to stretch one's imagination to call this a Spitzoid nevus. It does fit the pattern because there is a central blue-white structure (*asterisk*) and there are asymmetrically located streaks (*arrows*) at the periphery. The pigment network is very atypical. It does not matter whether this is called Spitzoid or not—it could be a melanoma and should be excised.

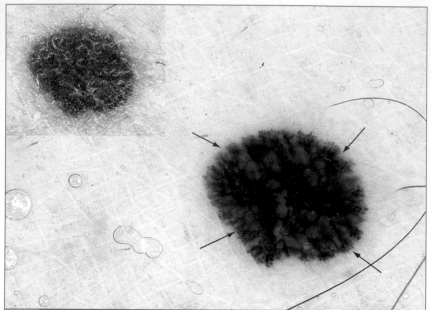

Fig. 296 Spitz nevus.

Here is another rather classic symmetrical starburst pattern. If this pattern is etched on the mind, it will be recognized immediately. This Spitz nevus has a darker central blotch partially covering a blue-white structure, and symmetrically located streaks (*arrows*) at all points along the periphery of the lesion.

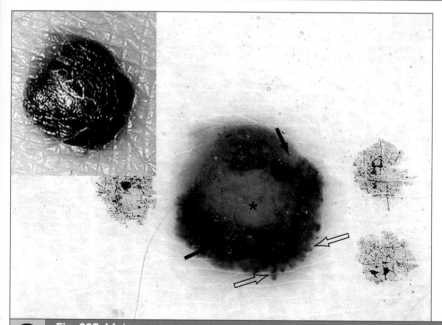

Fig. 297 Melanoma.

This is a Spitzoid melanoma with a centrally located blue-white structure (*asterisk*), a horseshoe-shaped dark blotch (*solid arrows*), and asymmetrically located streaks (*open arrows*) at the periphery. Pink color—beware.

Special nevi

General principles

- Special nevi are defined as benign melanocytic nevi that exhibit a rather specific constellation of features resulting often in a targetoid or iris-like appearance.
- The group of nevi with special features includes Sutton nevi, Meyerson nevi, traumatized nevi, recurrent nevi, combined nevi, and cockade nevi.

- Special nevi can be clinically easily diagnosed, and in most cases, dermoscopy simply confirms the clinical diagnosis.
- A special history of injury or incomplete surgical removal provides further clues for the diagnosis of traumatized and recurrent nevi.
- Special rules have been established for the management of special nevi.

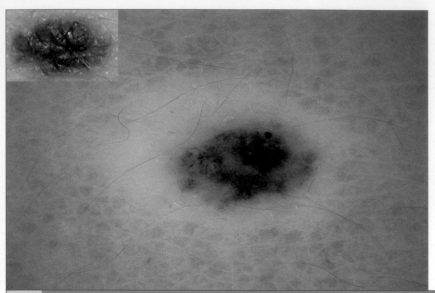

Fig. 298 Sutton nevus (halo nevus).

Sutton nevi, also termed "halo nevi," are benign melanocytic nevi clinically characterized by a peripheral rim (halo) of depigmentation. Dermoscopically, the central nevus component typically reveals a benign globular, structureless brown, or reticular pattern, whereas the peripheral ring is white and structureless. If appearing during young adolescence, no further treatment is warranted and we raise the green flag. Look carefully at the other nevi of your patient. Usually you will find a few more Sutton nevi.

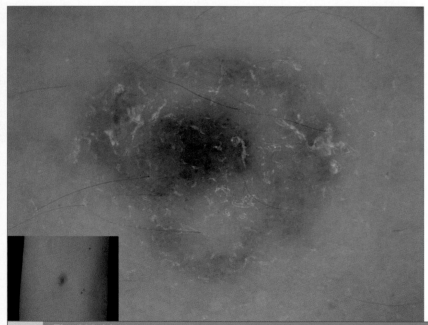

Fig. 299 Meyerson nevus.

Meyerson nevus, also termed "eczematous nevus," is characterized by the development of an eczematous halo around one or more pigmented nevi. Because the eczematous inflammation results in an unclear clinical and dermoscopic appearance, reevaluation after a short cycle of topical antibiotic or steroid treatment is recommended. In the case of persisting or recurrent inflammation or if atypical features are present, excision is recommended. In this case, the halo resolved following a short term of topical steroid treatment, and therefore the lesion was not excised.

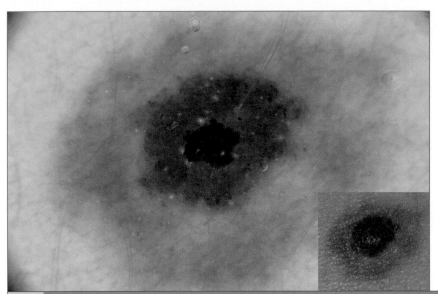

Fig. 300 Hemosiderotic targetoid nevus.

Traumatized nevi, also termed "irritated or hemosiderotic targetoid nevi," are characterized by the sudden onset of a peripheral purple rim after injury to a preexisting nevus. Typically, traumatized nevi are nodular or papillomatous, and patients refer to a recent history of injury. Dermoscopically, the central nevus component appears blurred and is often covered by a hemorrhagic crust typically surrounded by a purple structureless rim as is the case here. Reevaluation after a couple of weeks is recommended to reassess the disappearance of the peripheral purple halo. Please do not forget that sometimes also melanomas may be traumatized.

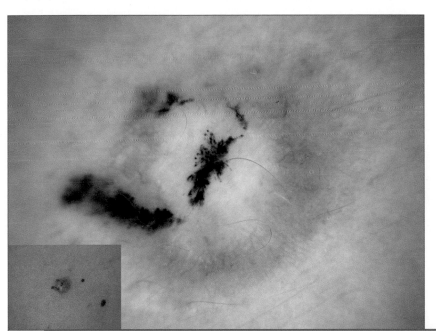

Fig. 301 Recurrent nevus.

Recurrent nevi are also often referred to as melanoma simulators both dermoscopically and histopathologically, and were historically termed "pseudomelanoma." They occur frequently in scars shortly after incomplete surgical removal (shave biopsies or saucerizations) or following a trauma. By dermoscopy, recurrent nevi exhibit centrally located irregular dots, globules and streaks, or, as in this special case, also several irregularly outlined brownish-black blotches. In cases with a confirmed previous histopathologic diagnosis of a nevus, no further treatment is warranted, while in all other cases, excision is mandatory. Pigmentation extending past the scar is also cause for concern, as at 9 o'clock in this lesion, so we recommended excision and were relieved by the diagnosis of a recurrent nevus.

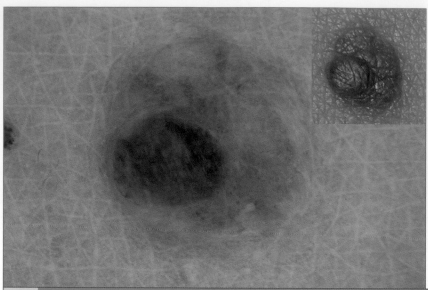

Fig. 302 Combined nevus.

Combined melanocytic nevi are defined as the histopathologic presence of two different types of benign melanocytic proliferations. They often have a clinically targetoid appearance (see also Fig. 300). Because of the presence of two populations of nevus cells, color variegations or more than one structure can be present. Dermoscopically, the most classic type is that of a blue nevus and a congenital nevus as demonstrated here. Please note the light-brown nearly structureless area on the right and the homogeneous blue-whitish roundish area on the left. Because combined nevi are rare, excision is generally recommended to rule out a melanoma within a preexisting nevus.

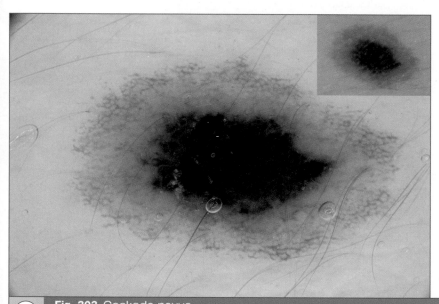

Fig. 303 Cockade nevus.

Cockade nevi are benign nevi characterized by a central pigmented, often papular portion that is surrounded by an inner depigmented and outer pigmented rim. The central portion typically shows a globular or cobblestone pattern, whereas the outer pigmented rim often shows a reticular pattern as nicely displayed here. Cockade nevi are benign and no further treatment is required. Of course, in case you are not familiar with this specific type of nevus, you may raise the orange flag and, depending on the specific location, a diagnostic excision or a second opinion consultation may be the way to go.

Multiple Clark (dysplastic) nevi

General principles

- Examining multiple nevi with dermoscopy is cost-effective and provides information about whether a patient has multiple high-risk or banal nevi.
- Most patients with multiple nevi have low-risk lesions, but this can be confirmed by checking them out with dermoscopy.
- Ask patients whether they have any new or changing nevi. Never ignore the patient's history.

- The "ugly duckling" pigmented skin lesion seen both clinically and with dermoscopy warrants a histopathologic diagnosis.
- If a patient has multiple high-risk-looking lesions with dermoscopy, excise one or two to make a dermoscopic-pathologic correlation.
- The true number of melanomas is small compared to the number of patients with multiple dysplastic nevi. The vast majority do not need to be excised but can be followed using digital systems to look for significant changes over time.

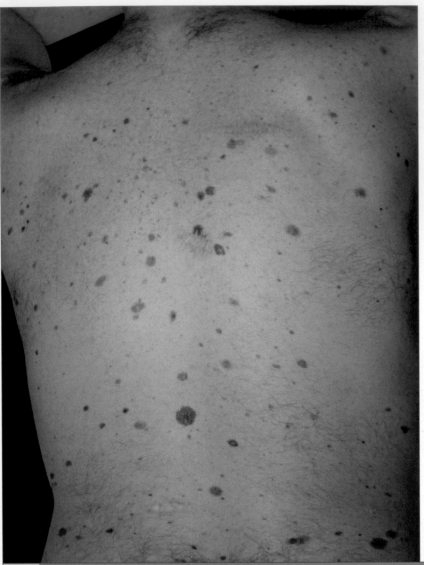

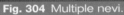

Fig. 304 Multiple nevi.

This is a stereotypical example of a person with multiple nevi. Clinically most look low risk, but he could have a melanoma. It is possible to examine most of these lesions rapidly with dermoscopy and obtain clues to point to high-risk lesions that do not look high risk clinically. These are usually the early melanomas where detection offers patients their best chances of survival. Dermoscopy opens up a new world of colors and structures that help in managing this common, difficult, and serious problem (see Figs. 305–308). In patients with many large atypical nevi, total body photography is useful in reducing the number of unnecessary excisions.

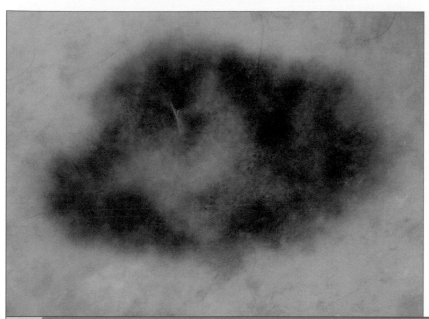

Fig. 305 Clark (dysplastic) nevus.

Here is an example of a dysplastic nevus from the individual shown in Fig. 304. A large central area of hypopigmentation, blue-whitish structures, atypical pigment network from 3–7 o'clock, and some irregular dots and globules are seen. In the realm of dysplastic nevi, dermoscopic findings do not always correlate with pathology. Very worrisome lesions often turn out to be mildly dysplastic, whereas relatively featureless lesions may be histopathologically severely dysplastic. This case is suitable for short-term monitoring.

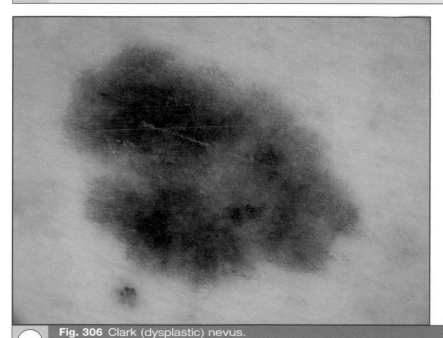

Fig. 306 Clark (dysplastic) nevus.

The mild asymmetry in structure is in keeping with the dermoscopic features of many other large nevi in this person, and no further specific management is recommended here.

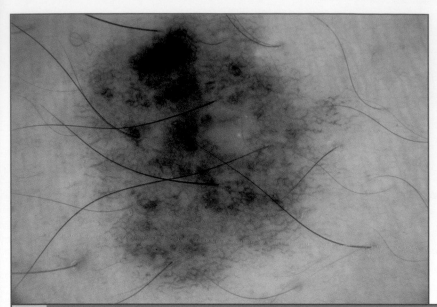

Fig. 307 Clark (dysplastic) nevus.

This is a third dermoscopic example of the patient with multiple large atypical nevi (or large dysplastic nevi) in Fig. 304. This lesion is characterized by a patchy reticular pattern with a black blotch at 12 o'clock and a hypopigmented area near the center, making us consider excision or short-term monitoring. It is very important to assess dermoscopically as many of these large nevi as possible in order to get a good understanding of the individual's lesion variability.

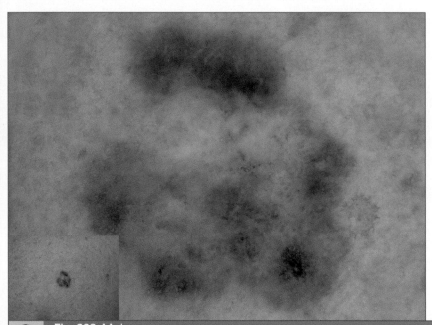

Fig. 308 Melanoma.

Here is the ugly duckling, however. This pinkish, relatively featureless lesion clearly differs from the others. Note the multifocal hypopigmentation verging on regression areas, peppering, increased vascularization, and foci of atypical pigment network. Excision is mandatory. Dermoscopy reveals high-risk lesions like these, which can otherwise easily be overlooked if the patient is examined with the naked eye. Melanomas will be missed less often if dermoscopy is mastered.

Follow-up of melanocytic lesions

General principles

- A high number of nevi, particularly when clinically atypical, is the strongest risk factor for the development of de novo melanoma. Early evolving melanomas are often not recognizable, as they are small, uniformly colored and regularly outlined, and consequently mistaken for an otherwise common nevus. Because most melanomas arise de novo, the main challenge in the management of patients with multiple, atypical nevi is the identification of initial melanomas hiding among a sea of nevi.
- Total-body photography and periodic digital dermoscopic monitoring improve the early recognition of melanoma, as it adds information about the evolution over time, which in turn assists in diagnosis. The premise behind digital follow-up is that stable lesions are biologically indolent and thus of no concern, whereas some of the new and/ or changing lesions may prove to be melanomas. These initial melanomas, if followed over months to years, will eventually manifest enough atypical clinical criteria allowing for their discovery.
- There are several follow-up protocols including short-term follow-up after 3 months, intermediate-term follow-up after 6–12 months, and long-term monitoring over years.
- However, for patient compliance, the first follow-up visit after baseline documentation should be scheduled after 3 months, and then, depending on the situation, every 6–12 months.
- With the exception of nevi in childhood or young adolescence, any lesion in adults showing even subtle changes after 3 months' follow-up, or with asymmetric enlargement accompanied by significant structural changes after 6–12 months, should be excised.
- Equivocal nodular or blue lesions must never be followed up but should be immediately excised at the time of visit. This is because, in the case of melanoma, the tumor will be already invasive, and even a 3 months' delay may worsen the prognosis.
- Growing nevi in childhood or young adolescence are characterized by a peripheral rim of globules or by peripheral streaks in the case of flat evolving pigmented Spitz/Reed nevi. When performing digital follow-up, it should be kept in mind that these nevi tend to enlarge symmetrically, the growth being at times accompanied by structural changes.

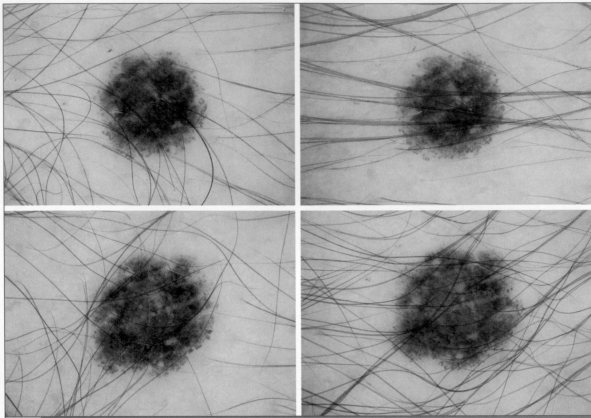

Fig. 309 Evolving nevus.

Evolving nevi are very common from puberty to middle age in people with numerous large acquired nevi and reveal a peripheral rim of globules. During follow-up, these nevi will symmetrically enlarge until the final disappearance of globules indicates stabilization of growth. These images come from a 25-year-old male, imaged every 6 months. Upper left is the baseline dermoscopic image, followed in the upper right and lower panels by images taken at 6, 12, and 18 months later. Follow-up after 6 months shows a minor, symmetric enlargement without significant structural changes (*upper right*). Follow-up of 12 months after baseline documentation shows a significant symmetric increase in size but no structural changes (*lower left*), while in the 18 month image the peripheral globules are beginning to disappear (*lower right*).

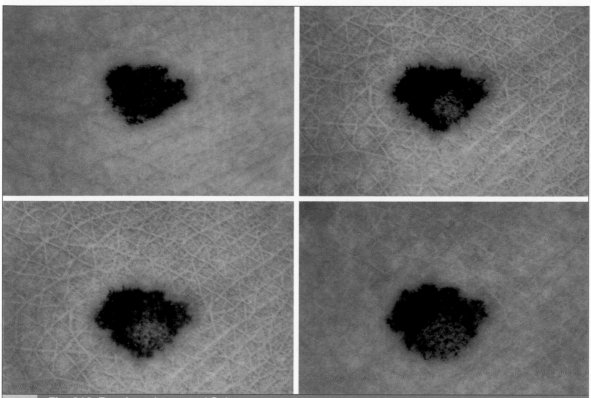

Fig. 310 Reed or pigmented Spitz nevus.

Reed nevi and pigmented Spitz nevi are rapidly growing nevi that may show a significant enlargement even after short-term follow-up of 3 months. Upper left: This baseline image of a pigmented Spitz nevus is located on the hand of an 8-year-old girl. Dermoscopically, it reveals a rather symmetric distribution of peripheral streaks. Upper right, lower left and right: Follow-up at intervals of 3 months shows more prominent streaks and a new blue-whitish zone. Digital follow-up of pigmented Spitz nevi could be considered optional in children, while excision is recommended after puberty.

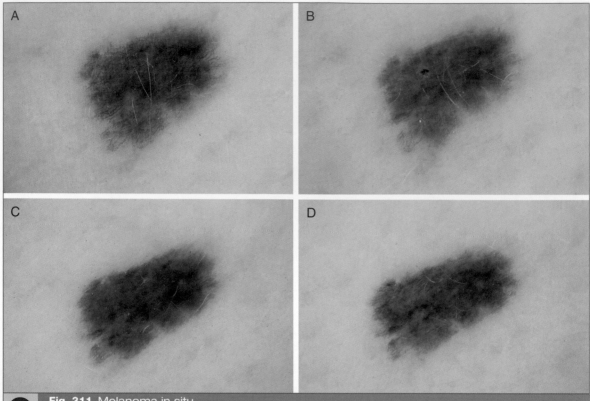

Fig. 311 Melanoma in situ.

This small melanoma is located on the leg of a 51-year-old woman with multiple nevi. The upper left image shows the melanoma at baseline, while the other images show the follow-up of the lesion every 3 months. Changes such as enlargement and darkening of the lesion and appearance of new structures such as irregular blotches can be seen. One problem of follow-up is that the size of the lesion can be influenced by the pressure and angle of the dermoscope on the skin. However, lesions that show structural changes, such as the new brown globules at the lower pole of the lesion in images C and D but not in A and B, after such short periods should always be excised.

Lesions with regression

General principles

- A bone-white color often represents scarring seen in regression.
- Do not confuse hypopigmentation with regression.
- A blue-white veil is a bluish ground glass–appearing area that can also be seen with regression.
- At times it is not possible to tell whether one is dealing with a white area of regression or a blue-white veil. These can now be diagnosed as blue-white structures.
- Blue-white structures are high-risk criteria seen in melanomas or Spitz nevi.
- Superficial spreading melanomas often have areas of regression.
- If even a hint of a blue-white structure is identified, it is better to err on the side of caution and make a histopathologic diagnosis.

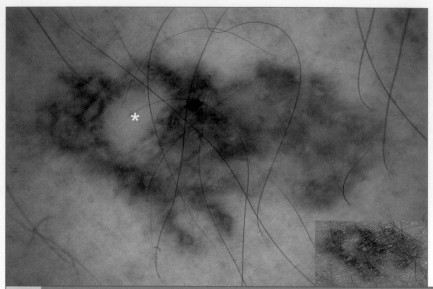

Fig. 312 Melanoma.

The white color in the left part of this lesion (*asterisk*) is slightly whiter than the surrounding skin; also adjacent to it are numerous blue structures corresponding to melanophages in the papillary dermis. Therefore by definition we interpret this as a regressive melanocytic proliferation. The significant asymmetry of color and structure points toward the diagnosis of a melanoma, and the beginner has to raise the red flag here. Histopathology revealed a superficial melanoma with focal regression.

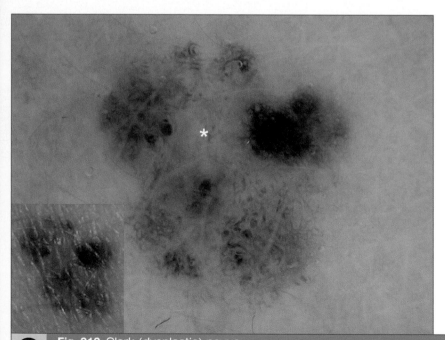

Fig. 313 Clark (dysplastic) nevus.

In contrast to Fig. 312, the light color (*asterisk*) is not light enough to be considered a regression area. However, there is clear-cut asymmetry in color and structure, and we raised the red flag and excised the lesion. Histopathology, however, showed only a Clark (dysplastic) nevus and not a superficial melanoma. This happens often, and the experienced dermoscopist knows very well that a linear correlation between dermoscopic and histopathologic dysplasia/atypia does not exist.

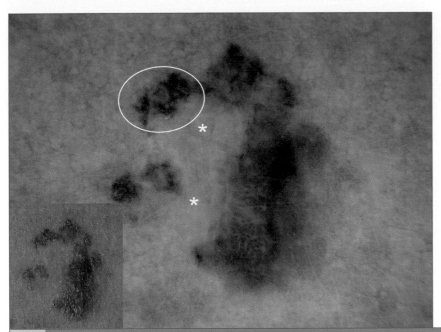

Fig. 314 Melanoma.

Asymmetry of color and structure—beware. There is a clearly evident white structure in the left part of this lesion (*asterisks*) corresponding to pronounced fibrosis in the papillary dermis histopathologically. In addition to the prominent asymmetry, there are remnants of an atypical pigment network (*circle*) visible at 11 o'clock. No doubt we raise the red flag and excise this regressive melanoma.

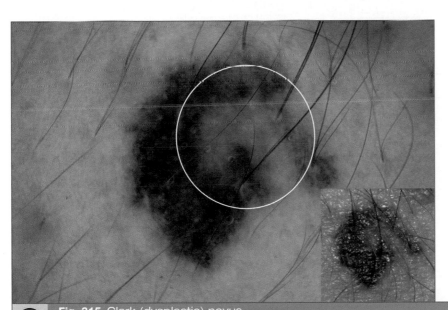

Fig. 315 Clark (dysplastic) nevus.

Is this a blue-whitish veil (*circle*) or a regression area characterized by white and blue areas representing fibrosis and melanosis? The asymmetry of this lesion is mostly due to this blue-white structure. A second pathologic opinion was requested when this was first diagnosed as a benign Clark (dysplastic) nevus. Always try to make a good dermoscopic-pathologic correlation. If there is divergence, get a second pathologic opinion. And remember, whatever the histopathologic diagnosis of this lesion will tell you, excision was the correct choice.

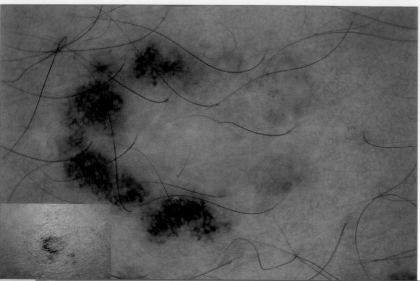

Fig. 316 Melanoma.

This slightly pinkish melanoma has a prominent central white structure extending to the upper right quadrant, which includes some peppering. This whitish area causes asymmetry of color and structure and, along with the rim of broadened pigment network from 6–12 o'clock, this lesion should be considered to be a melanoma until proven otherwise. Consequently, we raised the red flag.

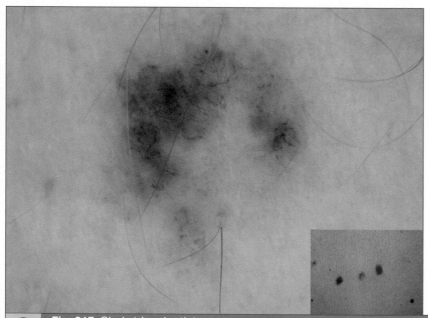

Fig. 317 Clark (dysplastic) nevus.

This only slightly asymmetric lesion is very difficult to diagnose. Although there are zones with white structures and also a few subtle granular blue-gray areas (also called peppering) in the upper left quadrant and center, the overall impression of this lesion is a benign regressive melanocytic proliferation, as no other melanoma-specific dermoscopic criteria can be found. Still we raised the red flag and performed a diagnostic excision. However, we did not challenge the diagnosis of a benign Clark (dysplastic) nevus.

Flat lesions on the face

General principles

- The clinical appearance and initial "gut" impressions should not be ignored when evaluating flat brown lesions on the head and neck.
- Do not confuse the follicular ostia of a melanocytic lesion with the milia-like cysts of a seborrheic keratosis. Many times you will not be able to tell the difference.

- Do not expect to see "classic" site-specific criteria. If there is a possible site-specific criterion, then consider it to be one.
- Many high-risk lesions on the head and neck area are relatively featureless. Look for subtle high-risk clues such as different shades of color asymmetrically located in the lesion.

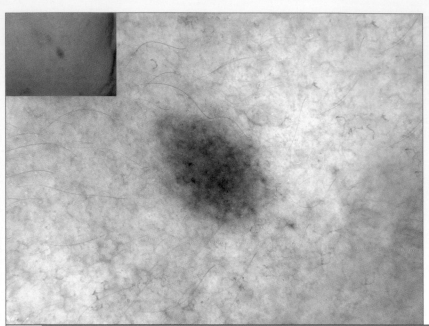

Fig. 318 Lentigo maligna on the cheek.

Are any site-specific, melanoma-specific criteria visible here? There are few asymmetrically pigmented follicular openings, no annular-granular structures, and no clear-cut rhomboidal structures. There are the beginnings of a gray pseudonetwork. The asymmetry of different shades of brown and gray color is another clue for this early type of lentigo maligna. Flat lesions on the face can now be diagnosed with confidence by reflectance confocal microscopy, providing a quasi-histological resolution. We raised the red flag here and performed a shave biopsy, which confirmed the diagnosis.

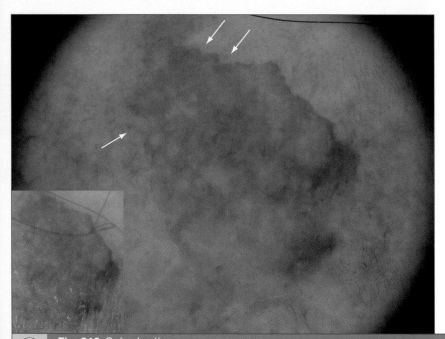

Fig. 319 Solar lentigo.

Is this a melanocytic or a nonmelanocytic lesion? There are no site-specific, melanoma-specific criteria present. However, there is a slight asymmetry of different shades of brown and gray. The concavity of the border's "moth-eaten" appearance (*arrows*) and the so-called jelly sign (brownish pigmentation appearing as a smear at the periphery of the lesion) are a clue to the correct diagnosis of solar lentigo. Because of the asymmetry in shape and color, the orange flag was raised and a diagnostic shave biopsy was performed.

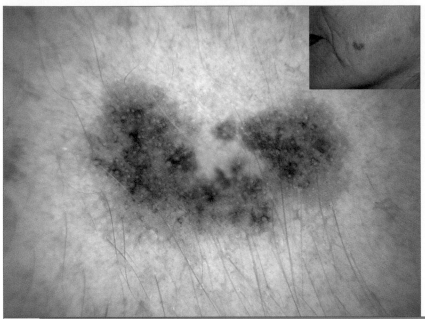

Fig. 320 Flat seborrheic keratosis.

This image shows asymmetry of color and structure with two site-specific, melanoma-specific criteria—asymmetrically pigmented follicular openings (for example, at 2 and 5 o'clock) and annular-granular structures at 8 o'clock. In this case, these high-risk criteria that led us to excise the lesion turned out to be a false positive.

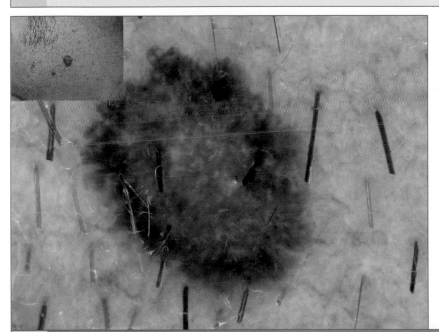

Fig. 321 Seborrheic keratosis.

This rather heavily pigmented lesion shows asymmetry of color and structure and a suggestion of rhomboidal structures around the periphery, which could also be interpreted as so-called fat finger-like structures. In addition, the hint of milia-like cysts in the upper center of the lesion allows the provisional diagnosis of a seborrheic keratosis. Because this lesion is clearly elevated, the differential diagnosis is lentigo maligna melanoma, so diagnostic biopsy is required.

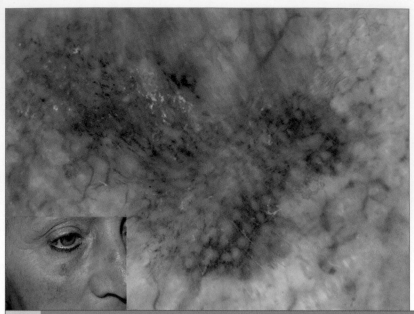

Fig. 322 Lichen planus-like keratosis.

It is necessary to develop a differential diagnosis for all dermoscopic criteria, and such knowledge is needed for difficult-to-diagnose lesions like this. There are multiple bluish dots and globules in the upper left pole of the lesion and near the periphery from 1–6 o'clock. They are annular-granular structures made up of melanophages. Melanophages can be seen in melanocytic, nonmelanocytic, benign, or malignant lesions. The differential diagnoses here include a lichen planus–like keratosis, a pigmented actinic keratosis, and a lentigo maligna. If reflectance confocal microscopy is not available, we recommend a diagnostic shave biopsy.

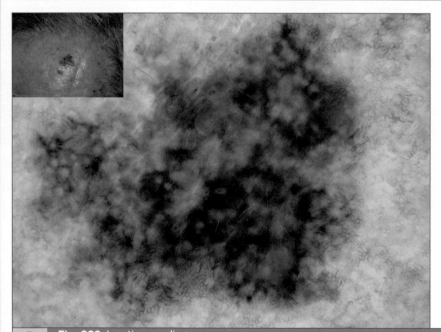

Fig. 323 Lentigo maligna.

This solitary heavily pigmented lesion on the forehead shows numerous classical rhomboidal structures particularly in its lower half. No doubt that the dermoscopically prominent asymmetry in color and structure here will lead even the novice to the diagnosis of lentigo maligna. Raise the red flag!

Nodular lesions on the face

General principles

- The differential diagnosis of pigmented and nonpigmented nodules on the face includes melanocytic, nonmelanocytic, benign, and malignant lesions. Quite often, the clinical appearance is nonspecific, and dermoscopy will help in making a clinical diagnosis.
- Nodules often have ridges and fissures. Do not confuse pigmentation in the fissures with an atypical pigment network.

- A macular component to a nodular lesion should raise the index of suspicion that the lesion could be high risk.
- A soft compressible nodule that can be easily moved from side to side favors low-risk pathology. Do not hesitate to palpate or squash lesions down and move them from side with the instrumentation used.
- The main differential diagnosis for nodular lesions on the face are nevi and basal cell carcinomas. Nodular melanoma is rarely found in this area. Do not forget squamous cell carcinomas including keratoacanthomas.

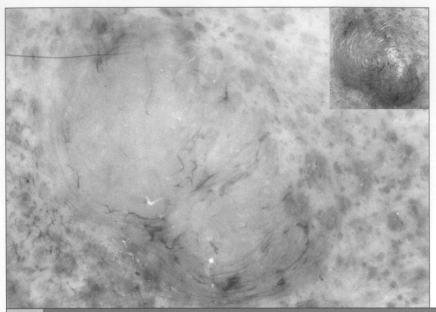

Fig. 324 Basal cell carcinoma.

A pigment network, dots and globules, and streaks are not seen, so consider this to be a nonmelanocytic lesion. Some nevi can have this dermoscopic picture but are usually soft and can be easily moved from side to side. Clinically this looks like a basal cell carcinoma. There are some larger vessels, but they are not the stereotypical arborizing ones. Rarely amelanotic melanoma looks like this.

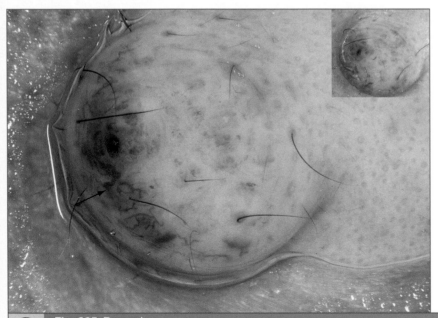

Fig. 325 Dermal nevus.

Pink color—beware. Soft, movable lesion—relax. Although there are definite arborizing vessels (*arrow*), the history and soft nodule point to benign pathology. If in doubt, cut it out. N.B. hairs are virtually never seen in a basal cell carcinoma.

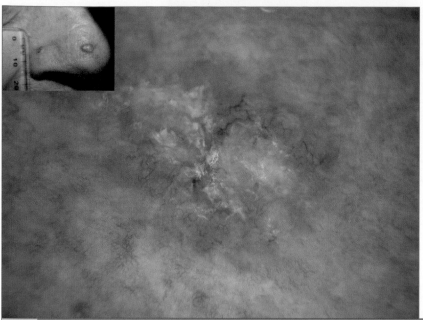

Fig. 326 Basal cell carcinoma.

In some cases, the clinico-dermoscopic correlation is crucial for the diagnosis. In this example, the pearly appearance of the nodule in the clinical image is very suspicious for a basal cell carcinoma. Closer scrutiny with dermoscopy reveals subtle but sharply in-focus arborizing vessels, allowing us to make the diagnosis of a basal cell carcinoma with confidence. The numerous scales in the center of the dermoscopic image make this diagnosis more difficult, pointing to the differential diagnosis of actinic keratosis.

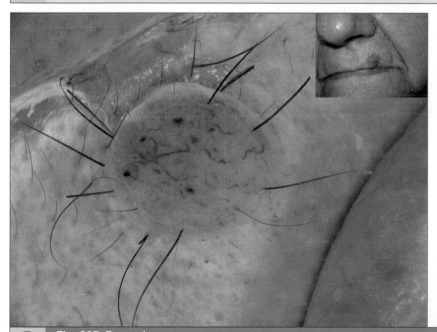

Fig. 327 Dermal nevus.

This is another example of the importance of clinico-dermoscopic correlation for diagnosing. The lesion in question is clearly a benign dermal nevus (Miescher nevus), characterized clinically by a dome-shaped smooth surface and numerous intra-lesional hairs. Dermoscopically, the not-in-focus arborizing vessels can lead the novice astray to the diagnosis of a nodular basal cell carcinoma. The few dark brown to black globules throughout the lesion most likely represent pigmented hair follicles.

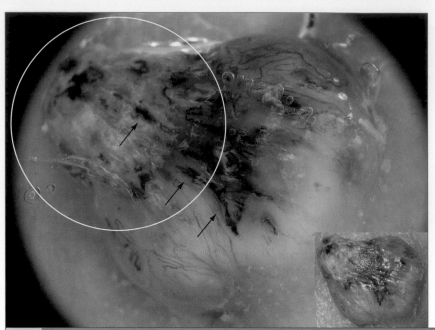

Fig. 328 Keratoacanthoma.

This nodular lesion clearly reveals a keratotic area (*circle*) and numerous dark-red to black streaks (*arrows*) simply representing hemorrhage. The clearly visible vessels display neither the characteristic arborizing architecture of nodular basal cell carcinomas nor the dotted or irregular linear vessels found in melanomas. The diffuse whitish coloration around the vessels favors a keratinocytic proliferation, and because of the overall asymmetry, we recommend raising the red flag here. The histopathologic diagnosis was keratoacanthoma, a distinct type of keratinocytic lesion that is interpreted nowadays by most (but not all!) pathologists as a specific variant of squamous cell carcinoma.

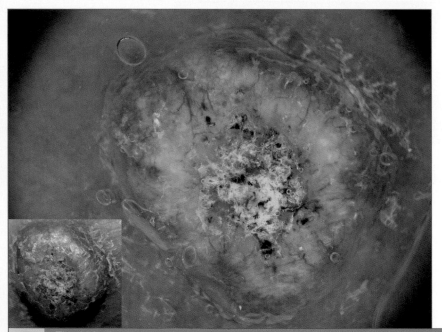

Fig. 329 Keratoacanthoma.

This lesion looks worrisome despite its relative symmetry of color and structure. There is a prominent central keratotic plug, and both a whitish and pinkish coloration can be seen. The vessels are not pathognomonic and together with the keratotic plug rule out a nodular melanoma and a nodular basal cell carcinoma with a high level of confidence. Raise the red flag and excise this lesion under the working diagnosis of keratoacanthoma or squamous cell carcinoma. Most pathologists will call the lesion squamous cell carcinoma, keratoacanthoma type.

Acral lesions

General principles

- Asymmetry of color and structure—rule out melanoma.
- Parallel ridge pattern = melanoma.
- Parallel furrow pattern = nevus.
- Lattice-like and fibrillar patterns = benign nevi.
- Purple color and variations of red color = blood.
- Blood can be found in nail apparatus and acral lentiginous melanomas; therefore, if blood is seen, always search for melanoma-specific criteria.

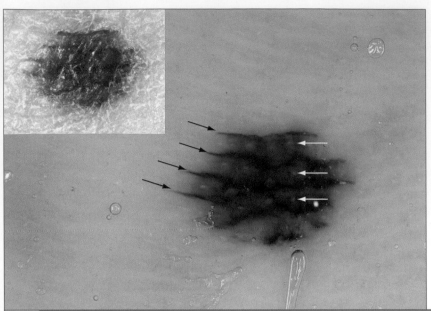

Fig. 330 Nevus.

Parallel ridge? Parallel furrow? The linear darker brown color is pigmentation in the furrows (*black arrows*). White dots, the "string of pearls" (*white arrows*), are always in the ridges. There is also a blue-white structure in the center of the lesion. Err on the side of caution and do a biopsy, and the dermoscopist will feel more confident the next time he or she sees a nevus that looks like this.

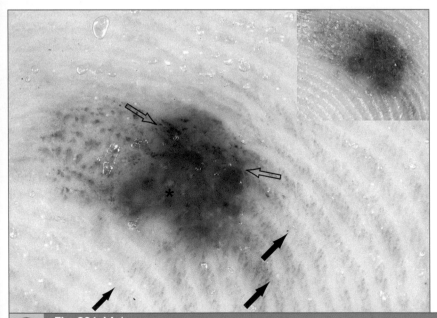

Fig. 331 Melanoma.

This lesion shows the parallel ridge pattern (*solid arrows*). There is also asymmetry of color and structure, atypical dots and globules (*open arrows*), and a blue-white structure (*asterisk*). This is a melanoma until proven otherwise.

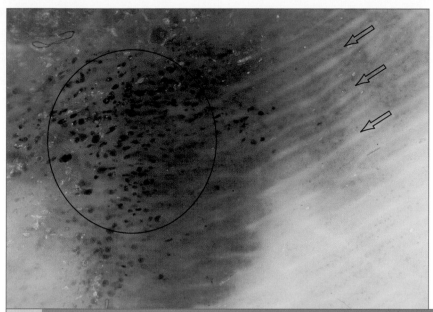

Fig. 332 Melanoma.

Parallel ridge? Parallel furrow? The string-of-pearls white dots of the sweat duct pores cannot be seen clearly, but this is the high-risk parallel ridge (*arrows*) pattern. If the dermoscopist is not sure what to do, the irregular dots and globules (*circle*) are worrisome enough by themselves to warrant a biopsy.

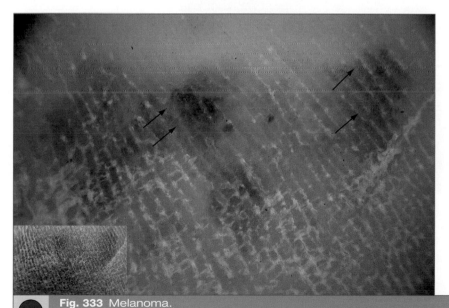

Fig. 333 Melanoma.

Parallel ridge? Parallel furrow? Does this look like the parallel furrow pattern of a benign nevus? Because of the scaly surface, the exact location of the parallel pigmented bands is difficult to determine. Closer scrutiny, however, reveals that the parallel pigmented bands (*arrows*) are separated only by thin whitish lines. The brownish color does not support at all hemorrhage or a vascular lesion. Despite the overall very subtle appearance of this lesion, we have to raise the red flag. Histopathology confirmed a melanoma in situ.

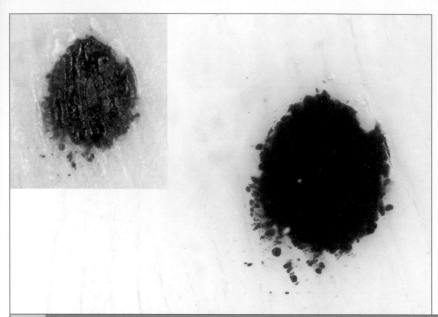

Fig. 334 Subcorneal hemorrhage.

Is the color here black or purple? It is purplish and amorphous (structureless); therefore it is blood. Take a needle and poke some out. Needling is a simple test to confirm that one is dealing with blood. Another clue that this is blood is the purplish dots adjacent to the lesion.

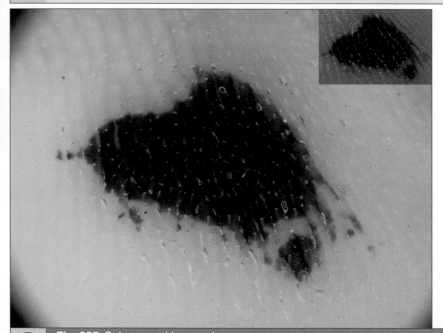

Fig. 335 Subcorneal hemorrhage.

This is the color of blood, but with a distinct pattern. Parallel ridge? Parallel furrow? Check the surrounding skin. Ridges are thicker than furrows. The blood is in both. The ridges are the darker lines. If unconvinced, needle out some of the dried blood. Take into consideration that usually your patients will not recall a trauma. Otherwise they would not seek your advice.

Pigmented lesions of the nails

General principles

- Dermoscopy makes the nail apparatus clearer.
- Nail-apparatus melanoma (NAM) accounts for 1–2% of melanomas in the lighter-skinned population and 15–20% of melanomas in darker-skinned people.
- Amelanotic NAM exists, so pink color—beware.

- High-risk dermoscopic criteria suggestive of NAM include asymmetry of color and structure, irregular pigmented bands, irregular blotches, irregular dots and globules, and Hutchinson's sign.
- Blood can be found in NAM, so look for high-risk criteria if you find blood in the nail.
- The chance of finding high-risk pathology in the pediatric population is low; therefore, a worrisome history might be more important than a high-risk dermoscopic appearance.

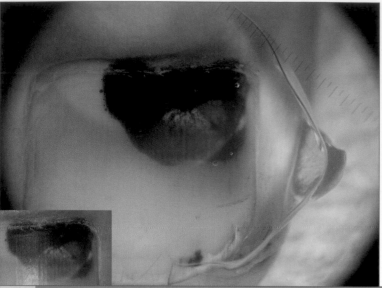

Fig. 336 Subungual hemorrhage.

This is a stereotypical example of a subungual hemorrhage (or subungual hematoma) characterized by a dark-red to black diffuse blotch revealing the color of dried blood. In addition, there is a tiny blotch at the distal end of the nail plate. Even if this patient cannot recall some form of trauma to the nail, we confidently raise the green flag here. Often, simple questions about hiking, other physical activities, or new shoes will prompt the patient to remember a potential trauma.

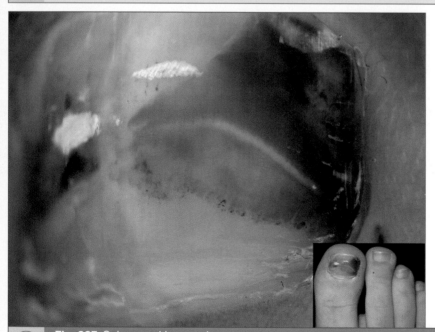

Fig. 337 Subungual hemorrhage.

This image shows another variation of the morphology seen with subungual hemorrhage. The purple color is important, and in this example we see several shades of red as well. The whitish areas are clearly related to the nature of the trauma. The hemorrhage is well demarcated and relatively structureless. We also see similarly colored dots and globules within the homogenous areas. We raise the green flag and can reassure the patient that this is not a subungual melanoma.

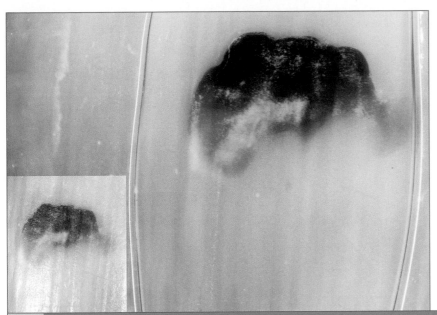

Fig. 338 Subungual hemorrhage.

The dark dried blood in this nail is well demarcated, featureless, and in the middle of the nail plate. It is growing out. Follow patients carefully to avoid missing subungual melanoma masquerading as blood.

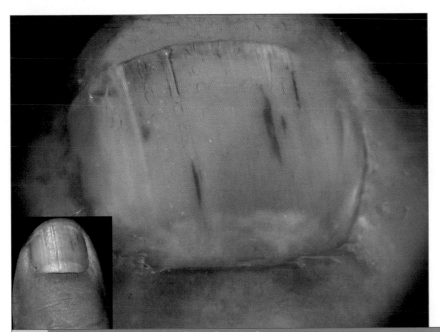

Fig. 339 Subungual splinter hemorrhage.

There are many faces of nail-apparatus hemorrhage. Clinico-dermoscopic correlations will lead us here in the correct direction, that these splinter hemorrhages are traumatically induced in a blue-collar worker. It is not a nail unit melanoma because the longitudinal striae do not extend the full length of the nail. Splinter hemorrhage can also occur in patients with endocarditis.

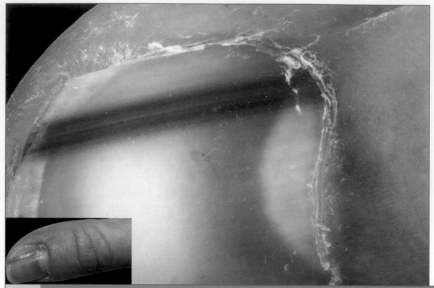

Fig. 340 Nail unit nevus.

The history of this lesion, age, and ethnicity of the patient needs to be considered together with the dermoscopic picture before deciding on the management of nail-apparatus pigmentation. In this case, there is rather uniform color and uniform linearity of the bands—a benign feature in most cases. As a rule, we recommend follow-up every six months in persons with linear nail pigmentation, particularly in cases that are not clear cut.

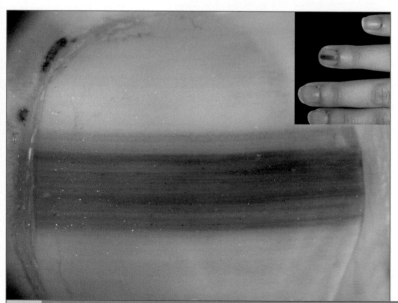

Fig. 341 Nail unit melanoma.

Even in a young patient, this broad pigmented band composed of many multicolored lines running the whole length of the nail are correlated with high-risk pathology. The different widths of the lines are a subtle additional feature for a nail unit melanoma. This is a stereotypical example of a high-risk nail-apparatus dermoscopic picture. Note the blotchy and multicolored pigmentation of the nail cuticle—a positive Hutchinson's sign.

Mucosal lesions

General principles

- Most pigmented lesions on mucosal surfaces are low risk.
- Determine whether the lesion is black, brown, blue, or red.
- Red-blue color—nonmelanocytic.
- Brown-black color—melanocytic.
- If a pigmented skin lesion looks worrisome clinically, shows asymmetry of color and structure, and has melanoma-specific criteria, it does not matter where on the body it is located. These criteria are high risk and warrant a histopathologic diagnosis.

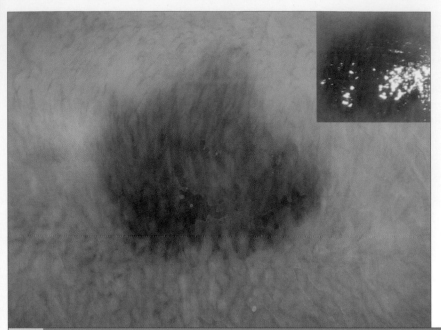

Fig. 342 Labial lentigo.

This pigmented lesion on the lower lip is characterized by curvilinear pigmented lines in the upper half and a reticular pattern in the lower half. There are two shades of brown. Carefully we raised the orange flag and recommended a diagnostic shave biopsy or a short-term follow-up to reassure no major changes. Histopathology then confirmed the diagnosis of a benign labial lentigo.

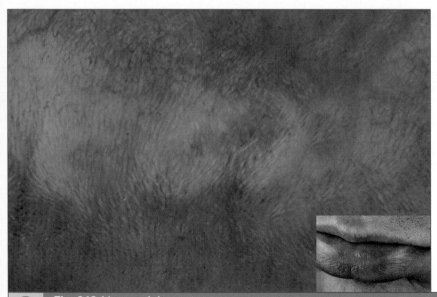

Fig. 343 Venous lake.

This is a stereotypical venous lake on the upper lip with a homogeneous purplish-blue color. The bluish clinical appearance may mislead novices, but once the lesion has been squashed down easily and the color disappears, the patient can be reassured that this is benign.

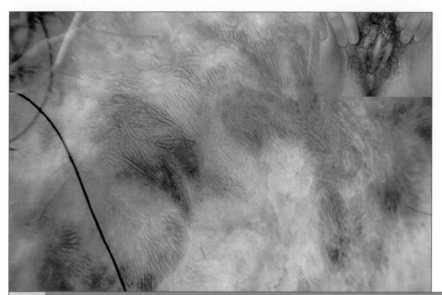

Fig. 344 Melanotic labial macules of the vulva.

This pigmented lesion was present on the superior part of the introitus vaginae of a 46-year-old woman. She just recently noticed the lesions and could not recall how long they were there. Dermoscopy reveals the characteristic features of a labial melanotic macule (or labial lentigo), characterized by numerous parallel and curvilinear brownish lines reminiscent of fingerprints. No melanoma-specific dermoscopic criteria were noted. Still, we performed a punch biopsy that confirmed the benign diagnosis and recommended annual follow-up visits.

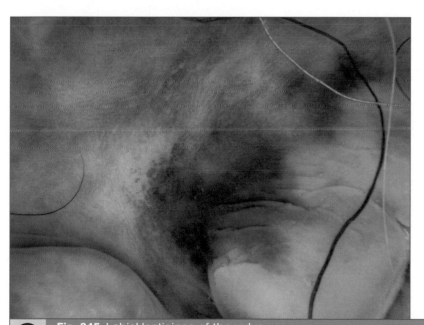

Fig. 345 Labial lentigines of the vulva.

This 75-year-old woman presented with several, confluent bluish-black macules and patches on the vulva and was concerned about a tendency of growth. Dermoscopically, a prominent asymmetry in shape and color was observed and also blue areas and a grayish hue became evident. No doubt that we raised the red flag here; however, we recommended punch biopsies from two or three patches to obtain a presurgical diagnosis. The histopathologic examination revealed features of benign labial lentigines of the vulva with a slight increase of melanocytes at the dermo-epidermal junction. Regular follow-up of patients such as this is crucial.

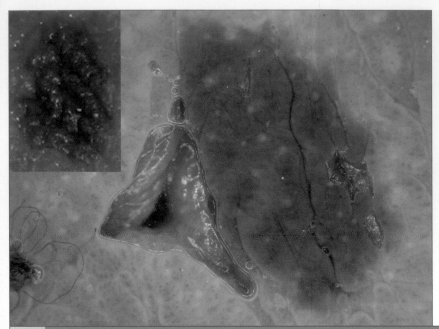

Fig. 346 Genital nevus.

This 15-year-old girl presented with a rather large, darkly pigmented lesion on her vulva with a stable clinical course. Dermoscopy exhibits a homogeneous brown-gray coloration with few intermingled whitish-yellowish dots. The latter can be observed also in the surrounding normal skin and represent sebaceous glands. Because of the bland history and the prominent homogeneous pattern, we recommend annual follow-up.

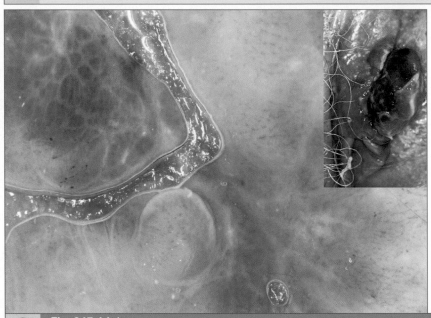

Fig. 347 Melanoma.

This is a melanoma of the vulva. No other diagnosis should come to mind on seeing this clinical and dermoscopic picture. This large asymmetrical lesion shows blue-white structures and irregular dots and globules.

Differential diagnostic value of blood vessels

General principles

- Blood vessels can be seen in melanocytic, nonmelanocytic, benign, and malignant lesions.
- Vessels can be seen with other criteria, or vessels may be the only criterion found in a lesion.
- Some vessels are associated with high-risk pathology and others with low-risk pathology.
- Pink lesions with vessels may be melanocytic, nonmelanocytic, benign, or malignant. The shape of the vessels may provide a clue to the correct diagnosis.

Melanocytic lesions

- Dermal nevi—comma-shaped vessels.
- Clark (dysplastic) nevi—comma-shaped and dotted vessels.
- Melanoma—dots and irregular linear vessels or milky-red areas.

Nonmelanocytic lesions

- Basal cell carcinoma—thick branching (arborizing) vessels.
- Seborrheic keratosis—hairpin vessels.
- Bowen's disease—small foci of dotted vessels that look like glomeruli in the kidney.

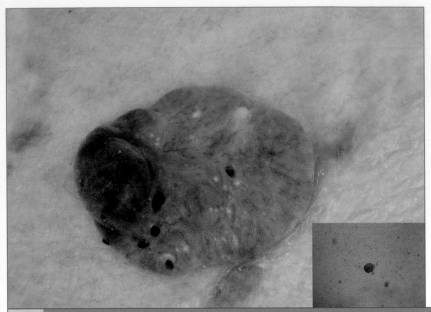

Fig. 348 Dermal nevus.

The correct diagnosis for this papillomatous dermal nevus is based on clinico-dermoscopic correlation and confirmed by the shape of the vessels. They are comma shaped. A few comedo-like openings and milia-like cysts are also present and an expected finding in papillomatous nevi. Do not confuse these vessels with the larger branching vessels seen in a basal cell carcinoma.

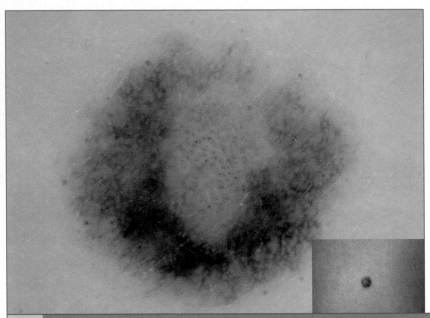

Fig. 349 Clark (dysplastic) nevus.

This lesion has a pigment network and a few dots and globules around the periphery; therefore, it is a melanocytic lesion. There is a combination of a few comma-shaped and many dotted vessels in the center of the lesion. This is an unusual Cark (dysplastic) nevus, and therefore we have excised this lesion.

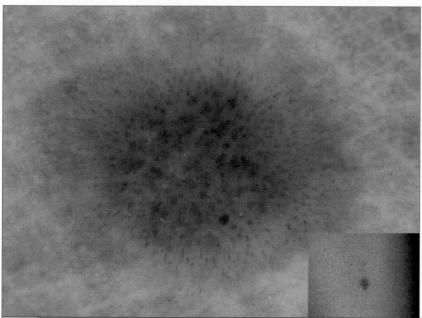

Fig. 350 Spitz nevus.

This pinkish lesion lacks pigmentation. Remember pink color—beware, so it could be high risk. It is a stereotypical example of a nonpigmented Spitz nevus with numerous large dotted vessels evenly distributed throughout the center of the lesion. Around the periphery are more linear irregular vessels. The color in this lesion is strikingly pink. Milky-red color dotted and linear irregular vessels are a high-risk pattern that can be seen in nonpigmented Spitz nevi and melanoma, so we raise a red flag here. It is not always possible to differentiate Spitz nevi from melanoma. A diagnostic excision with a margin of 5 mm is indicated to rule out an amelanotic melanoma.

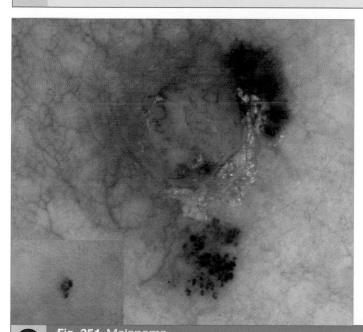

Fig. 351 Melanoma.

This lesion displays striking asymmetry of brown-gray-blue globules at 5–6 o'clock, streaks at 1–2 o'clock, and a central pinkish nodule (*circle*) characterized by polymorphic vessels, including linear irregular and hairpin vessels, underpinning the diagnosis of melanoma. The overall irregularity and vascular pattern visible here is not compatible with the diagnosis of a seborrheic keratosis or a basal cell carcinoma.

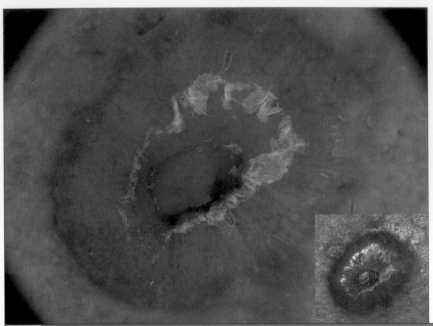

Fig. 352 Melanoma.

This is a rather dramatic "featureless" amelanotic melanoma with a delicate gray-brownish peripheral ring. This ring as well as the paracentral scaling has no diagnostic significance at all. Overall the lesion is raised and shows a milky-red color with fine irregular linear vessels. Milky-red color—beware!

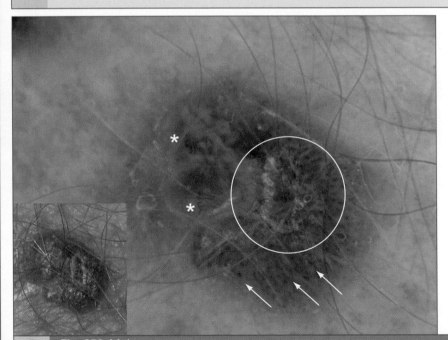

Fig. 353 Melanoma.

A keratotic area (*circle*) does not make this a seborrheic keratosis, nor does it rule out a melanoma. Dotted (*arrows*) and irregular linear vessels (*asterisks*) are usually not seen within a seborrheic keratosis. Dotted vessels and linear-irregular vessels are the most common combination of vascular pattern in melanoma, and a red flag must be always raised.

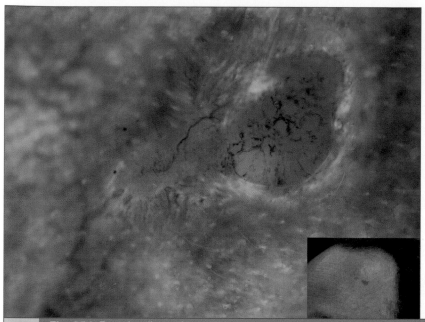

Fig. 354 Basal cell carcinoma.

This is a commonly seen basal cell carcinoma without pigment. The blood vessels, which are thick and branching, point to the correct diagnosis, although this is not the most exciting example of arborizing vessels. The vessels are superficial and are therefore in focus. If the vessels are deeper in the lesion, they would be blurred and out of focus. If so, think amelanotic melanoma.

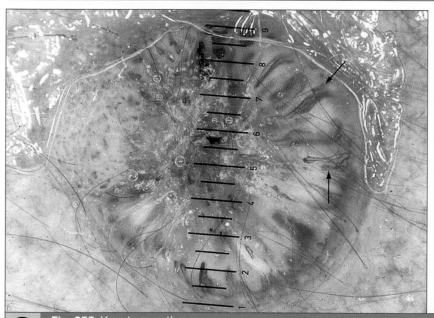

Fig. 355 Keratoacanthoma.

If there could be one, then this is a classic keratoacanthoma with hairpin-shaped vessels (*arrows*) and a white background. The white color is not always scarring seen with regression but in this case represents hyperkeratosis seen in keratinizing tumors. White color can be seen in melanocytic, nonmelanocytic, benign, and malignant lesions. The central crust plus the history and clinical appearance all help in determining the management of this lesion.

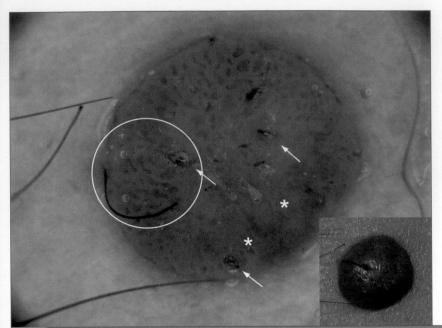

Fig. 356 Seborrheic keratosis.

This is an irritated, smoothly polished seborrheic keratosis. Note that only few comedo-like openings (*arrows*) are visible. The gray color (*asterisks*) represents pigmentary incontinence probably secondary to inflammation and gives this lesion a worrisome look. Numerous hairpin vessels (not exclusively within the circle) can be identified and are suggestive for a seborrheic keratosis. Still, we raised the orange flag and performed a diagnostic shave biopsy.

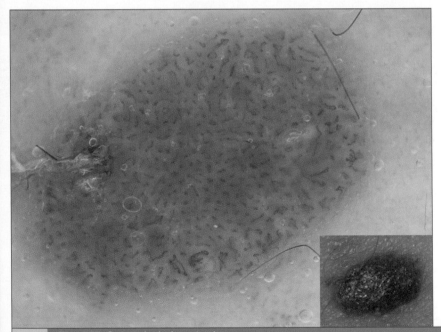

Fig. 357 Seborrheic keratosis.

This is another example of a rather unusual nonpigmented seborrheic keratosis characterized by numerous dotted, linear irregular, and some hairpin-shaped vessels. Such a polymorphic vascular pattern may well be observed also in an amelanotic melanoma. So we raised the orange flag and were happy to hear that histopathologically this lesion only represented an acanthotic type of seborrheic keratosis as we originally suspected.

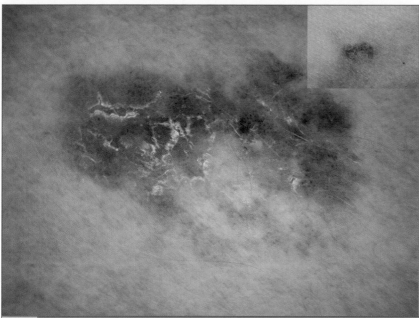

Fig. 358 Bowen disease.

Pigmented Bowen disease is a difficult clinical and dermoscopic diagnosis to make. Here we see well-circumscribed round areas of red dotted vessels in combination with scales, and several clusters of brownish and a few gray dots in the pigmented area of the lesion.

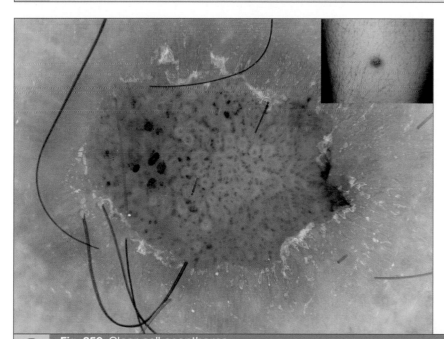

Fig. 359 Clear cell acanthoma.

Clinically, a nodular pink lesion with superficial ulceration surrounded by a brownish rim is highly suspicious for hypomelanotic nodular melanoma. However, dermoscopy reveals classical features of a clear cell acanthoma, composed of strings of pearls in a characteristic polygonal pattern. Based on these dermoscopic features, the diagnosis of clear cell acanthoma nowadays can be made with confidence.

Amelanotic and partially pigmented melanoma

General principles

- Amelanotic or hypomelanotic melanomas often present clinically unequivocal.
- The history of growth or change is of uppermost importance.
- Use the EGF rule: *E*levated *F*irm *G*rowing lesions are suspicious.
- Study carefully the vessels in pink lesions.
- Vessels are in many cases the only clue for the correct diagnosis.
- The dermoscopic examination of amelanotic or hypomelanotic lesions should follow a stepwise algorithm assessing the morphology of the vascular pattern, the architectural arrangement of vessels, and the presence of additional dermoscopic criteria.

- Dotted and linear irregular vessels are suggestive of melanomas or, in more general terms, two or more different morphologic types of vessels should raise your suspicion for a melanoma.
- Many amelanotic and hypomelanotic melanomas display atypical, polymorphic vessels.
- The arrangement of vessels in amelanotic or hypomelanotic melanomas is asymmetric and irregular.
- Frequently you find remnants of pigmentation in amelanotic melanomas (of course, then the term "hypomelanotic melanoma" is more appropriate).
- Search for residual pigment network structures, brown or blue blotches, and/or brown, gray, or black dots/globules.
- Histopathology is obligatory in lesions displaying dotted, linear irregular, or polymorphic vessels or exhibiting a milky-red color.

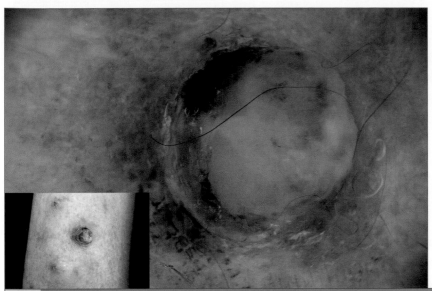

Fig. 360 Melanoma.

By default, this is a melanocytic lesion because it lacks criteria for any other lesion such as a basal cell carcinoma or squamous cell carcinoma. Don't be led astray by the history of a recent trauma and call this a pyogenic granuloma. There are large white blotches and pink and dark brown to black hues. There is also asymmetry of color and structure, with dark irregular botches at 10–12 o'clock and irregular streaks at 7–8 o'clock. There are also dotted vessels in the upper pole of the lesion. An ulcerated nodular lesion like this one always needs to be excised urgently.

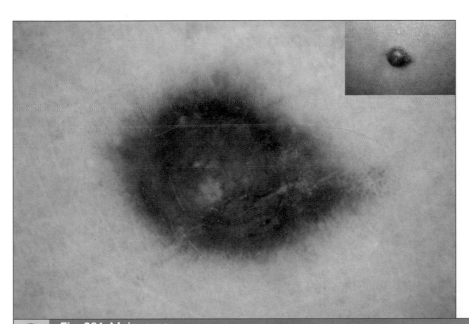

Fig. 361 Melanoma.

Based on the clinical appearance of this pinkish nodule with a peripheral rim of pigmentation, the differential diagnoses include a dermatofibroma, a desmoplastic nevus, or an amelanotic melanoma. Sometimes dermoscopy does not provide the expected ultimate answer. There are some subtle irregular linear vessels in the center of the lesion and there is a prominent grayish ring around the central red area, but these criteria are not really diagnostic. Still, pink color—beware. And never monitor a nodular lesion if you are not 100% sure about its benign nature.

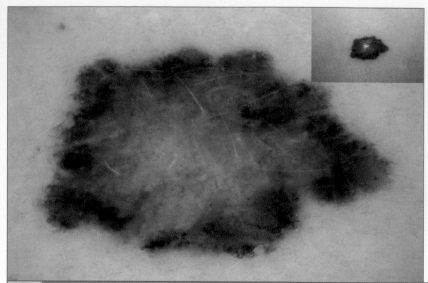

Fig. 362 Melanoma.

This is a clear-cut example of a melanoma clinically and dermoscopically. The central hypopigmented nodule of this melanoma should not be confused with the central white patch of a dermatofibroma. The broad peripheral rim of pigmentation is characterized by areas with a broadened pigment network, irregular streaks, and brownish to black dots.

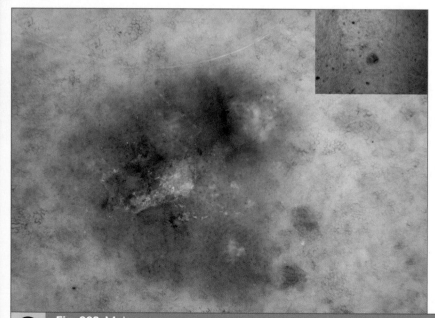

Fig. 363 Melanoma.

This is a subtle and difficult case. Pink color—beware. Is this an ugly duckling lesion? Look to see if the patient has other similar lesions. It is less worrisome if so. The tiny red dots of the melanoma-specific vascular pattern at 4–6 o'clock can be seen. In addition, there are subtle gray areas present in several parts of the lesion. The grayish and pink colors in this lesion plus the dotted vascular pattern are sufficient clues to warrant diagnostic excision.

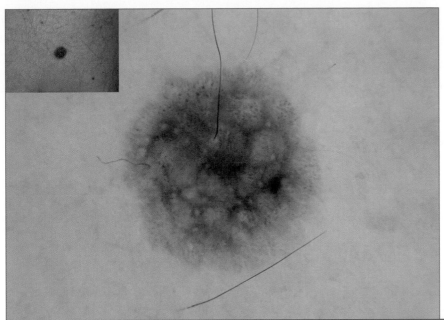

Fig. 364 Melanoma.

The differential diagnoses here include an irritated nevus or a hypomelanotic melanoma. This hypopigmented lesion is characterized dermoscopically by subtle asymmetry in color and structure, with irregularly scattered gray dots among the brown dots. Note the relatively pronounced pinkish coloration and dotted vessels clearly visible with dermoscopy. This lesion was excised and diagnosed histopathologically as superficial melanoma.

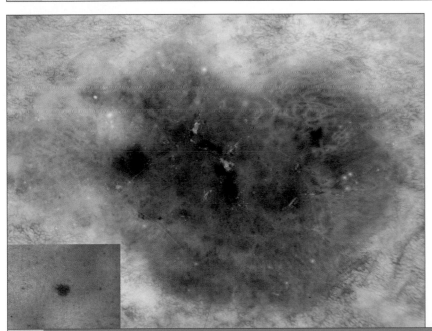

Fig. 365 Melanoma.

Based on clinico-dermoscopic correlation, there is no doubt that this is a high-risk lesion. Dermoscopically, there are several blue-gray areas embedded in a pinkish background coloration. The grayish blotch at 9 o'clock is clearly visible clinically. Theoretically, the differential diagnosis here represents an unusual combined nevus. Raise the red flag and act accordingly.

Dermoscopy tests

General principles

Several features such as scales, crusts, or inflammation may cause uncertainty in the dermoscopic diagnosis of skin lesions. On these occasions, simple dermoscopic tests may aid you to obtain the correct diagnosis.

Tape test

A nevus often raising concern is the so-called black or hypermelanotic nevus. The reason is its dark color and a more or less centrally located black blotch covering most of the nevus. The black blotch correlates histopathologically to pigmented parakeratosis of an otherwise conventional junctional nevus. Yet, this pigmented scale (or black blotch) can be easily removed by a tape or plaster, which allows the recognition of the underlying otherwise regular network. The tape test therefore facilitates the nevus diagnosis.

Scrape test

The differential diagnosis of acral lesions showing a parallel ridge pattern is between acral melanoma and subcorneal hemorrhage. In doubtful cases, the scrape test can be performed. Simply scrape the cornified layer with a scalpel, and if this scraping results in the removal of the pigment, a diagnosis of subcorneal hemorrhage can be made with confidence.

Blanching test

Clark nevi, particularly in subjects with fair skin types or when located on seborrheic areas of the trunk, may at times reveal erythema, which does not allow the proper recognition of the pigmented structures. In such a case, the blanching test by applying pressure on the nevus with the dermoscope may be helpful. This will result in the disappearance of the erythema, which in turn allows a better visualization of the pigmented structures.

The Wobble sign

During the dermoscopic examination of a nodular pigmented skin lesion, the dermoscope can be maintained fixed at the surface of the skin. If the device is slightly moved horizontally, parallel to the surface, a dynamic approach is added. The lesion sticks to the dermoscope and follows its movement. In the cases of papillomatous dermal nevi, the lesion follows the movement of the dermoscope, leaving back the surrounding skin. The static pattern of the nevus itself is dissociated, and deeper structures having a fleshy consistency seem to move under the superficial component. In contrast, melanoma tends to be firm and fixed to the skin and is therefore not easily moveable.

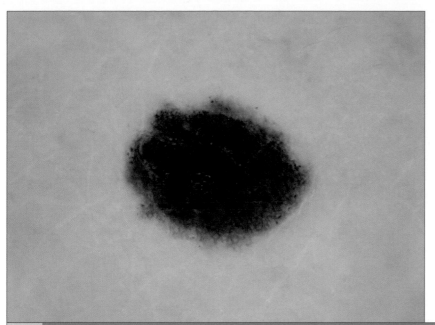

Fig. 366 Tape test.

This heavily hyperpigmented nevus, also called black nevus, is characterized by a centrally located dark black blotch covering large parts of the nevus.

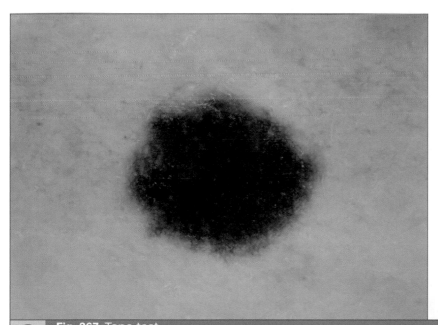

Fig. 367 Tape test.

The same nevus as shown in Fig. 366 after removal of the dark scale with tape. The regular pigmented network throughout the lesion is now much more evident.

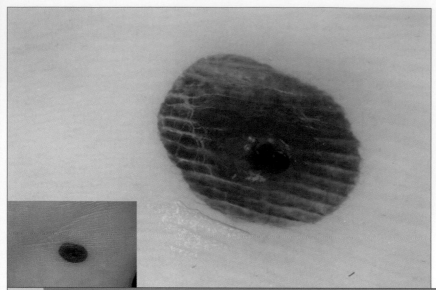

Fig. 368 Scrape test.

Subcorneal hemorrhage revealing a parallel ridge pattern. The sharp demarcation and red color already point toward the correct diagnosis.

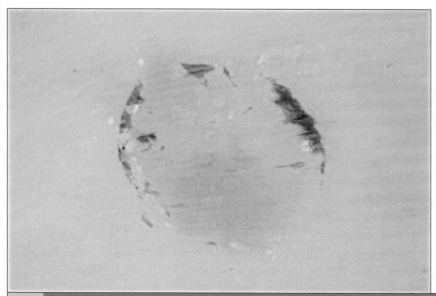

Fig. 369 Scrape test.

The same hemorrhage as seen in Fig. 368 just a few minutes later, after nearly complete removal of the blood with a scalpel.

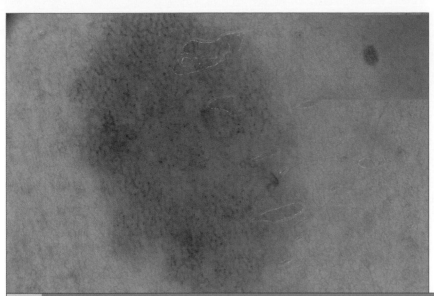

Fig. 370 Blanching test.

Dermoscopy of this pinkish Clark nevus reveals a background erythema, dotted vessels, and some shades of light-brown color.

Fig. 371 Blanching test.

The same nevus as seen in Fig. 370 under pressure. The erythema and dotted vessels have mostly disappeared and a regular light-brown network surrounding a central structureless area becomes visible.

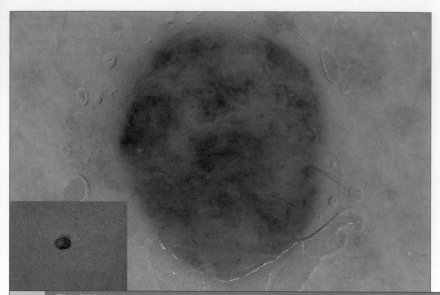

Fig. 372 Wobble sign.

Dermoscopic static view of a slightly papillomatous dermal nevus showing shades of brown and gray color and vascular patterns.

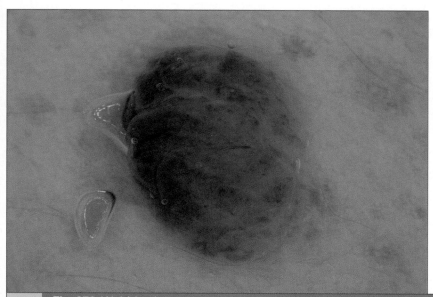

Fig. 373 Wobble sign.

Movement of the dermoscope allows the visualization of the right lateral base of the papillomatous dermal nevus.

Further reading

Akasu R, Sugiyama H, Araki M, et al. Dermatoscopic and videomicroscopic features of melanocytic plantar nevi. *Am J Dermatopathol.* 1996;18:10–18.

Altamura D, Avramidis M, Menzies SW. Assessment of the optimal interval for and sensitivity of short-term sequential digital dermoscopy monitoring for the diagnosis of melanoma. *Arch Dermatol.* 2008;144:502–506.

Altamura D, Menzies SW, Argenziano G, et al. Dermatoscopy of basal cell carcinoma: morphologic variability of global and local features and accuracy of diagnosis. *J Am Acad Dermatol.* 2010;62:67–75.

Alvarez Martinez D, Boehncke WH, Kaya G, et al. Recognition of early melanoma: a monocentric dermoscopy follow-up study comparing de novo melanoma with nevus-associated melanoma. *Int J Dermatol.* 2018;57:692–702.

Annessi G, Bono R, Abeni D. Correlation between digital epiluminescence microscopy parameters and histopathological changes in lentigo maligna and solar lentigo: a dermoscopic index for the diagnosis of lentigo maligna. *J Am Acad Dermatol.* 2017;76:234–243.

Arevalo A, Altamura D, Avramidis M, et al. The significance of eccentric and central hyperpigmentation, multifocal hyper/hypopigmentation, and the multicomponent pattern in melanocytic lesions lacking specific dermoscopic features of melanoma. *Arch Dermatol.* 2008;144:1440–1444.

Argenyi ZB. Dermoscopy (epiluminescence microscopy) of pigmented skin lesions. Current status and evolving trends. *Dermatol Clin.* 1997;15:79–95.

Argenziano G, Catricalà C, Ardigo M, et al. Seven-point checklist of dermoscopy revisited. *Br J Dermatol.* 2011;164:785–790.

Argenziano G, Fabbrocini G, Carli P, et al. Epiluminescence microscopy for the diagnosis of doubtful melanocytic skin lesions. Comparison of the ABCD rule of dermatoscopy and a new 7-point checklist based on pattern analysis. *Arch Dermatol.* 1998;134:1563–1570.

Argenziano G, Ferrara G, Francione S, et al. Dermoscopy—the ultimate tool for melanoma diagnosis. *Semin Cutan Med Surg.* 2009;28:142–148.

Argenziano G, Kittler H, Ferrara G, et al. Slow-growing melanoma: a dermoscopy follow-up study. *Br J Dermatol.* 2010;162:267–273.

Argenziano G, Mordente I, Ferrara G, et al. Dermoscopic monitoring of melanocytic skin lesions: clinical outcome and patient compliance vary according to follow-up protocols. *Br J Dermatol.* 2008;159:331–336.

Argenziano G, Puig S, Zalaudek I, et al. Dermoscopy improves accuracy of primary care physicians to triage lesions suggestive of skin cancer. *J Clin Oncol.* 2006;24:1877–1882.

Argenziano G, Scalvenzi M, Staibano S, et al. Dermatoscopic pitfalls in differentiating pigmented Spitz naevi from cutaneous melanomas. *Br J Dermatol.* 1999;141:788–793.

Argenziano G, Soyer HP, Chimenti S, et al. Dermoscopy of pigmented skin lesions: results of a consensus meeting via the internet. *J Am Acad Dermatol.* 2003;48:679–693.

Argenziano G, Soyer HP. Dermoscopy of pigmented skin lesions—a valuable tool for early diagnosis of melanoma. *Lancet Oncol.* 2001;2:443–449.

Argenziano G, Zalaudek I, Corona R, et al. Vascular structures in skin tumors: a dermoscopy study. *Arch Dermatol.* 2004;140:1485–1489.

Argenziano G, Zalaudek I, Ferrara G, et al. Proposal of a new classification system for melanocytic naevi. *Br J Dermatol.* 2007;157:217–227.

Argenziano G, Zalaudek I, Ferrara G, et al. Dermoscopy features of melanoma incognito: indications for biopsy. *J Am Acad Dermatol.* 2007;56:508–513.

Arzberger E, Curiel-Lewandrowski C, Blum A, et al. Teledermoscopy in high-risk melanoma patients: a comparative study of face-to-face and teledermatology visits. *Acta Derm Venereol.* 2016;96:779–783.

Bafounta ML, Beauchet A, Aegerter P, et al. Is dermoscopy (epiluminescence microscopy) useful for the diagnosis of melanoma? Results of a meta-analysis using techniques adapted to the evaluation of diagnostic tests. *Arch Dermatol.* 2001;137:1343–1350.

Bassoli S, Kyrgidis A, Ciardo S, et al. Uncovering the diagnostic dermoscopic features of flat melanomas located on the lower limbs. *Br J Dermatol.* 2018;178:e217–e218.

Bauer J, Metzler G, Rassner G, et al. Dermatoscopy turns histopathologists attention to the suspicious area in melanocytic lesions. *Arch Dermatol.* 2001;137:1338–1340.

Benvenuto-Andrade C, Dusza SW, Agero AL, et al. Differences between polarized light dermoscopy and immersion contact dermoscopy for the evaluation of skin lesions. *Arch Dermatol.* 2007;143:329–338.

Binder M, Puespoeck-Schwarz M, Steiner A, et al. Epiluminescence microscopy of small pigmented skin lesions: short-term formal training improves the diagnostic performance of dermatologists. *J Am Acad Dermatol.* 1997;36:197–202.

Binder M, Schwarz M, Winkler A, et al. Epiluminescence microscopy. A useful tool for the diagnosis of pigmented skin lesions for formally trained dermatologists. *Arch Dermatol.* 1995;131:286–291.

Biondo G, Gnone M, Sola S, et al. Dermoscopy of a Spark's nevus. *Dermatol Pract Concept.* 2018;8:126–128.

Boespflug A, Debarbieux S, Depaepe L, et al. Association of subungual melanoma and subungual squamous cell carcinoma: a case series. *J Am Acad Dermatol.* 2018;78:760–768.

Bollea-Garlatti LA, Galimberti GN, Galimberti RL. Lentigo Maligna: keys to dermoscopic diagnosis. *Actas dermosifiliogr.* 2016;107:489–497.

Bombonato C, Pampena R, Franceschini C, et al. Sclerosing nevus with pseudomelanomatous features: dermoscopic and confocal aspects. *J Eur Acad Dermatol Venereol.* 2019;33:525–532. https://doi.org/10.1111/jdv.15284.

Bories N, Dalle S, Debarbieux S, et al. Dermoscopy of fully regressive cutaneous melanoma. *Br J Dermatol.* 2008;158:1224–1229.

Borve A, Dahlen Gyllencreutz J, Terstappen K, et al. Smartphone teledermoscopy referrals: a novel process for improved triage of skin cancer patients. *Acta Derm Venereol.* 2015;95:186–190.

Bowling J, Argenziano G, Azenha A, et al. Dermoscopy key points: recommendations from the International Dermoscopy Society. *Dermatology.* 2007;214:3–5.

Braun RP, Gaide O, Oliviero M, et al. The significance of multiple blue-grey dots (granularity) for the dermoscopic diagnosis of melanoma. *Br J Dermatol.* 2007;157:907–913.

Braun RP, Rabinovitz HS, Kopf AW, et al. Pattern analysis. A two-step procedure for the dermoscopic diagnosis of melanoma. *Clin Dermatol.* 2002;20:236–239.

Braun RP, Rabinovitz H, Kopf AW, et al. Dermoscopic diagnosis of seborrheic keratosis. *Clin Dermatol.* 2002;20:270–272.

Braun RP, Rabinovitz H, Tzu JE, et al. Dermoscopy research—an update. *Semin Cutan Med Surg.* 2009;28:165–171.

Bruce AF, Mallow JA, Theeke LA. The use of teledermoscopy in the accurate identification of cancerous skin lesions in the adult population: a systematic review. *J Telemed Telecare.* 2018;24:75–83.

Carli P, de Giorgi V, Chiarugi A, et al. Addition of dermoscopy to conventional naked-eye examination in melanoma screening: a randomized study. *J Am Acad Dermatol.* 2004;50:683–689.

Carli P, De Giorgi V, Crocetti E, et al. Improvement of malignant/benign ratio in excised melanocytic lesions in the 'dermoscopy era': a retrospective study 1997–2001. *Br J Dermatol.* 2004;150:687–692.

Carli P, De Giorgi V, Giannotti B. Dermoscopy and early diagnosis of melanoma: the light and the dark. *Arch Dermatol.* 2001;137:1641–1644.

Carli P, De Giorgi V, Naldi L, et al. Reliability and inter-observer agreement of dermoscopic diagnosis of melanoma and melanocytic naevi. *Dermoscopy Panel. Eur J Cancer Prev.* 1998;7:397–402.

Carli P, Massi D, DeGiorgi V, et al. Clinically and dermoscopically featureless melanoma: when prevention fails. *J Am Acad Dermatol.* 2002;46:957–959.

Carrera C, Marchetti MA, Dusza SW, et al. Validity and reliability of dermoscopic criteria used to differentiate nevi from melanoma: a web-based International Dermoscopy Society study. *JAMA Dermatol.* 2016;152:798–806.

Carrera C, Marghoob AA. Discriminating nevi from melanomas: clues and pitfalls. *Dermatol Clin.* 2016;34:395–409.

Carrera C, Scope A, Dusza SW, et al. Clinical and dermoscopic characterization of pediatric and adolescent melanomas: multicenter study of 52 cases. *J Am Acad Dermatol.* 2018;78:278–288.

Carrera C, Segura S, Aquilera P, et al. Dermoscopic clues for diagnosing melanomas that resemble seborrheic keratosis. *JAMA Dermatol.* 2017;153:544–551.

Chatterjee M, Neema S. Dermoscopy of pigmentary disorders in brown skin. *Dermatol Clin.* 2018;36:473–485.

Coates SJ, Kvedar J, Granstein RD. Teledermatology: from historical perspective to emerging techniques of the modern era: part II: emerging technologies in teledermatology, limitations and future directions. *J Am Acad Dermatol.* 2015;72:577–586.

Conforti C, Giuffrida R, de Barros MH, et al. Dermoscopy of a single plaque on the face: an uncommon presentation of cutaneous sarcoidosis. *Dermatol Pract Concept.* 2018;8:174–176.

Consensus Net Meeting on Dermoscopy www.dermoscopy.org Consensus Net Meeting on Dermoscopy (CNMD) 2000 Unifying concepts of Dermoscopy.

Cunha DG, Kassuga-Roisman LEBP, Silveira LKCB, et al. Dermoscopic features of clear cell acanthoma. *An Bras Dermatol.* 2018;93:449–450.

Dahlen Gyllencreutz J, Johansson Backman E, Terstappen K, et al. Teledermoscopy images acquired in primary health care and hospital settings—a comparative study of image quality. *J Eur Acad Dermatol Venereol.* 2018;32:1038–1043.

Dahlen Gyllencreutz J, Paoli J, Bjellerup M, et al. Diagnostic agreement and interobserver concordance with teledermoscopy referrals. *J Eur Acad Dermatol Venereol.* 2017;31:898–903.

de Giorgi V, Massi D, Salvini C, et al. Thin melanoma of the vulva: a clinical, dermoscopic-pathologic case study. *Arch Dermatol.* 2005;141:1046–1047.

Debarbieux S, Ronger-Salve S, Dalle S, et al. Dermoscopy of desmoplastic melanoma: report of six cases. *Br J Dermatol.* 2008;159:360–363.

Desai A, Ugorji R, Khachemoune A. Acral melanoma foot lesions. Part 2: clinical presentation, diagnosis, and management. *Clin Exp Dermatol.* 2018;43:117–123.

Di Brizzi EV, Moscarella E, Piana S, et al. Clinical and dermoscopic features of pleomorphic dermal sarcoma. *Australas J Dermatol.* 2019;60:e153–e154. https://doi.org/10.1111/ajd.12924.

Di Stefani A, Campbell TM, Malvehy J, et al. Shiny white streaks: an additional dermoscopic finding in melanomas viewed using contact polarised dermoscopy. *Australas J Dermatol.* 2010;51:295–298.

Dolianitis C, Kelly J, Wolfe R, et al. Comparative performance of 4 dermoscopic algorithms by nonexperts for the diagnosis of melanocytic lesions. *Arch Dermatol.* 2005;141:1008–1014.

Dupuy A, Dehen L, Bourrat E, et al. Accuracy of standard dermoscopy for diagnosing scabies. *J Am Acad Dermatol.* 2007;56:53–62.

Eminovic N, de Keizer NF, Wyatt JC, et al. Teledermatologic consultation and reduction in referrals to dermatologists: a cluster randomized controlled trial. *Arch Dermatol.* 2009;145:558–564.

Esteva A, Kuprel B, Novoa RA, et al. Dermatologist-level classification of skin cancer with deep neural networks. *Nature.* 2017;542:115–118.

Felder S, Rabinovitz H, Oliviero M, et al. Dermoscopic differentiation of a superficial basal cell carcinoma and squamous cell carcinoma in situ. *Dermatol Surg.* 2006;32:423–425.

Ferrara G, Argenyi Z, Argenziano G, et al. The influence of clinical information in the histopathologic diagnosis of melanocytic skin neoplasms. *PLoS ONE.* 2009;4:e5375.

Ferrara G, Argenziano G, Soyer HP, et al. Dermoscopic and histopathologic diagnosis of equivocal melanocytic skin lesions: an interdisciplinary study on 107 cases. *Cancer.* 2002;95:1094–1100.

Ferrara G, Argenziano G, Soyer HP, et al. The spectrum of Spitz nevi: a clinicopathologic study of 83 cases. *Arch Dermatol.* 2005;141:1381–1387.

Ferrara G, Gianotti R, Cavicchini S, et al. Spitz nevus, Spitz tumor, and spitzoid melanoma: a comprehensive clinicopathologic overview. *Dermatol Clin.* 2013;31:589–598.

Ferrara G, Giorgio CM, Zalaudek I, et al. Sclerosing Nevus with pseudomelanomatous features (nevus with regression-like fibrosis): clinical and dermoscopic features of a recently characterized histopathologic entity. *Dermatology.* 2009;219:202–208.

Ferrara G, Soyer HP, Malvehy J, et al. The many faces of blue nevus: a clinicopathologic study. *J Cutan Pathol.* 2007;34:543–551.

Ferrari A, Buccini P, Covello R, et al. The ringlike pattern in vulvar melanosis: a new dermoscopic clue for diagnosis. *Arch Dermatol.* 2008;144:1030–1034.

Finnane A, Dallest K, Janda M, et al. Teledermatology for the diagnosis and management of skin cancer: a systematic review. *JAMA Dermatol.* 2017;153:319–327.

Friedman RJ, Rigel DS, Silverman MK, et al. Malignant melanoma in the 1990's: the continued importance of early detection and the role of physician examination and self-examination of the skin. *CA Cancer J Clin.* 1991;41:201–226.

Giacomel J, Zalaudek I. Dermoscopy of superficial basal cell carcinoma. *Dermatol Surg.* 2005;31:1710–1713.

Giacomel J, Lallas A, Zalaudek I, et al. Dermoscopic "signature" pattern of pigmented and nonpigmented lentigo maligna. *J Am Acad Dermatol.* 2014;70. e33–e35.

González-Ramírez RA, Guerra-Segovia C, Garza-Rodríguez V, et al. Dermoscopic features of acral melanocytic nevi in a case series from Mexico. *An Bras Dermatol.* 2018;93:665–670.

Gori A, Oranges T, Janowska A, et al. Clinical and dermoscopic features of lichenoid keratosis: a retrospective case study. *J Cutan Med Surg.* 2018;22:561–566.

Grin CM, Friedman KP, Grant-Kels JM. Dermoscopy: a review. *Dermatol Clin.* 2002;20:641–646.

Grob JJ, Bonerandi JJ. The 'ugly duckling' sign: identification of the common characteristics of nevi in an individual as a basis for melanoma screening. *Arch Dermatol.* 1998;134:103–104.

Grover C, Kharghoria G, Bhattacharya SN. Linear nail bed dyschromia: a distinctive dermoscopic feature of nail lichen planus. *Clin Exp Dermatol.* 2019;44:697–699. https://doi.org/10.1111/ced.13809.

Haenssle HA, Korpas B, Hansen-Hagge C, et al. Selection of patients for long-term surveillance with digital dermoscopy by assessment of melanoma risk factors. *Arch Dermatol.* 2010;146:257–264.

Haenssle HA, Korpas B, Hansen-Hagge C, et al. Seven-point checklist for dermatoscopy: performance during 10 years of prospective surveillance of patients at increased melanoma risk. *J Am Acad Dermatol.* 2010;62:785–793.

Haenssle HA, Krueger U, Vente C, et al. Results from an observational trial: digital epiluminescence microscopy follow-up of atypical nevi increases the sensitivity and the chance of success of conventional dermoscopy in detecting melanoma. *J Invest Dermatol.* 2006;126:980–985.

Hofmann-Wellenhof R, Blum A, Wolf IH, et al. Dermoscopic classification of atypical melanocytic nevi (Clark nevi). *Arch Dermatol.* 2001;137:1575–1580.

Horsham C, Loescher LJ, Whiteman DC, et al. Consumer acceptance of patient-performed mobile teledermoscopy for the early detection of melanoma. *Br J Dermatol.* 2016;175:1301–1310.

Hue L, Makhloufi S, Sall N'Diaye P, et al. Real-time mobile teledermoscopy for skin cancer screening targeting an agricultural population: an experiment on 289 patients in France. *J Eur Acad Dermatol Venereol.* 2016;30:20–24.

Husein-ElAhmed H. Sclerodermiform basal cell carcinoma: how much can we rely on dermatoscopy to differentiate from non-aggressive basal cell carcinomas? Analysis of 1256 cases. *An Bras Dermatol.* 2018;93:229–232.

Inui S, Nakajima T, Nakagawa K, et al. Clinical significance of dermoscopy in alopecia areata: analysis of 300 cases. *Int J Dermatol.* 2008;47:688–693.

Iyatomi H, Oka H, Celebi M, et al. Computer-based classification of dermoscopy images of melanocytic lesions on acral volar skin. *J Invest Dermatol.* 2008;128:2049–2054.

Jaimes N, Chen L, Dusza SW, et al. Clinical and dermoscopic characteristics of desmoplastic melanomas. *JAMA Dermatol.* 2013;149:413–421.

Jaimes N, Marghoob AA, Rabinovitz H, et al. Clinical and dermoscopic characteristics of melanomas on nonfacial chronically sun-damaged skin. *J Am Acad Dermatol.* 2015;72:1027–1035.

Janda M, Loescher LJ, Soyer HP. Enhanced skin self-examination: a novel approach to skin cancer monitoring and follow-up. *JAMA Dermatol.* 2013;149:231–236.

Johr RH. Pink lesions. *Clin Dermatol.* 2002;20:189–296.

Kalkhoran S, Milne O, Zalaudek I, et al. Historical, clinical, and dermoscopic characteristics of thin nodular melanoma. *Arch Dermatol.* 2010;146:311–318.

Kenet RO, Kang S, Kenet BJ, et al. Clinical diagnosis of pigmented lesions using digital epiluminescence microscopy. Grading protocol and atlas. *Arch Dermatol.* 1993;129:157–174.

Kenet RO, Kenet BJ. Risk stratification. A practical approach to using epiluminescence microscopy/dermoscopy in melanoma screening. *Dermatol Clin.* 2001;19:327–335.

Kim GW, Shin K, You HS, et al. Dermoscopic "landscape painting patterns" as a clue for labial melanotic macules: an analysis of 80 cases. *Ann Dermatol*. 2018;30:331–334.

Kittler H. Early recognition at last. *Arch Dermatol*. 2008;144:533–534.

Kittler H, Binder M. Follow-up of melanocytic skin lesions with digital dermoscopy: risks and benefits. *Arch Dermatol*. 2002;138:1379.

Kittler H, Guitera P, Riedl E, et al. Identification of clinically featureless incipient melanoma using sequential dermoscopy imaging. *Arch Dermatol*. 2006;142:1113–1119.

Kittler H, Marghoob AA, Argenziano G, et al. Standardization of terminology in dermoscopy/dermatoscopy: results of the third consensus conference of the International Society of Dermoscopy. *J Am Acad Dermatol*. 2016;74:1093–1106.

Kittler H, Pehamberger H, Wolff K, et al. Follow-up of melanocytic skin lesions with digital epiluminescence microscopy: patterns of modifications observed in early melanoma, atypical nevi, and common nevi. *J Am Acad Dermatol*. 2000;43:467–476.

Kittler H, Pehamberger H, Wolff K, et al. Diagnostic accuracy of dermoscopy. *Lancet Oncol*. 2002;3:159–165.

Kittler H, Seltenheim M, Dawid M, et al. Frequency and characteristics of enlarging common melanocytic nevi. *Arch Dermatol*. 2000;136:316–320.

Kolm I, Di Stefani A, Hofmann-Wellenhof R, et al. Dermoscopy patterns of halo nevi. *Arch Dermatol*. 2006;142:1627–1632.

Kreusch JF. Vascular patterns in skin tumors. *Clin Dermatol*. 2002;20:248–254.

Lallas A, Apalla Z, Ioannides D, et al. Update on dermoscopy of Spitz/Reed naevi and management guidelines by the International Dermoscopy Society. *Br J Dermatol*. 2017;177:645–655.

Lallas A, Argenziano G, Moscarella E, et al. Diagnosis and management of facial pigmented macules. *Clin Dermatol*. 2014;32:94–100.

Lallas A, Longo C, Manfredini M, et al. Accuracy of dermoscopic criteria for the diagnosis of melanoma in situ. *JAMA Dermatol*. 2018;154:414–419.

Lallas A, Tschandl P, Kyrgidis A, et al. Dermoscopic clues to differentiate facial lentigo maligna from pigmented actinic keratosis. *Br J Dermatol*. 2016;174:1079–1085.

Lallas A, Zalaudek I, Apalla Z, et al. Management rules to detect melanoma. *Dermatology*. 2013;226:52–60.

Lee DW, Kim DY, Hong JH, et al. Correlations between histopathologic and dermoscopic findings in Korean actinic keratosis. *Microsc Res Tech*. 2019;82:12–17. https://doi.org/10.1002/jemt.23043.

Lee JH, Lim Y, Park JH, et al. Clinicopathologic features of 28 cases of nail matrix nevi (NMNs) in Asians: comparison between children and adults. *J Am Acad Dermatol*. 2018;78:479–489.

Lee KJ, Finnane A, Soyer HP. Recent trends in teledermatology and teledermoscopy. *Dermatol Pract Concept*. 2018;8:214–223.

Lin J, Koga H, Takata M, et al. Dermoscopy of pigmented lesions on mucocutaneous junction and mucous membrane. *Br J Dermatol*. 2009;161:1255–1261.

Lipoff JB, Scope A, Dusza SW, et al. Complex dermoscopic pattern: a potential risk marker for melanoma. *Br J Dermatol*. 2008;158:821–824.

Liu W, Liu JW, Ma DL. Dermoscopic patterns of spitz nevi—reply. *JAMA*. 2018;319:194.

Lombardi M, Pampena R, Borsari S, et al. Dermoscopic features of Basal cell carcinoma on the lower limbs. A Chameleon! *Dermatology*. 2018;233:482–488.

Lorentzen HF, Weismann K, Larsen FG. Structural asymmetry as a dermatoscopic indicator of malignant melanoma: a latent class analysis of sensitivity and classification errors. *Melanoma Res*. 2001;11:495–501.

Lorentzen HF, Weismann K, Secher L, et al. The dermatoscopic ABCD rule does not improve diagnostic accuracy of malignant melanoma. *Acta Derm Venereol*. 1999;79:469–472.

Lozano-Masdemont B, Polimón-Olabarrieta I, Marinero-Escobedo S, et al. Rosettes in actinic keratosis and squamous cell carcinoma: distribution, association to other dermoscopic signs and description of the rosette pattern. *J Eur Acad Dermatol Venereol*. 2018;32:48–52.

Malvehy J, Puig S. Dermoscopic patterns of benign volar melanocytic lesions in patients with atypical mole syndrome. *Arch Dermatol*. 2004;140:538–544.

Malvehy J, Puig S, Argenziano G, et al. Dermoscopy report: proposal for standardization. Results of a consensus meeting of the International Dermoscopy Society. *J Am Acad Dermatol*. 2007;57:84–95.

Manahan MN, Soyer HP, Loescher LJ, et al. A pilot trial of mobile, patient-performed teledermoscopy. *Br J Dermatol*. 2015;172:1072–1080.

Marchetti MA, F Codella NC, Dusza SW, et al. Results of the 2016 International Skin Imaging Collaboration International Symposium on Biomedical Imaging challenge: comparison of the accuracy of computer algorithms to dermatologists for the diagnosis of melanoma from dermoscopic images. *J Am Acad Dermatol*. 2018;78:270–277.

Marghoob AA, Braun R. Proposal for a revised 2-step algorithm for the classification of lesions of the skin using dermoscopy. *Arch Dermatol*. 2010;146:426–428.

Marghoob AA, Scope A. The complexity of diagnosing melanoma. *J Invest Dermatol*. 2009;129:11–13.

Marghoob AA, Terushkin V, Dusza SW, et al. Dermatologists, general practitioners, and the best method to biopsy suspect melanocytic neoplasms. *Arch Dermatol*. 2010;146:325–328.

Martinez Leborans L, Garcias Ladaria J, Oliver Martinez V, et al. Extrafacial lentigo maligna: a report on 14 cases and a review of the literature. *Actas Dermosifiliogr*. 2016;107:e57–e63.

Massone C, Hofmann-Wellenhof R, Ahlgrimm-Siess V, et al. Melanoma screening with cellular phones. *PLoS ONE*. 2007;2:e483.

Mayer J. Systematic review of the diagnostic accuracy of dermatoscopy in detecting malignant melanoma. *Med J Aust*. 1997;167:206–210.

Mazzella C, Costa C, Cappello M, et al. Difficult to diagnose small cutaneous melanoma metastases mimicking angiomas: utility of dermoscopy. *Int J Dermatol*. 2018;57:1085–1087.

Menzies SW. A method for the diagnosis of primary cutaneous melanoma using surface microscopy. *Dermatol Clin*. 2001;19:299–305.

Menzies SW, Crotty KA, Ingvar C, et al. *An Atlas of Surface Microscopy of Pigmented Skin Lesions: Dermoscopy*. McGraw-Hill;2003.

Menzies SW, Emery J, Staples M, et al. Impact of dermoscopy and short-term sequential digital dermoscopy imaging for the management of pigmented lesions in primary care: a sequential intervention trial. *Br J Dermatol.* 2009;161:1270–1277.

Menzies SW, Gutenev A, Avramidis M, et al. Short-term digital surface microscopic monitoring of atypical or changing melanocytic lesions. *Arch Dermatol.* 2001;137:1583–1589.

Menzies SW, Ingvar C, Crotty KA, et al. Frequency and morphologic characteristics of invasive melanomas lacking specific surface microscopic features. *Arch Dermatol.* 1996;132:1178–1182.

Menzies SW, Ingvar C, McCarthy WH. A sensitivity and specificity analysis of the surface microscopy features of invasive melanoma. *Melanoma Res.* 1996;6:55–62.

Menzies SW, Kreusch J, Byth K, et al. Dermoscopic evaluation of amelanotic and hypomelanotic melanoma. *Arch Dermatol.* 2008;144:1120–1127.

Menzies SW, Westerhoff K, Rabinovitz H, et al. Surface microscopy of pigmented basal cell carcinoma. *Arch Dermatol.* 2000;136(8):1012–1016.

Micali G, Lacarrubba F. Dermatoscopy: instrumental update. *Dermatol Clin.* 2018;36:345–348.

Micali G, Verzì AE, Quattrocchi E, et al. Dermatoscopy of common lesions in pediatric dermatology. *Dermatol Clin.* 2018;36:463–472.

Micantonio T, Neri L, Longo C, et al. A new dermoscopic algorithm for the differential diagnosis of facial lentigo maligna and pigmented actinic keratosis. *Eur J Dermatol.* 2018;28:162–168.

Moscarella E, Lallas A, Longo C, et al. Performance of the "if in doubt, cut it out" rule for the management of nodular melanoma. *Dermatol Pract Concept.* 2017;7:1–5.

Mun JH, Jo G, Darmawan CC, et al. Association between Breslow thickness and dermoscopic findings in acral melanoma. *J Am Acad Dermatol.* 2018;79:831–835.

Navarrete-Dechent C, Bajaj S, Marchetti MA, et al. Association of shiny white blotches and strands with nonpigmented basal cell carcinoma: evaluation of an additional dermoscopic diagnostic criterion. *JAMA Dermatol.* 2016;152:546–552.

Niederkorn A, Ahlgrimm-Siess V, Fink-Puches R, et al. Frequency, clinical and dermoscopic features of benign papillomatous melanocytic naevi (Unna type). *Br J Dermatol.* 2009;161:510–514.

Noor O, Nanda A, Rao BK. A dermoscopy survey to assess who is using it and why it is or is not being used. *Int J Dermatol.* 2009;48:951–952.

Oliveria SA, Geller AC, Dusza SW, et al. The Framingham school nevus study: a pilot study. *Arch Dermatol.* 2004;140:545–551.

Ozdemir F, Errico MA, Yaman B, et al. Acral lentiginous melanoma in the Turkish population and a new dermoscopic clue for the diagnosis. *Dermatol Pract Concept.* 2018;8:140–148.

Pagnanelli G, Soyer HP, Argenziano G, et al. Diagnosis of pigmented skin lesions by dermoscopy: web-based training improves diagnostic performance of non-experts. *Br J Dermatol.* 2003;148:698–702.

Pan Y, Gareau DS, Scope A, et al. Polarized and nonpolarized dermoscopy: the explanation for the observed differences. *Arch Dermatol.* 2008;144:828–829.

Papageorgiou C, Apalla Z, Variaah G, et al. Accuracy of dermoscopic criteria for the differentiation between superficial basal cell carcinoma and Bowen's disease. *J Eur Acad Dermatol Venereol.* 2018;32:1914–1919. https://doi.org/10.1111/jdv.14995.

Pehamberger H, Binder M, Steiner A, et al. In vivo epiluminescence microscopy: improvement of early diagnosis of melanoma. *J Invest Dermatol.* 1993;100(suppl):356–625.

Pehamberger H, Steiner A, Wolff K. In vivo epiluminescence microscopy of pigmented skin lesions. I. Pattern analysis of pigmented skin lesions. *J Am Acad Dermatol.* 1987;17:571–583.

Pellacani G, Cesinaro AM, Longo C, et al. Microscopic in vivo description of cellular architecture of dermoscopic pigment network in nevi and melanomas. *Arch Dermatol.* 2005;141:147–154.

Peris K, Ferrari A, Argenziano G, et al. Dermoscopic classification of Spitz/Reed nevi. *Clin Dermatol.* 2002;20:259–262.

Peris K, Maiorino A, Di Stefani A, et al. Brown globules in lentigo maligna (LM): a useful dermoscopic clue. *J Am Acad Dermatol.* 2016;75:429–430.

Piccolo V, Russo T, Agozzino M, et al. Dermoscopy of cutaneous lymphoproliferative disorders: where are we now? *Dermatology.* 2018;234:131–136.

Piccolo V, Russo T, Moscarella E, et al. Dermatoscopy of vascular lesions. *Dermatol Clin.* 2018;36:389–395.

Piraccini BM, Alessandrini A, Starace M. Onychoscopy: dermoscopy of the nails. *Dermatol Clin.* 2018;36:431–438.

Pizzichetta MA, Kittler H, Stanganelli I, et al. Pigmented nodular melanoma: the predictive value of dermoscopic features using multivariate analysis. *Br J Dermatol.* 2015;173:106–114.

Pizzichetta MA, Kittler H, Stanganelli I, et al. Dermoscopic diagnosis of amelanotic/hypomelanotic melanoma. *Br J Dermatol.* 2017;177:538–540.

Pizzichetta MA, Talamini R, Marghoob AA, et al. Negative pigment network: an additional dermoscopic feature for the diagnosis of melanoma. *J Am Acad Dermatol.* 2013;68:552–559.

Pizzichetta MA, Talamini R, Piccolo D, et al. The ABCD rule of dermatoscopy does not apply to small melanocytic skin lesions. *Arch Dermatol.* 2001;137:1376–1378.

Pizzichetta MA, Talamini R, Stanganelli I, et al. Amelanotic/hypomelanotic melanoma: clinical and dermoscopic features. *Br J Dermatol.* 2004;150:1117–1124.

Pollock JL. Dermoscopic patterns of Spitz Nevi. *JAMA.* 2018;319:194.

Pralong P, Bathelier E, Dalle S, et al. Dermoscopy of lentigo maligna melanoma: report of 125 cases. *Br J Dermatol.* 2012;167:280–287.

Puig S, Argenziano G, Zalaudek I, et al. Melanomas that failed dermoscopic detection: a combined clinicodermoscopic approach for not missing melanoma. *Dermatol Surg.* 2007;33:1262–1273.

Rabinovitz H, Kopfa AW, Katz B. *Dermoscopy: A Practical Guide. CD ROM Version* MMA Worldwide Group Inc; Miami, 1999.

Rajpara SM, Botello AP, Townend J, et al. Systematic review of dermoscopy and digital dermoscopy/artificial intelligence for the diagnosis of melanoma. *Br J Dermatol.* 2009;161:591–604.

Ramji R, Valdes-Gonzalez G, Oakley A, et al. Dermoscopic 'chaos and clues' in the diagnosis of melanoma in situ. *Australas J Dermatol*. 2018;59:201–205.

Ribero S, Moscarella E, Ferrara G, et al. Regression in cutaneous melanoma: a comprehensive review from diagnosis to prognosis. *J Eur Acad Dermatol Venereol*. 2016;30:2030–2037.

Robinson JK, Nickoloff BJ. Digital epiluminescence microscopy monitoring of high-risk patients. *Arch Dermatol*. 2004;140:49–56.

Rogers T, Marino ML, Dusza SW, et al. A clinical aid for detecting skin cancer: the triage amalgamated dermoscopic algorithm (TADA). *J Am Board Fam Med*. 2016;29:694–701.

Ronger S, Touzet S, Ligeron C, et al. Dermoscopic examination of nail pigmentation. *Arch Dermatol*. 2002;138:1327–1333.

Rosado B, Menzies S, Harbauer A, et al. Accuracy of computer diagnosis of melanoma: a quantitative meta-analysis. *Arch Dermatol*. 2003;139:361–367.

Rosendahl C, Cameron A, McColl I, et al. Dermatoscopy in routine practice—'chaos and clues'. *Aust Fam Physician*. 2012;41:482–487.

Rubegni P, Sbano P, Burroni M, et al. Melanocytic skin lesions and pregnancy: digital dermoscopy analysis. *Skin Res Technol*. 2007;13:143–147.

Ry TH, Kye H, Choi JE, et al. Features causing confusion between basal cell carcinoma and squamous cell carcinoma in clinical diagnosis. *Ann Dermatol*. 2018;30:64–70.

Saida T, Koga H. Dermoscopic patterns of acral melanocytic nevi: their variations, changes, and significance. *Arch Dermatol*. 2007;143:1423–1426.

Saida T, Oguchi S, Ishihara Y. In vivo observation of magnified features of pigmented lesions on volar skin using video macroscope. Usefulness of epiluminescence techniques in clinical diagnosis. *Arch Dermatol*. 1995;131:298–304.

Saida T, Oguchi S, Miyazaki A. Dermoscopy for acral pigmented skin lesions. *Clin Dermatol*. 2002;20:279–285.

Salerni G, Carrera C, Lovatto L, et al. Benefits of total body photography and digital dermatoscopy ("two-step method of digital follow-up") in the early diagnosis of melanoma in patients at high risk for melanoma. *J Am Acad Dermatol*. 2012;67:e17–27.

Salerni G, Teran T, Alonso C, et al. The role of dermoscopy and digital dermoscopy follow-up in the clinical diagnosis of melanoma: clinical and dermoscopic features of 99 consecutive primary melanomas. *Dermatol Pract Concept*. 2014;4:39–46.

Salerni G, Teran T, Puig S, et al. Meta-analysis of digital dermoscopy follow-up of melanocytic skin lesions: a study on behalf of the International Dermoscopy Society. *J Eur Acad Dermatol Venereol*. 2013;27:805–814.

Salopek TG, Kopf AW, Stetanoto CM, et al. Differentiation of atypical moles (dysplastic nevi) from early melanoma by dermoscopy. *Dermatol Clin*. 2001;19:337–345.

Scalvenzi M, Costa C, De Fata Salvatores G, et al. Clinical and dermoscopic features of Spitz naevus by sex, age and anatomical site: a study of 913 Spitz naevi. *Br J Dermatol*. 2018;179:769–770.

Schiffner R, Schiffner-Rohe J, Vogt T, et al. Improvement of early recognition of lentigo maligna using dermatoscopy. *J Am Acad Dermatol*. 2000;42:25–32.

Seidenari S, Pellacani G. Surface microscopy features of congenital nevi. *Clin Dermatol*. 2002;20:263–267.

Seidenari S, Pellacani G, Martella A, et al. Instrument-, age- and site-dependent variations of dermoscopic patterns of congenital melanocytic naevi: a multicentre study. *Br J Dermatol*. 2006;155:56–61.

Silipo V, De Simone P, Mariani G, et al. Malignant melanoma and pregnancy. *Melanoma Res*. 2006;16:497–500.

Skvara H, Teban L, Fiebiger M, et al. Limitations of dermoscopy in the recognition of melanoma. *Arch Dermatol*. 2005;141:155–160.

Soyer HP, Argenziano G, Chimenti S, et al. Dermoscopy of pigmented skin lesions. *Eur J Dermatol*. 2001;11:270–277.

Soyer HP, Argenziano G, Ruocco V, et al. Dermoscopy of pigmented skin lesions (Part II). *Eur J Dermatol*. 2001;11:483–498.

Soyer HP, Argenziano G, Talamini R, et al. Is dermoscopy useful for the diagnosis of melanoma? *Arch Dermatol*. 2001;137:1361–1363.

Soyer HP, Argenziano G, Zalaudek I, et al. Three-point checklist of dermoscopy. A new screening method for early detection of melanoma. *Dermatology*. 2004;208:27–31.

Soyer HP, Hofmann-Wellenhof R, Massone C, et al. Ozdemir F, et al. telederm.org: freely available online consultations in dermatology. *PLoS Med*. 2005:e87–e92.

Soyer HP, Kenet RO, Wolf IH, et al. Clinicopathological correlation of pigmented skin lesions using dermoscopy. *Eur J Dermatol*. 2000;10:22–28.

Soyer HP, Massone C, Ferrara G, et al. Limitations of histopathologic analysis in the recognition of melanoma: a plea for a combined diagnostic approach of histopathologic and dermoscopic evaluation. *Arch Dermatol*. 2005;141:209–211.

Soyer HP, Smolle J, Hodl S, et al. Surface microscopy. A new approach to the diagnosis of cutaneous pigmented tumors. *Am J Dermatopathol*. 1989;11:1–10.

Soyer HP, Smolle J, Leitinger G, et al. Diagnostic reliability of dermoscopic criteria for detecting malignant melanoma. *Dermatology*. 1995;190:25–30.

Spinks J, Janda M, Soyer HP, et al. Consumer preferences for teledermoscopy screening to detect melanoma early. *J Telemed Telecare*. 2016;22:39–46.

Starace M, Dika E, Fanti PA, et al. Nail apparatus melanoma: dermoscopic and histopathologic correlations on a series of 23 patients from a single centre. *J Eur Acad Dermatol Venereol*. 2018;32:164–173.

Stefanaki C, Soura E, Stergiopoulou A, et al. Clinical and dermoscopic characteristics of congenital melanocytic naevi. *J Eur Acad Dermatol Venereol*. 2018;32:1674–1680.

Steiner A, Binder M, Schemper M, et al. Statistical evaluation of epiluminescence microscopic criteria for melanocytic pigmented skin lesions. *J Am Acad Dermatol*. 1993;29:581.

Steiner A, Pehamberger H, Binder M, et al. Pigmented Spitz nevi: improvement of the diagnostic accuracy by epiluminescence microscopy. *J Am Acad Dermatol*. 1992;27:697–701.

Steiner A, Pehamberger H, Wolff K. In vivo epiluminescence microscopy of pigmented skin lesions. II. Diagnosis of small pigmented skin lesions and early detection of malignant melanoma. *J Am Acad Dermatol*. 1987;17:584–591.

Stolz W, Braun-Falco O, Bilek P, et al. *Color Atlas of Derma-toscopy*. 2nd ed. Blackwell Scientific Publications: Berlin, Germany; 2002.

Stolz W, Schiffner R, Burgdorf WH. Dermatoscopy for facial pigmented skin lesions. *Clin Dermatol*. 2002;20:276–278.

Suh KS, Park JB, Kim JH, et al. Dysplastic nevus: clinical features and usefulness of dermoscopy. *J Dermatol*. 2019;46:e76–e77. https://doi.org/10.1111/1346-8138.14583.

Tanaka M, Sawada M, Kobayashi K. Key points in dermo-scopic differentiation between lentigo maligna and solar lentigo. *J Dermatol*. 2011;38:53–58.

Tiodorovic-Zivkovic D, Argenziano G, Lallas A, et al. Age, gender, and topography influence the clinical and dermoscopic appearance of lentigo maligna. *J Am Acad Dermatol*. 2015;72:801–808.

Tripp JM, Kopf AW, Marghoob AA, et al. Management of dys-plastic nevi: a survey of fellows of the American Academy of Dermatology. *J Am Acad Dermatol*. 2002;46:674–682.

Uzuncakmak TK, Akay BN, Ozkanli S. Different dermoscopic features of clonal seborrhoeic keratoses. *Br J Dermatol*. 2019;180:197–198. https://doi.org/10.1111/bjd.17087.

van der Heijden JP, de Keizer NF, Bos JD, et al. Teledermatol-ogy applied following patient selection by general prac-titioners in daily practice improves efficiency and quality of care at lower cost. *Br J Dermatol*. 2011;165:1058–1065.

van der Rhee JI, Bergman W, Kukutsch N. The impact of dermoscopy on the management of pigmented lesions in everyday clinical practice of general dermatologists: a prospective study. *Br J Dermatol*. 2010;162:563–567.

Vestergaard ME, Macaskill P, Holt PE, et al. Dermoscopy com-pared with naked eye examination for the diagnosis of primary melanoma: a meta-analysis of studies performed in a clinical setting. *Br J Dermatol*. 2008;159:669–676.

Wang SQ, Marghoob AA, Scope A. Principles of dermoscopy and dermoscopic equipment. In: Marghoob AA, Malvehy J, Braun RP, eds. *Atlas of Dermoscopy*. 2nd ed. London: Informa Healthcare; 2012:3–9.

Warshaw EM, Lederle FA, Grill JP, et al. Accuracy of teleder-matology for nonpigmented neoplasms. *J Am Acad Dermatol*. 2009;60:579–588.

Warshaw EM, Lederle FA, Grill JP, et al. Accuracy of teleder-matology for pigmented neoplasms. *J Am Acad Dermatol*. 2009;61:753–765.

Weber P, Tschandl P, Sinz C, et al. Dermatoscopy of neoplas-tic skin lesions: recent advances, updates, and revisions. *Curr Treat Options Oncol*. 2018;19:56.

Westerhoff K, McCarthy WH, Menzies SW. Increase in the sensitivity for melanoma diagnosis by primary care physicians using skin surface microscopy. *Br J Dermatol*. 2000;143:1016–1020.

Wolf I. Dermoscopic diagnosis of vascular lesions. *Clin Der-matol*. 2002;20:273–275.

Wolff K. Why is epiluminescence microscopy important? *Recent Results Cancer Res*. 2002;160:125–132.

Wolner ZJ, Yelamos O, Liopyris K, et al. Enhancing skin cancer diagnosis with dermoscopy. *Dermatol Clin*. 2017;35:417–437.

Wolner ZJ, Bajaj S, Flores E, et al. Variation in dermoscopic features of basal cell carcinoma as a function of ana-tomical location and pigmentation status. *Br J Dermatol*. 2018;178:e136–e137.

Wozniak-Rito A, Zalaudek I, Rudnicka L. Dermoscopy of ba-sal cell carcinoma. *Clin Exp Dermatol*. 2018;43:241–247.

Wozniak-Rito AM, Rudnicka L. Bowen's disease in dermosco-py. *Acta Dermatovenerol Croat*. 2018;26:157–161.

Wu X, Oliveria SA, Yagerman S, et al. Feasibility and efficacy of patient-initiated mobile teledermoscopy for short-term monitoring of clinically atypical nevi. *JAMA Dermatol*. 2015;151:489–496.

Yadav S, Vossaert KA, Kopf AW, et al. Histopathologic corre-lates of structures seen on dermoscopy (epiluminescence microscopy). *Am J Dermatopathol*. 1993;15:297–305.

Yélamos O, Braun RP, Liopyris K, et al. Dermoscopy/derma-toscopy and dermatopathology correlates of cutaneous neoplasms. *J Am Acad Dermatol*. 2019;80:341–363.

Yélamos O, Braun RP, Liopyris K, et al. Usefulness of dermoscopy/dermatoscopy to improve the clinical and histopathologic diagnosis of skin cancers. *J Am Acad Dermatol*. 2018. pii: S0190-9622(18)32728-2.

Yélamos O, Navarrete-Dechent C, Marchetti MA, et al. 2018 Clinical and dermoscopic features of cutaneous BAP1 inactivated melanocytic tumors: results of a multicenter case-control study by the International Dermoscopy Society (IDS). *J Am Acad Dermatol*. 2019;80:1585–1593.

Zaballos P, Blazquez S, Puig S, et al. Dermoscopic pattern of intermediate stage in seborrhoeic keratosis regressing to lichenoid keratosis: report of 24 cases. *Br J Dermatol*. 2007;157:266–272.

Zaballos P, Daufí C, Puig S, et al. Dermoscopy of solitary angiokeratomas: a morphological study. *Arch Dermatol*. 2007;143:318–325.

Zaballos P, Gómez-Martín I, Martin JM, et al. Dermoscopy of adnexal tumors. *Dermatol Clin*. 2018;36:397–412.

Zaballos P, Llambrich A, Cuéllar F, et al. Dermoscop-ic findings in pyogenic granuloma. *Br J Dermatol*. 2006;154:1108–1111.

Zaballos P, Puig S, Llambrich A, et al. Dermoscopy of der-matofibromas: a prospective morphological study of 412 cases. *Arch Dermatol*. 2008;144:75–83.

Zalaudek I, Argenziano G, Di Stefani A, et al. Dermoscopy in general dermatology. *Dermatology*. 2006;212:7–18.

Zalaudek I, Argenziano G, Ferrara G, et al. Clinically equiv-ocal melanocytic skin lesions with features of regres-sion: a dermoscopic-pathological study. *Br J Dermatol*. 2004;150:64–71.

Zalaudek I, Argenziano G, Leinweber B, et al. Dermoscopy of Bowen's disease. *Br J Dermatol*. 2004;150:1112–1116.

Zalaudek I, Argenziano G, Mordente I, et al. Nevus type in dermoscopy is related to skin type in white persons. *Arch Dermatol*. 2007;143:351–356.

Zalaudek I, Argenziano G, Soyer HP, et al. Three-point check-list of dermoscopy: an open internet study. *Br J Dermatol*. 2006;154:431–437.

Zalaudek I, Docimo G, Argenziano G. Using dermoscopic criteria and patient-related factors for the manage-ment of pigmented melanocytic nevi. *Arch Dermatol*. 2009;145:816–826.

Zalaudek I, Giacomel J, Argenziano G, et al. Dermoscopy of facial nonpigmented actinic keratosis. *Br J Dermatol*. 2006;155:951–956.

Zalaudek I, Giacomel J, Cabo H, et al. Entodermoscopy: a new tool for diagnosing skin infections and infestations. *Dermatology*. 2008;216:14–23.

Zalaudek I, Hofmann-Wellenhof R, Soyer HP, et al. Naevogenesis: new thoughts based on dermoscopy. *Br J Dermatol*. 2006;154:793–794.

Zalaudek I, Kittler H, Marghoob AA, et al. Time required for a complete skin examination with and without dermoscopy: a prospective, randomized multicenter study. *Arch Dermatol.* 2008;144:509–513.

Zalaudek I, Kreusch J, Giacomel J, et al. How to diagnose nonpigmented skin tumors: a review of vascular structures seen with dermoscopy Part I. Melanocytic skin tumors. *J Am Acad Dermatol.* 2010;63:361–374.

Zalaudek I, Kreusch J, Giacomel J, et al. How to diagnose nonpigmented skin tumors: a review of vascular structures seen with dermoscopy Part II. Nonmelanocytic skin tumors. *J Am Acad Dermatol.* 2010;63:377–386.

Zalaudek I, Manzo M, Savarese I, et al. The morphologic universe of melanocytic nevi. *Semin Cutan Med Surg.* 2009;28:149–156.

Zampino MR, Corazza M, Costantino D, et al. Are melanocytic nevi influenced by pregnancy? A dermoscopic evaluation. *Dermatol Surg.* 2006;32:1497–1504.

Index

Note: Page numbers followed by "f" indicate figures, "t" indicate tables, and "b" indicate boxes.